Dermal Exposure Related to Pesticide Use

A C S   S Y M P O S I U M   S E R I E S **273**

Dermal Exposure Related to Pesticide Use

Discussion of Risk Assessment

Richard C. Honeycutt, EDITOR
CIBA-GEIGY

Gunter Zweig, EDITOR
University of California, Richmond

Nancy N. Ragsdale, EDITOR
Department of Agriculture

Based on a symposium sponsored by
the Division of Pesticide Chemistry
at the 187th Meeting
of the American Chemical Society,
St. Louis, Missouri,
April 8–13, 1984

American Chemical Society, Washington, D.C. 1985

Library of Congress Cataloging in Publication Data

Dermal exposure related to pesticide use.
(ACS symposium series, ISSN 0097-6156; 273)

Includes bibliographies and indexes.

1. Agricultural laborers—Diseases and hygiene—
Congresses. 2. Pesticides—Toxicology—Congresses.
3. Skin—Permeability—Congresses.

I. Honeycutt, Richard C., 1945-   . II. Zweig,
Gunter. III. Ragsdale, Nancy, 1938-   . IV. American
Chemical Society. Division of Pesticide Chemistry.
V. American Chemical Society. Meeting (187th: St.
Louis, Mo.) VI. Series.

RC965.A5D47   1985   616.5   84-28361
ISBN 0-8412-0898-0

ACS Symposium Series

M. Joan Comstock, *Series Editor*

Advisory Board

FOREWORD

The ACS SYMPOSIUM SERIES was founded in 1974 to provide a medium for publishing symposia quickly in book form. The format of the Series parallels that of the continuing ADVANCES IN CHEMISTRY SERIES except that, in order to save time, the papers are not typeset but are reproduced as they are submitted by the authors in camera-ready form. Papers are reviewed under the supervision of the Editors with the assistance of the Series Advisory Board and are selected to maintain the integrity of the symposia; however, verbatim reproductions of previously published papers are not accepted. Both reviews and reports of research are acceptable, because symposia may embrace both types of presentation.

CONTENTS

TRENDS IN EXPOSURE ASSESSMENT
AND PROTECTION

INTEGRATION OF EXPERIMENTAL DATA

PREFACE

I T IS GENERALLY RECOGNIZED that a potential health risk exists for agricultural workers (applicators, mixer-loaders, harvesters, and field workers) who are exposed to pesticides. Thus, since 1980, various symposia, including the one upon which this book is based, have been held to examine various parameters involved in the risk assessment of these workers due to dermal exposure from pesticides.

Although an abundance of literature has been published on the assessment of agricultural worker exposure, none integrates the three disciplines necessary for a complete risk assessment for field workers exposed to pesticides. These disciplines are dermal absorption, field exposure studies, and toxicology–risk assessment. This volume deals with these three disciplines and shows how they are integrated into a complete risk assessment for agricultural workers from dermal exposure to pesticides.

The book is divided into five sections, each dealing with specific topics of risk assessment. The first section deals with the most recent views on dermal absorption of chemicals through human skin and experimental methods and techniques on how to arrive at quantitative absorption data using animal models or in vitro systems. The diversity of methodology presented in this section reflects the quickly evolving state of the art in this field.

The second and third sections are descriptions and results of field studies with emphasis on methodology and specific compounds or specific applicator sites. The fourth section deals with trends in exposure assessment and protection and reflects some of the more creative approaches and research dealing with predicting exposure and protecting workers against exposure. Chapters 25, 26, and 27 deal with predicting exposure levels for agricultural workers.

Although such predictive techniques would be generally welcomed by regulators, industrial scientists, and academicians, the contradictory nature of some of the material in these three chapters reflects the current status of such research, i.e., the final answer on predictive techniques and a generic data base is not in yet. Much discussion is needed before moving from these first generation data bases to a common, functional, well-received second generation data base.

Furthermore, section four is a discussion of mathematical models and the use of fluorescent tracers in conjunction with television imagery, techniques that are seen by most researchers in the field to have the potential to replace older, more cumbersome, and less precise exposure evaluation techniques. The areas of the social impact of drift (unintentional exposure) and the use of protective clothing to eliminate exposure are addressed in this section, and they will be extremely important areas for exposure–risk-assessment research in the future.

The last section is a discussion of the use of experimental data to arrive at risk assessment as recommended by states such as California, Canadian governmental regulatory agencies, and industry. These parties share a common goal, namely to make the workplace safe for agricultural workers who are exposed to pesticides through normal work activities.

It is apparent from these last chapters that risk assessment for agricultural workers from dermal exposure to pesticides is an extremely complex technique that is evolving rapidly and will require considerable future resources for it to be refined to a fine science.

The editors of this volume, who were also the organizers of the symposium, want to thank all the contributors who gave so generously of their time and experience, and who made this publication a valuable tool for scientists, administrators, and others charged with establishing rules and regulations for the safe use of pesticides. We would also like to thank our symposium session chairpersons, Joe Reinert (EPA), Rhoda Wang (CDFA), Tom Fuhremann (Monsanto), Richard Moraski (EPA), and James Adams (EPA) for their contributions in making this symposium a success.

RICHARD C. HONEYCUTT
CIBA-GEIGY

GUNTER ZWEIG
University of California, Richmond

NANCY RAGSDALE
Department of Agriculture

November 1984

INTRODUCTION

THE TWO BASIC DETERMINANTS of human health hazard for toxic chemicals, including pesticides, are exposure (or dosage) and toxicity (or effect). Information on both these determinants of hazard is necessary in arriving at a risk assessment for a particular pesticide or pesticide usage. The exposure parameter is particularly important for agricultural workers because of their relatively greater contact with pesticides than is true for the general population.

A preponderance of past and current health-related research on pesticide chemicals has emphasized study of acute and chronic toxicity, teratology and reproductive effects, genotoxicity, including mutagenic and carcinogenic effects, neurotoxicity, and other modalities of toxicity. Study of these effects undoubtedly represents a most important and necessary step in defining the human health hazard of these agents. However, in order to complete the risk assessment process, it is also necessary to have information on the exposure, or dosage, involved.

Exposure to pesticides may occur through ingestion, by inhalation, and from skin contact. The major route of importance for the general population is through ingestion in food and water. Agricultural workers who have contact with pesticides in their occupation are exposed by the dermal and inhalation routes. Previous studies have shown that for most outdoor, field-type applications of pesticides dermal exposure is greater than respiratory exposure even when appropriate allowance is made for the greater speed and completeness of absorption by the inhalation pathway. Thus, the decision to target the symposium upon which this book is based to dermal exposure seems appropriate for agricultural workers.

Two general types of methods are available for estimating human exposure to pesticides. First, direct entrapment methods involve the use of some mechanism to entrap the toxic material as it comes in contact with the person during an exposure period. The amount of entrapped toxicant, as determined by chemical analysis, is then a direct measure of the particular exposure under study. Further calculations using the kinetics of dermal absorption for the compound and formulation under study are required to arrive at the actual absorbed dose. For the oral and inhalation routes, exposure and absorbed dose are more closely equivalent than for the dermal route. However, for precise data, absorption must be taken into account for these routes, also. Second, indirect methods are based on measurement of some effect of the compound on the exposed individual (such as blood cholinesterase level) or determination of the compound or its breakdown product(s) in the tissues or excreta (such as DDT in blood or p-nitrophenol in urine).

In comparing these methods, the direct entrapment procedures give the advantage of providing an absolute value for a discrete exposure even within a sequence of repetitive exposures to the same pesticide. They can also be used to differentiate the relative contributions of oral, dermal, and respiratory exposure to the total exposure picture.

This book provides an up-to-the-minute picture of the current status of research on measurement and risk assessment of dermal pesticide exposure for agricultural workers. The chapters also provide an insight into some newer areas (applications of mathematical models, use of fluorescent tracer materials, and extrapolation from a computer data base of generic pesticide exposure data) that will undoubtedly be receiving increased attention in the future.

WILLIAM F. DURHAM
Environmental Protection Agency
Research Triangle Park, North Carolina

December 1984

DERMAL ABSORPTION

Percutaneous Absorption: Interpretation of In Vitro Data and Risk Assessment

C. G. TOBY MATHIAS[1,2], ROBERT S. HINZ[3], RICHARD H. GUY[3], and HOWARD I. MAIBACH[1]

[1] Department of Dermatology, School of Medicine, University of California Medical Center, San Francisco, CA 94143
[2] Department of Medicine, Northern California Occupational Health Center, San Francisco General Hospital, San Francisco, CA 94110
[3] Departments of Pharmacy and Pharmaceutical Chemistry, School of Pharmacy, University of California Medical Center, San Francisco, CA 94143

Assessment of risk based on in vitro percutaneous absorption data depends on characterization of total penetrating amounts and of kinetic parameters which define the time course of absorption. Methods for determining these parameters have been reviewed. A pharmacokinetic model, which has the broad capability to predict not only the time course of absorption, but also the amounts accumulating within skin and remaining on the skin surface to be absorbed will be presented. Our results suggest that when a solid substance is deposited on the skin surface from a volatile solvent, a fraction of the applied dose is rapidly solubilized into the skin; faster absorption of this initially solubilized fraction is facilitated.

Assessment of risk upon cutaneous exposure to chemical substances requires analysis of three separate aspects of toxicology: 1) the quantitative amount of exposure; 2) the quantitative degree of percutaneous absorption following exposure; and 3) measurement of a biological effect following absorption. This paper will address the second of these aspects.

Percutaneous absorption may be measured in vivo or it may be determined in vitro using excised skin mounted in glass diffusion cells. The most frequently used approaches employ radiolabelled compounds. The validity of in vitro measurements relies on the assumption that no metabolism occurs in skin, and that absorption into the receptor fluid of the diffusion cells approximates absorption from dermal tissue into blood in vivo. These assumptions are generally unproven, and in vitro measurements ultimately require confirmation in vivo. These limitations notwithstanding, in vitro studies still provide substantially useful information, and a variety of methods have been developed. The first section of this paper will focus on the general interpretation of in vitro data and its application to risk assessment.

0097–6156/85/0273–0003$06.00/0
© 1985 American Chemical Society

An ideal predictive description of the percutaneous absorption
process should include not only the ability to predict the time
course of the penetration process through the skin and absorption
into the systemic circulation, but also an ability to predict the
residual amounts remaining both on the skin surface and within the
skin which are still available for absorption. In the latter half
of this paper, a potentially useful pharmacokinetic model, which has
this broad predictive capability, will be presented, together with
data suggesting that solid substances deposited on the skin surface
in volatile solvents are partially solubilized before the solvent
has evaporated; more rapid absorption of the solubilized fraction is
then likely.

Interpretation of Data

Percutaneous absorption studied in vitro is normally characterized
either by a permeability constant or by the time course of the
penetration process. Direct measurements of absorption require
intermittent sampling of fluid contained in the receptor half of a
diffusion cell. Permeability constants are frequently calculated by
removing and assaying microaliquots of receptor fluid at various
intervals during the early time course of absorption ("static"
diffusion cell technique), until steady state (ss) flux is obtained;
the permeability coefficients are then derived according to Fick's
First Law of Diffusion:

$$flux(ss) = A \cdot P \cdot Co \qquad (1)$$

where P denotes the permeability coefficient, Co is the concentration gradient (assumed equal to the initial concentration in the
donor half of the diffusion cell), and A is the surface area of skin
contacted by the penetrant.

If the receptor fluid is not replaced, the concentration in the
receptor phase of the diffusion cell will eventually equilibrate
with the donor phase concentration, at which point further net
absorption will cease. Thus, this technique is unsatisfactory for
measuring the complete time course of absorption. This limitation
may be overcome by intermittently emptying the receptor fluid and
replacing with "fresh" solution in order to maintain "sink"
conditions ("dynamic" diffusion cell technique).

Techniques which utilize continuously perfused, "dynamic"
diffusion cells maintain "sink" conditions, and serial samples may
be collected in automated fraction collectors. When these samples
are added, the cumulative amount removed ("excreted") from the
diffusion cell as a function of time is obtained. This is not
identical to cumulative absorption, which is the sum of the amount
excreted (EXC) plus the residual amount (RA) still remaining in the
diffusion cell. Thus, the continuous perfusion technique is limited
by the ability of the resulting cumulative excretion curve to
approximate the true cumulative percutaneous absorption curve. Two
methods of approximation may be employed. Both depend on an
understanding of the kinetic parameters which define the diffusion
cell system being utilized.

Provided that there is rapid, homogenous mixing, the volume of
receptor fluid "cleared" (clearance, Cl) of absorbed compound may be

related to the actual volume (V) of the receptor phase of the
diffusion cell with a constant of elimination (Ke) by the following
equation (1)

$$Cl = Ke \cdot V \tag{2}$$

In this situation, Cl is analogous to flow rate through the
diffusion cell. This relationship has been verified in our
laboratory by injecting 2 μmol of benzoic acid through excised human
skin into the receptor half of a diffusion cell (V=10 ml), and
subsequently perfusing the cell at a rate of 5 ml per hour. Here,
Ke predicted by Equation 2 is 0.50 hr^{-1}. The concentrations of
collected samples were plotted semilogarithmically, and a linear fit
obtained by regression analysis (Figure 1). Measured Ke can be
related to the slope (-0.22 hr^{-1}) of this resulting line by the
equation (2)

$$slope = -Ke/2.303 \tag{3}$$

and was calculated to be 0.51 hr^{-1}, which is indistinguishable from
the prediction of Equation 2.

The cumulative excretion curve generated with continuously
perfused diffusion cells may approximate the true percutaneous
absorption curve as the value of Ke becomes larger, provided that
absorption into the diffusion cell is the rate limiting step. Ke
may be increased by increasing the flow rate, decreasing receptor
phase volume, or both, as indicated by Equation 2. Figure 2 is a
series of computer generated curves, employing different values of
Ke, which relate the time course of cumulative excretion to
cumulative absorption, where the absorption constant (Ka) has been
arbitrarily fixed at 0.05 hr^{-1}. Assuming first order absorption
into the receptor phase, with the skin as a rate limiting membrane
only, the true time course of cumulative absorption (ABS) is
described by a monoexponential function

$$ABS = Xo \ (1-exp(-Ka \cdot t)) \tag{4}$$

where Xo is the total dose available for absorption. Inspection of
Figure 2 reveals that the initial rise of the absorption curve is
essentially linear until 10-15% of the available dose has been
absorbed.

The cumulative excretion curves depicted in Figure 2 are
described by the equation

$$EXC = Xo[1-Ke \cdot exp(-Ka \cdot t)/(Ke-Ka) - Ka \cdot exp(-Ke \cdot t)/(Ka-Ke)] \tag{5}$$

The profiles demonstrate that when Ke is only slightly larger than
Ka, a substantial lag occurs before peak flux (rate of rise of the
cumulative excretion curve) is obtained. As Ke increases, the term
$exp(-Ke \cdot t)$ approaches 0 more quickly, and Equation 5 reduces to
Equation 4. We may effect a reduction of Equation 5 to Equation 4
by assuming that this exponential approaches 0 when it is 95%
complete, i.e.,

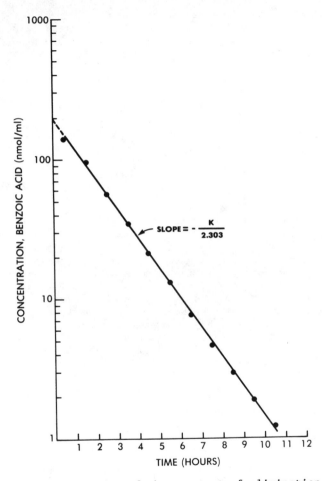

Figure 1. Determination of the constant of elimination (Ke).

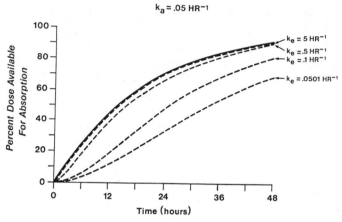

Figure 2. Relationship of cumulative excretion curves (broken lines) to the cumulative absorption curve (solid line).

$$\exp(-Ke \cdot t) = .05 \qquad\qquad (6)$$

Solving Equation 6 for t, we obtain

$$t \simeq 3/Ke \qquad\qquad (7)$$

Once this value of t has been exceeded, the reduction to Equation 4 has been effected and the remainder of the cumulative excretion curve is dependent on the absorption process only. Thus, as the value of Ke increases, the excretion curve approximates the absorption curve more closely.

If a reliable estimate of P is to be obtained from a cumulative excretion curve generated by a continuously perfused, "dynamic" diffusion cell, data points must be selected after the value of t defined by Equation 7 has been surpassed (when the shape of the excretion curve becomes dependent on absorption only), but before 10-15% of the total available dose has been absorbed (i.e., during the "steady state" period of absorption). Inspection of Figure 2 demonstrates that data points selected before or after these boundary conditions may lead to determinations of P which are falsely low.

Excretion data may also be transformed to approximate the true cumulative absorption (3). This method involves plotting excretion rates (determined from the collected samples) against time, and calculating the area under the resulting curve (AUC). These excretion rates are assumed to approximate the instantaneous rates at the midpoint of the sample collection intervals (4), and must be appropriately plotted along the time axis. AUC thus approximates total cumulative excretion to the midpoint (in time) of the last collected sample. Figure 3 depicts typical excretion rate data for benzoic acid (4.8 μmol deposited in acetone over 3.14 cm^2 of excised human skin, Ke=0.5 hr^{-1}). Using an analogous midpoint approximation, the concentration of the last collected sample is assumed to approximate the concentration of the residual receptor phase at the midpoint of the sample collection interval. The residual amount (RA) left in the diffusion cell is determined by multiplying the approximated concentration by the receptor volume. An approximated cumulative absorption curve may thus be generated from excretion rate data by adding RA to AUC for each collected sample, and P subsequently determined in the usual fashion.

Figure 4 compares the cumulative absorption curve for benzoic acid (4.8 μmol deposited in acetone over 3.14 cm^2 of excised human skin) approximated by this technique, compared to the true absorption curve obtained by manually emptying a diffusion cell at hourly intervals, then refilling with "fresh" solution to maintain sink conditions. The results are essentially identical.

The time course of the penetration process may be reasonably predicted from P (derived from any of the methods discussed above) according to Equation 1, assuming that Co never changes significantly over the period of observation ("infinite" dose). This situation may be obtained when the skin is exposed for a short period of time or to a large volume per unit surface area, such as immersion in a tank of solution. When the concentration in contact with the skin is likely to change over the period of exposure,

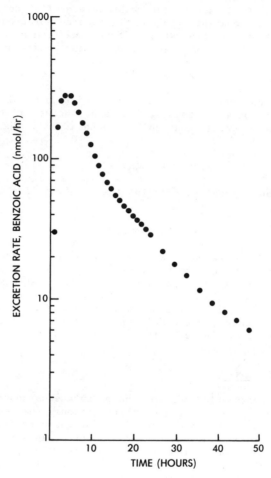

Figure 3.   Excretion rate data for benzoic acid, utilizing
midpoint approximations.

("finite dose", e.g., small volumes of solution saturating
clothing), P alone is insufficient to describe the penetration time
course. Here, the kinetics are more appropriately characterized by
Ka, the first order absorption rate constant.

A potentially useful mathematical relationship between P and Ka
may be derived. Cl is a constant which relates flux out of a
compartment to the concentration of the cleared solution. Cl may be
used to describe the initial steady state flux from an externally
applied solution through skin according to the relationship (1)

$$\text{flux(ss)} = Cl \cdot Co \qquad (8)$$

As defined in Equation 2, Cl is also related to the volume of the
cleared solution by a constant, which is analogous to Ka in this
situation. Substituting Equation 2 into Equation 8, the new
equation becomes:

$$\text{flux(ss)} = Ka \cdot V \cdot Co \qquad (9)$$

Setting Equation 9 equal to Equation 1 and solving for Ka, the
relationship

$$Ka = A \cdot P/V \qquad (10)$$

is obtained. Thus, the complete time course of the penetration
process may be characterized by transforming P into Ka and utilizing
Equation 4. It should be emphasized that this relationship is
applicable only when the substance contacting the skin is in
solution, and an initial value of Co is known. When a solid
substance is deposited on the skin from a volatile solvent, no
initial Co (or V) can be determined and P cannot be obtained.

Pharmacokinetic Model

An ideal pharmacokinetic model of the percutaneous absorption
process should be capable of describing not only the time course of
penetration through skin and into blood (or receptor fluid in a
diffusion cell), but also the time course of disappearance from the
skin surface and accumulation (reservoir effect) of penetrant within
the skin membrane. Neither Fick's First Law of Diffusion nor a
simple kinetic model considering skin as a rate limiting membrane
only is satisfactory, since neither can account for an accumulation
of penetrant within skin. To resolve this dilemma, we have analyzed
the in vitro time course of absorption of radiolabeled benzoic acid
(a rapid penetrant) and paraquat (a poor penetrant) through hairless
mouse skin using a linear three compartment kinetic model (Figure
5). The three compartments correspond to the skin surface (where
the initial dose is deposited), the skin itself (considered as a
separate compartment), and the receptor fluid in the diffusion
cell. The initial amount deposited on the skin surface is
symbolized by X10, and K12 and K23 are first order rate constants.

Both compounds were studied at equivalent doses of 1 μmol per
cm^2, deposited in approximately 16 μl per cm^2 of an appropriate

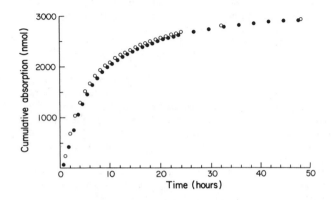

Figure 4. Cumulative absorption of benzoic acid, comparing the curve approximated by the AUC + RA technique (closed circles) to the true absorption curve (open circles).

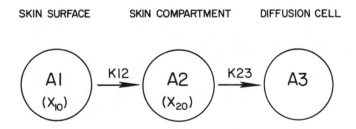

Figure 5. Linear 3 compartment pharmacokinetic model, considering the skin as a separate compartment. See text for explanation of symbols.

volatile solvent (acetone in the case of benzoic acid, methanol in
the case of paraquat). Evaporation of solvent from the skin surface
was allowed to occur at ambient conditions and was usually complete
within 3-4 minutes. Continuously perfused diffusion cells (receptor
volume = 10 ml) were utilized (3). The rate of perfusion was 10 ml
per hour, and samples were collected every 30-60 minutes.
Cumulative absorption curves were approximated using the AUC + RA
method from excretion rate data as described above. The total dose
available for absorption was considered to be the sum of all the
amounts recovered from skin surface washings, tissue digestion, and
cumulative absorption through skin (see below).
        The mathematical solution of the pharmacokinetic model depicted
by Figure 5 is described by Equation 5, where K12 and K23 are first
order rate constants analogous to Ka and Ke, respectively. This
solution was applied to the data and "best fit" parameters estimated
by iterative computational methods. The "fit" of the data to the
kinetic model was analyzed by least squares nonlinear regression
analysis (5).
        The suitability of the model in describing the percutaneous
penetration process was established by the following experiments.
1)   The input function (amount remaining on the skin surface for
      absorption over time) was determined by rinsing the skin
      surface with distilled water (3 consecutive rinses of 10-15
      seconds each) at various time periods after the initial
      application: 1/2 hr, 1 hr, 2 hr, 4 hr, 8 hr, 24 hr, and 48
      hr. Analysis of the recovered amounts by iterative
      computational estimation allowed "best fit" parameters
      describing this process to be obtained.
2)   The output function characterizing the movement of penetrant
      from the skin compartment into the receptor fluid of the
      diffusion cell was determined as follows. Thirty minutes after
      initial application, the skin surface was rinsed as described
      above to remove any surface residual. The diffusion cell was
      emptied, rinsed and refilled with fresh solution. All
      radiolabel recovered over the next 12 hours was assumed to have
      originated from the "filled" skin compartment, rather than the
      skin surface. "Best fit" parameters were obtained by
      computational methods as before.
        Having determined the kinetic parameters of the simulation by
the input and output function experiments, the appropriateness of
the kinetic model was confirmed by measuring the total amounts which
had both penetrated through and accumulated within the skin at
various time intervals. These data were obtained as part of the
same experiments to determine the input function. Following skin
washing to remove surface residual, the amount remaining within the
skin was determined by subsequent digestion in a tissue solubilizer
(Soluene 350, Packard Instruments, Downers Grove, IL). The
resulting data were compared to values predicted by the
pharmacokinetic model, using the parameters determined by the input
and output function experiments.
        Results of the input function experiments for both benzoic acid
and paraquat indicate that the residual amounts recovered from the
skin surface over time are best described by a monoexponential
function (Figure 6), with a fraction of the applied dose having

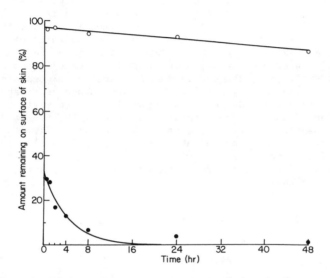

Figure 6.   Amounts of benzoic acid (closed circles) and
             paraquat (open circles) on the skin surface
             remaining to be absorbed, as a function of time.

disappeared completely from the surface at an rapid rate within the
first half hour. Each data point represents the average of 4
separate samples of hairless mouse skin. This suggests that the
volatile solvent vehicle may influence the percutaneous absorption
process, either solubilizing part of the applied dose in the
superficial skin surface lipid layer, before it has evaporated
(making it available for faster absorption), or possibly by carrying
a fraction of the applied dose into the skin compartment as a
portion of the solvent itself penetrates the skin.

The kinetic model depicted in Figure 5 may adequately account
for this rapid disappearance from the skin surface if it is assumed
that a fraction of the applied dose (X20) immediately partitions
into the skin compartment at time zero (r^2 for benzoic acid=0.95, r^2
for paraquat=0.97). Although the amount of paraquat (a poor
penetrant), which may rapidly solubilize into the skin compartment
is rather small (3%), the corresponding fraction for benzoic acid
appears to be quite large (77%). The slower phase of disappearance
from the skin surface depicted in Figure 6 may then reflect
dissolution of the residual applied substance (X10) from a dried
solid phase on the skin surface as a limiting step. Average K12
values for this slow phase of absorption were 0.25 hr^{-1} for benzoic
acid and 2×10^{-3} hr^{-1} for paraquat.

Results of the output function experiments for benzoic acid are
summarized in Table I.

Table I. Output Function Parameter Estimates for Benzoic Acid

Skin Sample #	F·X20(%)	K23/hr^{-1} (SE)	R^2
1	100	.68 (.007)	.83
2	100	.62 (.005)	.93
3	100	.28 (.002)	.91
AVE	100	.53 (.21)	

These indicate that the entire amount remaining to be absorbed from
the skin compartment after surface washing may be reasonably
described by a monoexponential function, with an average K23 value
of 0.53 hr^{-1}. On the other hand, a monoexponential function does
not adequately account for the entire dose of paraquat remaining to
be absorbed, and suggests that a substantial amount of paraquat may
bind to skin and be unavailable for absorption. The amount of
absorbed paraquat which may be reasonably described by a
monoexponential output function (F·X20) is only about 10% (assuming
irreversible binding), with an average K23 value of 0.82 hr^{-1} (Table
II).

The "best fit" parameter estimates obtained from the input and
output function experiments for both benzoic acid and paraquat are
summarized in Table III.

Table II. Output Function Parameter Estimates for Paraquat

Skin Sample #	F·X20(%) (SE)	K23/hr^{-1} (SE)	R^2
1	12.5 (.43)	0.59 (.009)	.73
2	10.8 (.28)	0.67 (.008)	.79
3	7.8 (.17)	1.20 (.19)	.49
AVE	10.4 (2.4)	.82 (.33)	

Table III. Summary of "Best Fit" Parameter Estimates

Penetrant	X10(%)(SE)	K12/hr^{-1}(SE)	X20(%)	F·X20(%)(SE)	K23/hr^{-1}(SE)
Benzoic acid	33.2(2.9)	0.23(.005)	76.8	100	0.53(.21)
Paraquat	96.9(0.5)	$2 \times 10^{-3}(2 \times 10^{-4})$	3.1	10.4(2.4)	0.82(.33)

Using these estimates, the kinetic model depicted in Figure 5 was applied to data describing the time course of penetration through skin (Figure 7) and accumulation within skin (Figure 8). Again, all data points represent average values obtained from 4 separate samples of hairless mouse skin. The solid lines represent values predicted by the model.

For benzoic acid, the "fit" of the kinetic model is in relatively good agreement with the observed data, without any consideration given for potential skin binding (r^2 for total penetration=0.94, r^2 for skin accumulation=0.83). In the case of paraquat, the binding observed in the output function experiments was assumed to be irreversible, and to occur only with X20. Although the early time courses are predicted reasonably well, the late time behavior is not (r^2 for total penetration=0.56, r^2 for skin accumulation=0.89). Further studies are in progress to consider potentially reversible binding for paraquat, which could account for these observations.

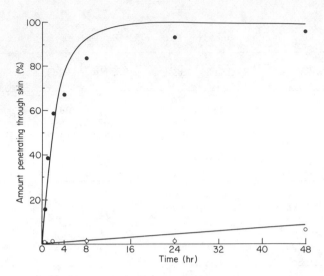

Figure 7.   Amounts of benzoic acid (closed circles) and
            paraquat (open circles) penetrating completely
            through skin as a function of time.

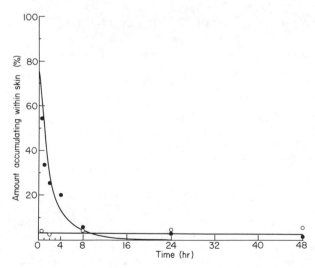

Figure 8.   Amounts of benzoic acid (closed circles) and
            paraquat (open circles) accumulating within the skin
            as a function of time.

Summary

The risk of an adverse systemic reaction following skin contact with
a potentially toxic chemical depends on the speed and total amount
of absorption through the skin. Several techniques have been
devised to measure these parameters across isolated skin mounted in
diffusion cells. The mathematical and kinetic relationships which
define the operation of these various systems have been reviewed. A
novel kinetic description of the penetration process has been
developed and applied to skin absorption measurements for benzoic
acid and paraquat. The results suggest that when these substances
are deposited on the skin surface in a volatile solvent, a portion
of the applied dose is rapidly solubilized into the skin and
available for fast absorption, while the remainder is absorbed more
slowly.

Acknowledgments

This work was supported, in part, by NIOSH grant OH–01830 (to
RHG). We thank Andrea Mazel for preparing the manuscript.

Literature Cited

1. Rowland, M.; Tozer, T.N. "Clinical Pharmacokinetics"; Lea and
    Febiger: Philadelphia, 1980; p. 84.
2. Gibaldi, M.; Perrier, D. "Pharmacokinetics"; Marcel Dekker: New
    York, 1975; pp. 2–6.
3. Mathias, C.G.T. Clin. Research 1983, 31, 586A.
4. Gibaldi, M.; Perrier, D. "Pharmacokinetics"; Marcel Dekker: New
    York, 1975; pp. 301–305.
5. Peck, C.; Barrett, B.B. J. Pharmacokin. Biopharm.·, 1979, 5,
    537.

RECEIVED November 27, 1984

Transdermal Absorption Kinetics
A Physicochemical Approach

RICHARD H. GUY[1], JONATHAN HADGRAFT[2], and HOWARD I. MAIBACH[3]

[1] Departments of Pharmacy and Pharmaceutical Chemistry, School of Pharmacy, University of California Medical Center, San Francisco, CA 94143
[2] Department of Pharmacy, University of Nottingham, Nottingham, NG7 2RD, United Kingdom
[3] Department of Dermatology, School of Medicine, University of California Medical Center, San Francisco, CA 94143

The development of a biophysically based model of chemical absorption via human skin is described. The simulation has been used to analyze the in vivo penetration kinetics of a broad range of molecular species. Four first-order rate constants are identified with the percutaneous absorption process: k_1 - penetrant diffusion through the stratum corneum; k_2 - transport across the viable epidermal tissue to the cutaneous microcirculation; k_3 - a retardation parameter which delays the passage of penetrant from stratum corneum to viable tissue; k_4 - the elimination rate constant of chemical from blood to urine. Interpretation of urinary excretion data following topical application is presented for 9 compounds. It is shown that the model has predictive potential based upon recognized cutaneous biology and penetrant physical chemistry, in particular the diffusive and partitioning properties of the substrate. Refinements and developments of the approach (e.g., to multiple exposure and competitive surface removal situations) are indicated and discussed.

Occupational disease, caused by skin contact with toxic substances, represents a major health problem in the United States (1). Dermal exposure of agricultural workers to pesticide agents, of course, is a particularly pertinent example of this problem. Prediction of the detrimental toxic effects of hazardous chemical exposure is difficult, however, because of the complexity of the percutaneous absorption process in man and a lack of any consistently identifiable relationship(s) between transport rate and chemical properties. In addition, the very diverse approaches, which have been used to measure skin penetration, further complicate the situation since the extrapolation of results to man in his workplace may involve questionable, non-validated assumptions. Our specific aim is to predict accurately the toxicokinetics of occupationally-encountered molecules (e.g., pesticides) absorbed across human skin in vivo. We present

here the application of a novel kinetic model (to analyze previously
published data) which suggests that the health hazard from cutaneous
exposure to toxic chemicals may be predicted correctly on the basis
of fundamental biological and physicochemical principles.

The Kinetic Model

The simulation is depicted in Figure 1 (2). The model is linear and
identifies four kinetic processes to describe a penetrant's transport
through, retention in, and removal from the skin and body.

k_1 characterizes transport of penetrant across the stratum
corneum and assumes negligible "vehicle" effects. Such an approach
is reasonable for skin contact with pure liquids and materials or
with volatile solvents which solubilize the potential penetrant.
More complicated vehicles or penetrant delivery systems will require
a separate input function to be added to the model. Because of the
passive nature of the stratum corneum barrier (3), we may relate k_1
to the substrate's diffusion coefficient (D_1) through this outermost
skin layer. Hence, in turn, k_1 can be shown to be penetrant
molecular weight (M) dependent via the Stokes-Einstein relationship
(4):

$$k_1 = C \cdot D_1 = C'(M)^{-1/3} \qquad (1)$$

where C and C' are constants. If k_1 is known for one or more substances, then its value for a new or different molecule may be evaluated using Equation 1 (assuming (i) that the transport mechanism
remains unaltered, and (ii) that the partial specific volumes of the
penetrants are approximately equivalent), i.e.,

$$k_1^u = k_1^k (M^k/M^u)^{1/3} \qquad (2)$$

where the superscripts u and k refer to the molecules whose k_1 values
are unknown and known, respectively. In this paper, we have utilized
an experimental estimate of k_1 for benzoic acid (5) to determine
k_1^u values for the other penetrants discussed.

k_2 describes penetrant diffusion through viable epidermal and
dermal tissue to the cutaneous blood vessels and systemic circulation. Again, we equate k_2 with the corresponding diffusion coefficient (D_2) and substrate molecular weight via an equation analogous
to Equation 1:

$$k_2 = C'' \cdot D_2 = C'''(M)^{-1/3} \qquad (3)$$

C'' and C''' are constants. Previous estimates of k_2 (2) have shown
that the rate constant reflects a diffusive process with $D_2 \approx 10^{-7}$
$cm^2 \; s^{-1}$, a value consistent with the perception of this tissue region
as an aqueous protein gel (6).

k_3 plays a decisive role in determining the final kinetic
profile by reflecting the competition for penetrant between hydrophobic stratum corneum and the more aqueous viable tissue. k_3 acts,
therefore, as a retardation rate constant (i.e., the greater k_3, the
longer the penetrant is held up in the horny layer and the slower it
partitions into the viable tissue). The magnitude of k_3 can, in this

way, signify the possibility of penetrant binding to skin or the likelihood of a "reservoir" effect (7). k_3 can, furthermore, correct for the simplistic relationship between k_1 and M. A high value of k_3, for example, may be used to imply very slow stratum corneum diffusion, because of increased interaction between penetrant and tissue. If such an assignation is accepted, then the ratio k_3/k_2 becomes a measure of an "effective partition coefficient" for the penetrant between stratum corneum and viable tissue. As is shown below, this interpretation provides important and significant predictive power to the simulation.

k_4 describes penetrant removal from the body once the chemical has reached the dermal vasculature. Compound in the cutaneous micro-circulation is not differentiated from that in the systemic pool. k_4 is equated, therefore, with the elimination rate constant (or combination of constants) that would be obtained if the penetrant were administered intravenously.

Four differential equations describe mathematically the model shown in Figure 1 (2). These expressions relate to the rates of change of penetrant concentration on and within the skin, in the blood and in the urine. Solution is straightforward and gives the following equation for ϕ_t, the amount of penetrant appearing in the urine as a function of time (t):

$$\phi_t = Fk_1 k_2 k_4 \ \{1/\alpha\beta k_1 - \exp(-k_1 t)/[k_1(k_1 - \alpha)(k_1 - \beta)] -$$

$$\exp(-\alpha t)/[\alpha(\alpha - \beta)(\alpha - k_1)] - \exp(-\beta t)/[\beta(\beta - k_1)(\beta - \alpha)]\} \qquad (4)$$

F is the fraction of the total amount of penetrant in contact with the skin at t=0 which eventually penetrates, and α and β satisfy the relationships:

$$\alpha\beta = k_2 k_4 \qquad (5)$$

$$(\alpha + \beta) = k_2 + k_3 + k_4 \qquad (6)$$

Equation 4 allows determination of % dose excreted per unit time for any specified times and we have made such calculations to coincide with the experimental data, which is interpreted below.

Data Interpretation

The kinetic model has been used to analyze percutaneous penetration rate data for nine molecules: aspirin, benzoic acid, caffeine, chloramphenicol, diethyltoluamide, nitrobenzene, salicylic acid (8) and the methyl and benzyl esters of nicotinic acid (9). Experimentally, the chemicals (^{14}C-labelled) were applied topically in acetone to the ventral forearm of human volunteers and the urinary excretion of radioactivity was then measured over a five day period; F values were thus determined directly. k_4 parameters for these molecules were also assessed by monitoring urinary excretion following intravenous administration of a ^{14}C-labelled dose (8). Typically, k_4 and F values are associated with a standard deviation of 10-15% (8). The experimental results are plotted in Figures 2-10; on each figure, calculated urinary excretion rates are also given

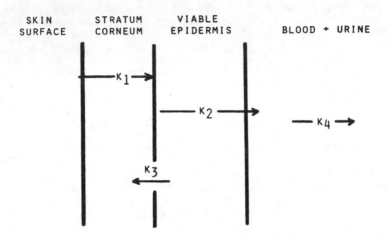

Figure 1.   The pharmacokinetic model.

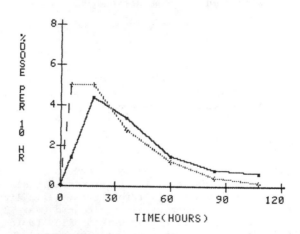

Figure 2.   Aspirin: comparison between experimental data (solid line) and theoretical prediction (broken line) based on the rate constants (k_1–k_4) given in Table I.

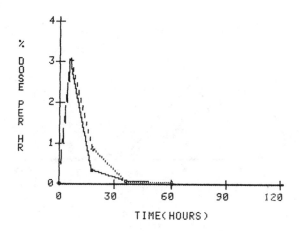

Figure 3. Benzoic acid: comparison between experimental data (solid line) and theoretical prediction (broken line) based on the rate constants (k_1-k_4) given in Table I.

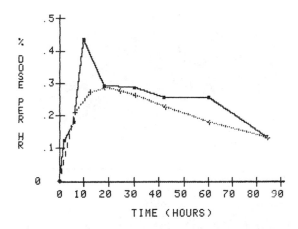

Figure 4. Benzyl nicotinate: comparison between experimental data (solid line) and theoretical prediction (broken line) based on the rate constants (k_1-k_4) given in Table I.

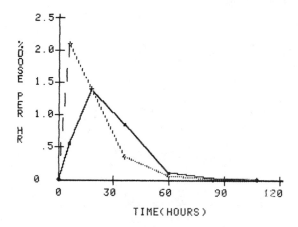

Figure 5. Caffeine: comparison between experimental data (solid line) and theoretical prediction (broken line) based on the rate constants (k_1-k_4) given in Table I.

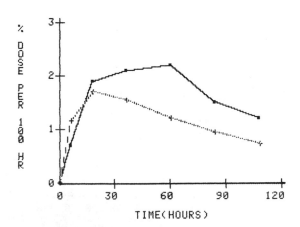

Figure 6. Chloramphenicol: comparison between experimental data (solid line) and theoretical prediction (broken line) based on the rate constants (k_1-k_4) given in Table I.

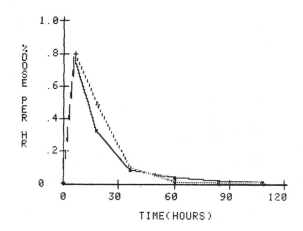

Figure 7. Diethyltoluamide: comparison between experimental data (solid line) and theoretical prediction (broken line) based on the rate constants (k_1-k_4) given in Table I.

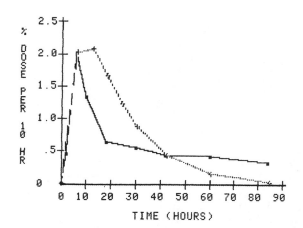

Figure 8. Methyl nicotinate: comparison between experimental data (solid line) and theoretical prediction (broken line) based on the rate constants (k_1-k_4) given in Table I.

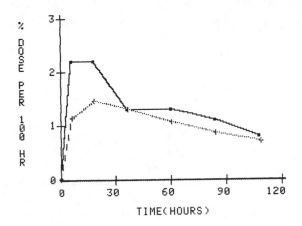

Figure 9. Nitrobenzene: comparison between experimental data (solid line) and theoretical prediction (broken line) based on the rate constants (k_1-k_4) given in Table I.

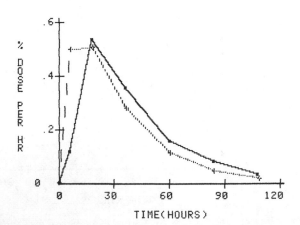

Figure 10. Salicylic acid: comparison between experimental data (solid line) and theoretical prediction (broken line) based on the rate constants (k_1-k_4) given in Table I.

which have been evaluated using Equation 4 and the values of $k_1 - k_4$ and F given in Table I.

Table I. Rate Parameters of the Kinetic Model for Nine Chemicals

Penetrant	F	$k_1(hr^{-1})$	$k_2(hr^{-1})$	$k_3(hr^{-1})$	$k_4(hr^{-1})$
Aspirin	0.22	0.16	2.6	15	0.17
Benzoic acid	0.43	0.18	2.9	5.0	0.59
Benzyl nicotinate	0.28	0.15	2.4	30	0.17
Caffeine	0.48	0.16	2.5	2.5	0.12
Chloramphenicol	0.02	0.13	2.1	21	0.12
Diethyltoluamide	0.17	0.16	2.5	1.5	0.17
Methyl nicotinate	0.06	0.18	2.8	5.0	0.17
Nitrobenzene	0.02	0.18	2.9	9.0	0.04
Salicylic acid	0.23	0.18	2.8	10	0.17

As stated above, k_4 and F were measured in vivo. k_1 and k_2 were determined (as discussed previously) from parameter estimates for benzoic acid (2) and application of appropriate molecular weight corrections (see Equation 2). The k_3 values presented are those which give, by repeated iteration, the best fits to the published experimental results, i.e., the calculated excretion rates shown in Figures 2-10. It follows that the accuracy of the k_3 rate constants parallels those of the experimentally measured k_4 and F values.

In Table II, for each penetrant, the k_3/k_2 ratio is listed together with the corresponding octanol/water partition coefficient (9-11); Figure 11 illustrates this information graphically.

Table II. Comparison Between the Estimated Ratio of k_3/k_2 and the Octanol-Water Partition Coefficient (K) for the Nine Penetrants Considered

Penetrant	k_3/k_2	K
Aspirin	5.8	16.2
Benzoic acid	1.7	74.1
Benzyl nicotinate	1.8	270
Caffeine	1.0	0.85
Chloramphenicol	10.0	13.8
Diethyltoluamide	0.6	2.50
Methyl nicotinate	1.8	11.5
Nitrobenzene	3.1	72.4
Salicylic acid	3.6	17.0

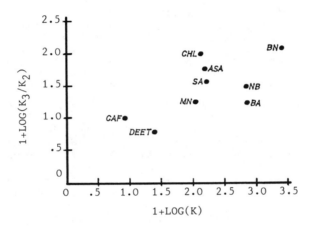

Figure 11. Comparison between the calculated k_3/k_2 ratio and the octanol-water partition coefficient (K) for each of the penetrants considered.

Discussion

Firstly, it is apparent that the simulation proposed can successfully
model penetration data for a very diverse range of chemical
moieties. The k_3/k_2 ratios span three orders of magnitude indicating
the markedly different stratum corneum/viable tissue affinities of
the penetrants considered. Further, the reasonable correlation
between k_3/k_2 and K (octanol/H_2O) provides support for the putative
biophysical significance of the model and suggests how k_3 (the most
experimentally inaccessible parameter) may be predicted for any
compound. We may also appreciate the power of k_3 in controlling the
kinetic profile for chemicals of relatively high stratum corneum
affinity. The sensitivity of k_3, therefore, permits careful modula-
tion of the time-course of a penetrant's behavior within the skin
and, subsequently, within the body.
    Thus, we have shown that a straightforward, linear, kinetic
model of percutaneous absorption may be identified and tested. The
approach contends that chemical ingress via the skin is controlled by
(A) the penetrant's diffusion velocities across stratum corneum and
viable tissue, and (B) its partitioning characteristics between these
two tissue layers. It appears that the former may be estimated from
molecular size and biological knowledge of the skin and that the
latter may be correlated to the octanol/water distribution coefficient. Hence, the predictive power of the model may prove to be
considerable and may allow reliable dermal exposure risks from new
and existing chemicals to be made. At this time, further validation
of the approach seems well-justified on the basis of the encouraging
results obtained so far. Equally, refinement and development of the
model is in progress; for example:-
[1] We have used the simulation to interpret the limited multiple-
exposure percutaneous penetration information which is currently
available (12). Results for hydrocortisone and malathion (13,14)
have been analyzed and the differences observed between the two
species have been shown to be consistent with the different physicochemical properties of the penetrants.
[2] The model has been developed to include the effect of competitive
surface loss processes on the kinetics of skin absorption (15). The
refinement is of relevance because surface removal is a common occurrence (through desquamation and abrasion) and because many cutaneous
hazards encountered in the workplace and environment are volatile and
hence subject to some degree of evaporation before penetration.
[3] The approach has been extended to include the possibility that
metabolism of penetrant may take place within the skin (16). Because
such biotransformations may activate or detoxify an absorbing
molecule, the subject deserves much further consideration.

Conclusion

The physicochemical approach to the prediction of transdermal absorption kinetics described in this paper offers a promising stategy for
the estimation of cutaneous exposure risk. The model is conceptually
straightforward yet sensitive to the biology of skin and to the
chemical and physical properties of the penetrant. Human, in vivo,
penetration data for a diverse array of absorbing molecules have been

successfully and consistently analyzed with the proposed simulation. Future developments have been identified and followed and indicate significant predictive potential for this pathway to the understanding of dermal toxicity induced by chemical hazards.

Nontechnical Summary

Skin exposure to toxic chemicals (including pesticides) represents a significant occupational and environmental health hazard. Prediction of cutaneous toxicity is difficult, however, because the kinetics of skin absorption in man are not easily estimated. In this paper, we discuss a mathematical model for the penetration of chemicals across the skin of humans. The simulation incorporates recognized aspects of cutaneous biology and pertinent physical chemical properties of the penetrant and calculates, on this basis, the transport kinetics of molecules into the body via the skin. Experimental penetration data for 9 chemicals of very diverse characteristics have been analyzed successfully using the physicochemical method. Many different types of absorption behavior, it appears, can be understood adequately with the single interpretive approach proposed. It seems reasonable to suggest that the model may offer a novel and facile means to predict dermal toxicity for a wide range of hazardous and potentially dangerous substances.

Acknowledgments

This work was supported by N.I.O.S.H. grant OH-01830-01 (RHG) and by travel grants (JH, RHG) from the The Wellcome Trust and The Burroughs-Wellcome Fund. We thank Andrea Mazel for manuscript preparation.

Literature Cited

1. "NIOSH Dermatology Program Announcement: Occupational Cutaneous Hazards and Diseases", U.S. Department of Health, Education and Welfare, 1980.
2. Guy, R. H.; Hadgraft, J.; Maibach, H. I. Internat. J. Pharmaceut. 1982, 11, 119.
3. Wester, R. C.; Maibach, H. I. Drug Metab. Rev. 1983, 14, 169.
4. Atkins, P. W. "Physical Chemistry"; Oxford University Press: Oxford, 1978; pp. 833-843.
5. Anjo, D. M.; Feldmann, R. J.; Maibach, H. I. In "Percutaneous Penetration of Steroids"; Mauvais-Jarvais, P.; Wepierre, J.; Vickers, C. F. H., Eds.; Academic: New York, 1980; pp. 31-51.
6. Scheuplein, R. J. J. Invest. Dematol. 1976, 67, 672.
7. Hadgraft, J. Internat. J. Pharmaceut. 1979, 2, 265.
8. Feldman, R. J.; Maibach, H. I. J. Invest. Dermatol. 1970, 51, 399.
9. Bucks, D. A. W.; Guy, R. H., unpublished results.
10. Leo, A.; Hansch, C.; Elkins, D. Chem. Rev. 1971, 71, 525.
11. Reifenrath, W., personal communication.
12. Guy, R. H.; Hadgraft, J.; Maibach, H. I. Internat. J. Pharmaceut. 1983, 17, 23.

13.   Wester, R. C.; Noonan, P. K.; Maibach, H. I.   Arch. Dermatol.
      1980, 116, 186.
14.   Wester, R. C.; Maibach, H. I.; Bucks, D. A. W.; Guy, R. H.
      Toxicol. Appl. Pharmacol. 1983, 68, 116.
15.   Guy, R. H.; Hadgraft, J.   J. Soc. Cosmet. Chem. 1984, 35, 103.
16.   Guy, R. H.; Hadgraft, J.   Internat. J. Pharmaceut. 1984, 20, 43.

RECEIVED September 11, 1984

In Vitro Methods for the Percutaneous Absorption of Pesticides

ROBERT L. BRONAUGH

Division of Toxicology, Food and Drug Administration, Washington, DC 20204

The primary barrier to the entry of chemicals through
skin is the upper layer of the epidermis, the stratum
corneum. The passive diffusion through this nonliving
tissue forms the rationale for using in vitro diffusion
cell systems to measure skin absorption. This
procedure has been validated in our laboratory and by
others by comparison with in vivo results. Compounds
that lack water solubility can present difficulties in
the standard in vitro method using an aqueous receptor
solution beneath the skin. This fluid must be modified
so that it is sufficiently lipophilic to allow
partitioning of the test compound from skin into the
diffusion cell receptor. We have used a nonionic
surfactant, oleth 20, to increase the absorption of
this type of compound without apparent damage to the
skin. The permeation (percent of applied dose) of the
hydrophobic pesticide DDT through human skin was 1.1%
with saline in the receptor and 4.5% using 6% oleth
20. These results with a model compound illustrate the
need to consider the solubility properties of a
compound in a percutaneous absorption study.

The results of a number of comparative studies (1-4) indicate that
the percutaneous absorption of chemicals can be measured accurately
by in vitro techniques. When discrepancies have been found between
in vivo and in vitro values, they are often the result of
experimental differences. Errors in the measurement of
percutaneous absorption are possible with in vivo techniques
because of the difficulties in observing absorption through skin by
measuring amounts of compound excreted in the urine and feces.

As with any technique, in vitro absorption measurements are
meaningful only when done with sound methodology and an awareness
of the potential problems and limitations. Probably the greatest
problem is in the measurement of absorption of compounds that are
insoluble in water. These compounds will not likely partition

freely into the aqueous diffusion cell receptor fluid routinely
used. A number of pesticides are subject to this pitfall because
of their poor water solubility.

Methods for in vitro absorption measurements will be presented,
including techniques for studying hydrophobic compounds. The
absorption of two pesticides with limited water solubility (DDT and
parathion) has been measured through excised human skin.

Diffusion Cell Methodology

In vitro percutaneous absorption experiments are sometimes
conducted with the principles of diffusion rigorously in mind. An
aqueous solution of the penetrant is applied on one side of the
skin and its diffusion followed into identical aqueous fluid on the
other side of the membrane. Stirring devices are used on both
sides of the membrane (2-chambered cell technique) (5). Currently,
skin absorption is frequently measured after application of the
test substance in a small amount of vehicle to the surface of the
skin. Permeation is followed by removal of aliquots from the
stirred solution in the receptor below the skin (1-chamber static
cell) (1, 6). This procedure more closely simulates the in vivo
situation because the skin is exposed to ambient conditions and is
not excessively hydrated as in the 2-chamber procedure.

A further refinement in absorption measurements is the use of a
perfusion fluid below the skin to take up penetrating substances
(7). Sampling is facilitated by collection of the effluent in
vials in a fraction collector. The flow-through diffusion cell is
a 1-chambered cell with many advantages. Automatic sampling allows
a savings of labor in addition to around-the-clock determination of
the absorption profile. Sink conditions are easily maintained even
in absorption studies where large amounts of nonradiolabeled
material are applied. A more physiological assessment of
percutaneous absorption might be obtained for compounds of limited
water solubility since the cells may serve to mimic the effect of
blood flow through the skin by taking up and carrying away the
absorbed compounds.

The volume of the receptor is critical. To completely remove
the material that has penetrated into the receptor in a given time,
the volume of fluid pumped into the cell must be many times the
volume of the receptor. This requires a small receptor volume so
that the volume of effluent from the cell is manageable.

The skin permeability of a hydrophobic fragrance material
(cinnamyl anthranilate) was examined using 1-chambered static
diffusion cell techniques (8). In vitro percutaneous absorption
measurements with rat skin using a normal saline receptor solution
resulted in values that were much lower than the corresponding in
vivo data for the compound. This difference is shown in the time
course for the absorption of cinnamyl anthranilate (Figure 1).

The effect of different receptor fluids on cinnamyl
anthranilate absorption was determined by comparing values obtained
at the end of 5 days (Table I). Only 12.7% of the compound
absorbed in vivo in the 5-day period was obtained in a
corresponding in vitro experiment using normal saline receptor
fluid and split-thickness rat skin. A 1.5% solution of the

nonionic surfactant oleth 20 (Volpo 20, Croda Inc., New York, NY)
enhanced by 3-fold the skin permeability to cinnamyl anthranilate;
the cortisone permeation determined simultaneously in the
dual-label experiment was not altered. When full-thickness rat
skin was used, no increase in cinnamyl anthranilate absorption was
obtained with the oleth 20, indicating the importance of removing
most of the dermal tissue. The optimal concentration of oleth 20
was 6%. A 5-fold increase in cinnamyl anthranilate permeation was
obtained without altering the permeation of the cortisone control.
    Rabbit serum and bovine serum albumin had no effect on the
integrity of the barrier, but they were also less effective in
increasing cinnamyl anthranilate absorption than oleth 20. A
methanol-water solution and 6% octoxynol 9 (Triton X-100, Rohm and
Haas Co., Philadelphia, PA) were equal to or superior to 6% oleth
20, but significant damage to the skin was indicated by the
increased cortisone permeation. A 6% solution of poloxamer 188 in
the receptor resulted in slight enhancement of both cinnamyl
anthranilate and cortisone permeation.
    Cinnamyl anthranilate absorption was evaluated in the
flow-through cell using saline or a solution of the nonionic
surfactant as the receptor fluid (7). With normal saline receptor

Table I. Effect of Diffusion Cell Conditions on the
Absorption of Cinnamyl Anthranilate (I) (Cortisone Control)[a]

Receptor Fluid	I, % Applied Dose Absorbed (5 days)	Cortisone Permeability Constant X 10^5 (cm/h)
Normal saline (4)[b]	5.0 ± 0.3	3.8 ± 0.7
1.5% Oleth 20 (4)[b]	5.4 ± 0.9	-
Normal saline (4)	5.8 ± 0.4	7.1 ± 0.5
1.5% Oleth 20 (10)	15.5 ± 1.2[c]	6.1 ± 0.5
6% Oleth 20 (8)	27.9 ± 1.8[c]	7.0 ± 0.9
20% Oleth 20 (8)	18.3 ± 1.8[c]	9.3 ± 0.9
Rabbit serum (4)	8.8 ± 0.6[c]	6.8 ± 0.8
3% Bovine serum albumin (4)	12.1 ± 1.2[c]	5.4 ± 0.2
50:50 Methanol-water (4)	27.1 ± 2.0[c]	17.2 ± 0.2[c]
1.5% Octoxynol 9 (4)	17.9 ± 1.1[c]	10.8 ± 0.5[c]
6% Octoxynol 9 (4)	38.4 ± 2.9[c]	14.5 ± 1.3[c]
6% Poloxamer 188 (4)	7.3 ± 1.3	9.8 ± 0.6[c]

[a]Values are the mean ± S.E. of the number of determinations in
parentheses. For most experiments, a 350-um section from the
surface of whole rat skin was prepared with a dermatome. Compounds
were applied to the skin in a petrolatum vehicle. In vivo
absorption of I was 45.6%.
[b]Whole skin.
[c]Significant increase when compared to results from saline
(dermatome section) by one-tailed Student's t-test, P <0.05.

fluid, absorption was significantly increased by the use of the
flow-through cell (Figure 2). However, the amount of absorption was
less than the similar values obtained with either type of cell when
6% oleth 20 was the receptor fluid.

Absorption of Pesticides

Percutaneous absorption measurements of a limited number of
pesticides have previously been reported. Permeation of DDT,
lindane, parathion, and malathion was measured in human volunteers
by Maibach and coworkers (9, 10). In vivo absorption values for the
same compounds were obtained for monkey, pig, and rabbit (11). The
dermal penetration of 14 pesticides in mice (12) and three
pesticides in rats (13) was measured by Shah and coworkers using in
vivo techniques.
   We have measured the absorption of radiolabeled DDT and
parathion through excised human abdominal skin using an in vitro
diffusion cell procedure. The poor water solubility properties of
these compounds (Table II) suggested that a nonionic surfactant
(oleth 20) would be necessary in the receptor fluid. The compounds
were applied to skin in an acetone vehicle at a concentration of
4 ug/cm^2. The surface of the skin was cleansed with acetone at 24
h to remove unabsorbed material. The absorption of the pesticides
was followed for a total of 7 days until the amount of compound
entering the receptor fluid was minimal (Figures 3 and 4).

Table II. Solubility Properties of Pesticides

Pesticide	Water Solubility (mg/L)	Octanol/Water Partition Coefficient[a]	Octanol Solubility (mg/L)
DDT	0.0001[b]	9500	9.5
Parathion	20[c]	2820	141

[a]Ref. 14.
[b]Ref. 15.
[c]Ref. 16.

The total absorption of both compounds was greater in
experiments with the oleth 20 receptor fluid (Table III) and so
these values were used as the absorption measurements. The
permeation of the least water-soluble compound, DDT, was increased
to the greatest extent (4-fold) with the use of the nonionic
surfactant. The absorption of parathion exceeded that of DDT, as
might have been predicted from the physical chemical properties of
the molecules. The compounds are of similar molecular weight, but
parathion has much greater oil and water solubility properties.

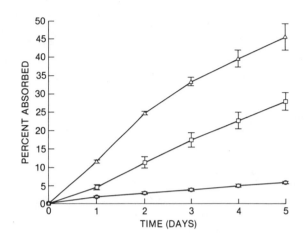

Figure 1.   Cinnamyl anthranilate absorption from a petrolatum
vehicle. △= in vivo; O= in vitro (saline in receptor); □= in
vitro (6% oleth 20 in receptor).

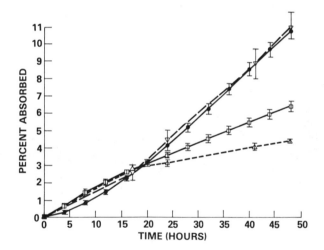

Figure 2.   Effect of cell type and receptor fluid on absorption
of cinnamyl anthranilate.   Cinnamyl anthranilate was applied to
the rat skin membrane in a petrolatum vehicle.   Receptor fluid
was either normal saline solution or 6% oleth 20 in water.
Absorption was expressed as the cumulative amount of compound
penetrating the skin.   Flow-through cell: □= normal saline, ●=
6% oleth 20; static cell: △= normal saline, ▽= 6% oleth 20.

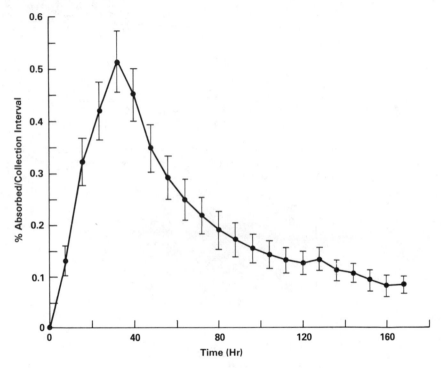

Figure 3.   DDT time-course of absorption through excised human
skin.   Collection interval = 8 h.

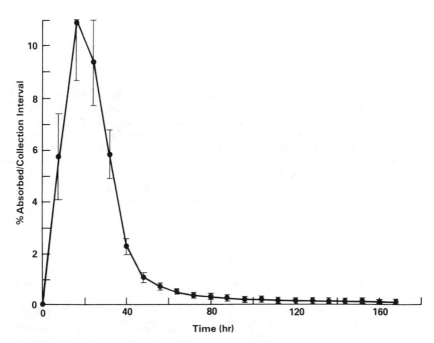

Figure 4.   Parathion time-course of absorption through excised human skin.   Collection interval = 8 h.

Table III. In Vitro Absorption of Pesticides - Human skin

	Applied Dose Absorbed[a] (%)	
Pesticide	Saline Solution	6% Oleth 20 Solution
DDT	1.1 + 0.1 (6)	4.5 + 0.6 (8)
Parathion	25.6 + 5.2 (6)	39.0 + 6.4 (8)

[a]Values are the mean + S.E. of the number of determinations in parentheses. The solutions refer to the fluid used in the diffusion cell receptor.

The previous in vivo human data initially appears to be in disagreement with our findings. Using a technique similar to ours (acetone vehicle, 4 ug compound/cm^2), the absorption of DDT and parathion was reported as 10.4 and 9.7%, respectively. However, parathion has been reported by the same investigators ([17]) to be absorbed more rapidly (18.5%) through abdominal skin, which is more comparable to our results (Table IV). The skin of the monkey has been reported to have permeability properties similar to those of human skin ([10]). In vivo monkey studies ([10]) have shown parathion to be absorbed much more rapidly than DDT (parathion = 30.3%, DDT = 1.5%).

Table IV. Absorption of Pesticides

	Applied Dose Absorbed (%)			
	Human			Monkey
Pesticide	In Vitro	In Vivo		In Vivo
DDT	4.5	10.4[a]		1.5[b,c]
Parathion	39.0	9.7[b]	18.5[d]	30.3[b]

[a]Ref. 10.
[b]Back skin, ref. 11.
[c]Not corrected by parenteral excretion method.
[d]Abdominal skin, ref. 17.

Conclusions

Percutaneous absorption studies using in vitro techniques appear to be of value in the assessment of pesticide absorption as well as with other types of compounds. As with any procedure, precautions may need to be taken in certain steps to ensure the accuracy of the data. For water-insoluble compounds, the lipophilicity of the receptor fluid may need to be increased (without damaging the integrity of the barrier). For all permeation studies with excised human skin, the barrier properties should be verified with a reference compound.

Nontechnical Summary

The measurement of the amount of absorption through the skin of chemicals that come in contact with its surface can be estimated using samples of skin that have been removed from human cadavers or nonliving animals. This is because the primary barrier to penetration through the skin is composed of nonliving tissue. Chemicals that are insoluble in water, however, are difficult to study using this procedure. Applied compounds may penetrate into the skin but do not enter the aqueous fluid beneath the skin in the diffusion cells. When this fluid was modified so that it was capable of dissolving water-insoluble compounds, more meaningful absorption values were obtained for the pesticide DDT.

Literature Cited

1. Franz, T.J. J. Invest. Dermatol. 1975, 64, 190-5.
2. Franz, T.J. Curr. Probl. Dermatol. 1978, 7, 58-68.
3. Bronaugh, R.L.; Stewart, R.F.; Congdon, E.R.; Giles, A.L., Jr. Toxicol. Appl. Pharmacol. 1982, 62, 474-80.
4. Bronaugh, R.L.; Maibach, H.I. J. Invest. Dermatol. 1984, submitted for publication.
5. Durrheim, H.; Flynn, G.L.; Higuchi, W.I.; Behl, C.R. J. Pharm. Sci. 1980, 69, 781-6.
6. Bronaugh, R.L.; Congdon, E.R.; Scheuplein, R.J. J. Invest. Dermatol. 1981, 76, 94-6.
7. Bronaugh, R.L.; Stewart, R.F. J. Pharm. Sci. 1984, in press.
8. Bronaugh, R.L.; Stewart, R.F. J. Pharm. Sci. 1984, in press.
9. Feldmann, R.J.; Maibach, H.I. Toxicol. Appl. Pharmacol. 1974, 28, 126-32.
10. Wester, R.C.; Maibach, H.I. In "Cutaneous Toxicity"; Drill, V.A., Ed.; Academic Press: New York, 1977; pp. 111-26.
11. Bartek, M.J.; LaBudde, J.A. In "Animal Models in Dermatology"; Maibach, H. Ed.; Churchill Livingstone: New York, 1975; pp. 103-19.
12. Shah, P.V.; Monroe, R.J.; Guthrie, F.E. Toxicol. Appl. Pharmacol. 1981, 59, 414-23.
13. Shah, P.V.; Guthrie, F.E. J. Invest. Dermatol. 1983, 80, 291-3.
14. Hansch, C.; Leo, A. "Substituent Constants for Correlation Analysis in Chemistry and Biology"; Wiley: New York, 1979.
15. Melnikov, N.N. "Chemistry of Pesticides"; Springer-Verlag: New York, 1971.
16. "Merck Index"; Merck & Co.: Rahway, NJ, 1976, 9th ed.
17. Maibach, H.l.; Feldmann, R.J., Arch. Environ. Health 1971, 23, 208-11.

RECEIVED September 12, 1984

Radiotracer Approaches to Rodent Dermal Studies

G. J. MARCO[1], B. J. SIMONEAUX[1], S. C. WILLIAMS[1], J. E. CASSIDY[1], R. BISSIG[2], and W. MUECKE[2]

[1] Agricultural Division, CIBA-GEIGY Corporation, Greensboro, NC 27409
[2] Agricultural Division, CIBA-GEIGY Ltd., Basel, Switzerland

With emphasis on safety evaluation applications, the use of radiotracers in rat and mouse dermal absorption studies are discussed. A multi-tiered experimental strategy is proposed containing judgement points providing skin absorption, tissue depletion and animal excretion rates in a cost effective manner. Techniques described include occlusive and non-occlusive treatments, sample preparations and data collection. Typical data is shown for herbicides and insecticides.

Our purpose for performing dermal treatment studies in the rat or mouse is to obtain data to better estimate the potential dermal penetration and rate of excretion of a compound for use in risk assessment evaluations and in monitoring worker dermal exposure. To obtain this goal, the following broad objectives can be stated:

1. To determine the rate of dermal absorption and penetration.
2. To determine levels of tissue deposition.
3. To determine mode and rate of excretion and tissue depletion.
4. To compare dermal and oral metabolism.
5. To determine a moiety relating to urinary metabolites for monitoring purposes.

While this paper introduces unique approaches to rodent dermal studies, other animals and man have been investigated using other procedures. Bartek et al (1) compared the rat, rabbit, pig and man. Hunziker et al (2) compared the Mexican hairless dog and man. A recent very good, extensive review on percutaneous absorption has been published by Wester and Maibach (3).

Strategy

These objectives can be met with the following experimental strategy containing judgement points to provide a variety of contingencies. Information obtained from either a previous oral

0097–6156/85/0273–0043$06.00/0

study or preliminary dermal study is normally necessary for the proper design of study details. Young adult rats of about 200 gm. are the animal of choice in this strategy. The radioactive dose (usually Carbon-14) is normally dissolved in an appropriate solvent at a concentration to permit a 100 µl dose on the marked area in order to provide uniform dosage distribution. In the preliminary study, one rat of each sex is treated at a high level (normally 10 mg/kg) and placed in closed glass cages and urine, feces, CO_2 and volatiles collected daily for 72 hours. At least 10 tissues are analyzed for total radioactive content. If total recovery is less than 90%, the carcass is also analyzed. However, an oral dose study can serve the same purpose.

Table I. Strategy for Rat Dermal Studies

Phase I (Absorption Kinetics)

3 male rats dosed 0.5 and 10 mg/kg per point.
Time points - 4, 8, 24 hours.
Excreta - 24 hour urine/feces - CO_2/volatiles optional.
Tissues - Treated skin, liver, kidney, plasma, RBC and carcass.
        - Other tissues based on retention information.

Phase II (Depletion Kinetics)

3 male rats per point dosed as in Phase I.
Minimum of 2 added points, maximum length of 7 days.
All other parameters the same as Phase I.

Phase III (Characterization of Urine Metabolites)

Chromatographic character of urine metabolites.
Select appropriate entity to analyze.

Phase IV (Extension of Study)

Add other sex, more rats/point, more points, etc., based on evaluation of data obtained in the previous three phases.

Phase I is done to observe absorption kinetics. Two groups of three male rats each per time point are chosen and treated at 0.5 and 10 mg/kg. Sacrifice time points are 4, 8 and 24 hours. Feces and urine are collected at least at 24 hours and CO_2 and volatiles only if more than 5% of the dose is collected in the preliminary or oral study or if the test material is volatile. Tissues analyzed are treated skin, liver, kidney, plasma, red blood cells and carcass. Other specific tissues are considered in addition if >0.5 ppm of total radioactivity is retained as seen from the preliminary study or >0.1 ppm from a previously done low single dose oral metabolism study (0.5 mg/kg after 7 days). However, these values are flags for decision rather than firm triggers.

Phase II is done to observe the depletion kinetics for tissue and excreta. Three male rats per sacrifice point, dosed in the same manner as Phase I are used. All other parameters of Phase I are duplicated. A minimum of two additional points are added when tissue and excretion kinetics are desired. However, the maximum study length is 7 days.

Phase III is done to characterize the urinary metabolites in order to devise a urine monitoring procedure. If an oral metabolism study has been done, the main metabolites are usually characterized and possibly identified. If the urinary metabolite patterns are similar in the oral and dermal study, a urinary method of metabolite analysis can be arrived at readily, if not already defined. Otherwise, converting the often observed multiple metabolites to one or two common entities is frequently desirable. The analytical method is of potential use in urine monitoring of workers.

Phase IV is a portion of the strategy that provides additional flexibility and judgement in extending the studies. Based on evaluation of the data obtained in the previous three phases, the second sex, more animals per point, more data points or other data may be desired. The original protocol can be written to include these additions or additions may be handled as amendments.

This experimental strategy provides a multitiered approach with Phases I and II the prime tiers. Use of this multitiered approach provides data sufficient for risk assessment estimates, yet is done in a time, materials and cost effective manner.

Techniques

In this section, the equipment and apparatus presently being used in our laboratory will be described. Two treatment modes are described. The radioactive chemical treated skin area may be covered (i.e., occlusive mode) or exposed to air (i.e., non-occlusive mode), depending upon the real world situation to be simulated.

The next series of figures show the steps presently used for the occlusive mode of treatment, first with a schematic of the dosage area. After shaving with an electric clipper and waiting 16 to 24 hours, the area is marked (Figure 1) and dose applied from a syringe (Figure 2a). An aluminum foil cover (Figure 2b) is applied and the entire area covered and secured with wide adhesive tape. At the end of treatment time, the tape is removed along with the foil, area wiped for unabsorbed material and the animal dissected for the tissues of interest.

For the non-occlusive approach several differences in treatment and animal handling were required. A technique was desired that would permit up to 7 days in the metabolism cages with minimum stress on the animal, access to feed and minimal cage contamination. The treatment area was further shaved with a microscreen faced electric shaver to provide minimum hair stub length. The next figure shows a schematic of the dosage area (Figure 3). In early studies, only one square was used, but presently the 5 square design is being used. A difference in the

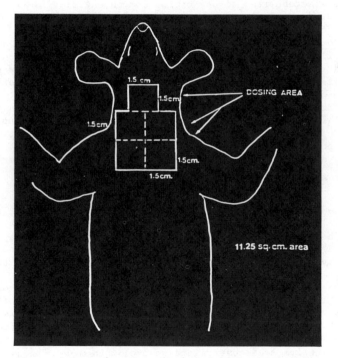

Figure 1.   Schematic of occlusive dermal treatment area.

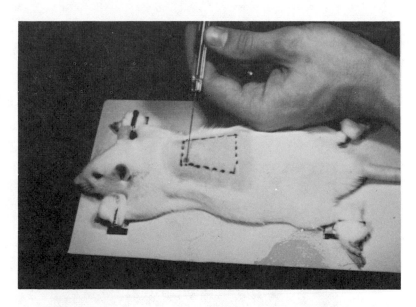

Figure 2 a.   Dose application by syringe in occlusive study.

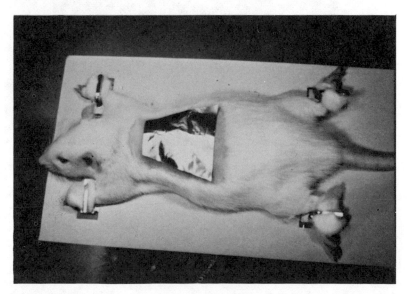

Figure 2 b.   Aluminum foil cover of treated area.

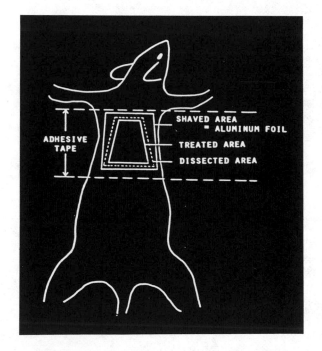

Figure 3.   Schematic of non-occlusive dermal treatment area.

techniques is in positioning of the treated area between the legs for occlusive, while beginning near the ear area for non-occlusive.

The next series of figures shows the non-occlusive approach with stainless steel jewelry chain shackles in place (Figure 4) and dose being applied to the marked area (Figure 5) with chain, wire connectors and template also shown. The shackles prevent scratching the dose area by the rear legs which could spread the dose undesirably. Scratching the dose by the front legs and rubbing treated area on cage walls has not been a problem. Also, syringes with teflon coating of plungers and needle tips were found to be best suited for dose application. Two other techniques for non-occlusive treatments have been reported. Knaak et al (3) used a polyethylene Queen Anne collar with neoprene template attached to the back. Bartek et al (1) used a non-occlusive foam pad device for large animals and restraining harness and collar for rats.

The length of the study is often set such that a skin absorption half-life is reached before study termination, but no longer than seven days (Phase II). At the end of treatment time, shackles are removed, animal is dissected for desired tissues and the treated skin area rinsed with the solvent used in the dose. While the rat is the animal of choice, the mouse (about 25 gm) is occasionally desired as the test animal. For the mouse, the sequence is the same but only one square (0.5 cm per side) is treated high on the back. Also, the jeweler's chain is sterling silver and much thinner.

The glass cage designs are shown next. The first (Figure 6a) is a close-up view of the occlusive treated rat with food provided by feed stick. Next (Figure 6b) shows the non-occlusive rat with powdered food in a cup. When properly mounted on a cart, a bank of four animals can be done simultaneously. Metal metabolism cages can also be used for added time points when CO_2 or volatiles are not collected. Finally, the mouse studies required a design different than for the rat, i.e., a glass cage shown in the next figure (Figure 7). The volatile and CO_2 traps shown are the same as for rat studies.

The CO_2 is trapped in 2N aqueous NaOH for both cages. The volatile trap contains no solution and is immersed in dry ice-acetone. The dry ice trap is generally rinsed with acetone. The dissected tissues are rinsed in water and ground to a homogeneous powder in liquid nitrogen. Most tissues are ground in a Bel-Arts Products micromill, adapted to remove the bottom blender cup for easier transfer of sample and cleaning. However, the smallest tissues are ground in a mortar, also in liquid nitrogen. The skin is so difficult to grind that it is dissolved in Beckman 450 Solubilizer. The urine and all the rinses and washes are aliquoted into Fischer ScintiVerse I. The dissolved skin solution is aliquoted into Beckman Ready-Solve MP. The Harvey combustion apparatus (both manual and automatic) is used for combustion of all the ground samples. The radioactive CO_2 is trapped directly into New England Nuclear Oxifluor-CO_2. The respiratory CO_2 trapped in the NaOH solution is released with acid solution and

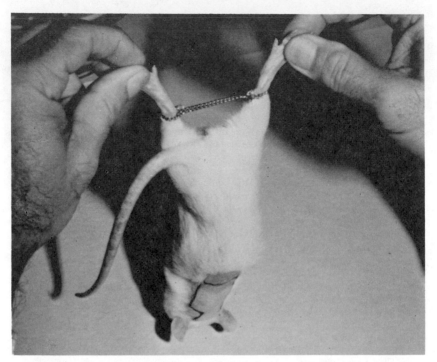

Figure 4.   Attachment of jewelry chain shackles for non-occlusive rat studies.

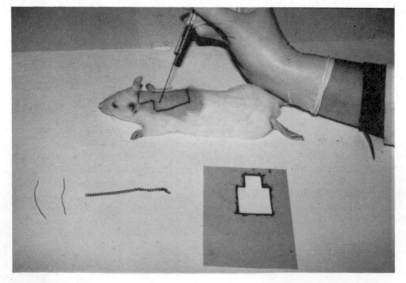

Figure 5.   Dose application by syringe in non-occlusive study.

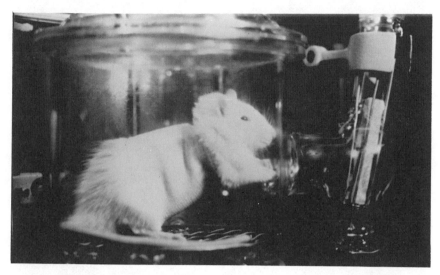

Figure 6 a.   Occlusive treated rat in glass cage.

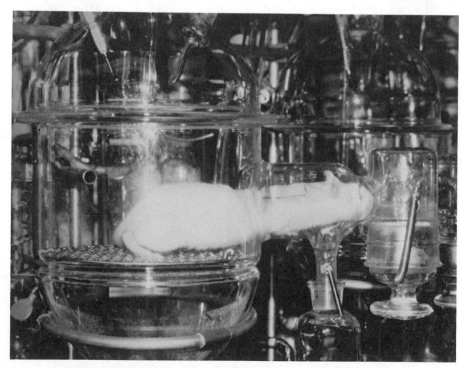

Figure 6 b.   Non-occlusive treated rat in glass cage.

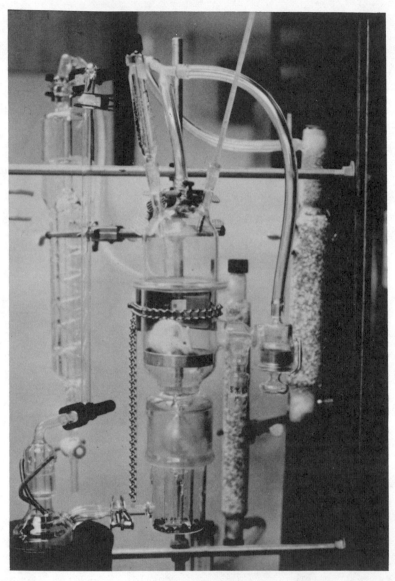

Figure 7.   Mouse glass metabolism cage.

retrapped in the Oxifluor for more effective counting. All the radioactive solutions are counted in a liquid scintillation counter.

All the balances and liquid scintillation counters are directly interfaced to a minicomputer network of Hewlett-Packard equipment including the HP-9800 and A Series. The schematic of the present system is shown (Figure 8) with only a portion of the network used for these dermal studies. This computer system is a modification of that previously reported (4). The tissues and excretion samples have the data reduced after the results of weighing and radioisotope counting are directly interfaced into the computer. Some tissues, such as plasma and red blood cells, have their total weights calculated from body weight using stored equations. To obtain a final summary sheet, some information needs to be hand entered in a program for formating the data. However, with the recent addition of the HP A600 to the network, sufficient capacity is available for preparing a program to automatically call in the various data files.

While the data generated by this proposed strategy can be reduced in a variety of ways, absorption and excretion kinetics are often useful. The skin absorption rate can be expressed as dose/area exposed/interval by the following calculation.

$$\text{mg/cm}^2/\text{hr.} = [\text{dose (mg)} - [\text{skin wash (mg)} + \text{dissolved skin (mg)} + \text{volatiles (mg)}]] \div \text{exposed area (cm}^2) \div \text{interval (hr.)}$$

The urine excretion rate can be expressed as excreted dose/area exposed/interval by the following calculation.

$$\text{mg/cm}^2/\text{hr.} = (\text{mg/ml urine} \times \text{urine volume}) \div \text{exposed area (cm}^2) \div \text{interval (hr.)}$$

Dividing either expression by the total dose in milligrams and multiplying by 100 will convert the expressions to percentages. The objectives of a particular study will establish which of the above expressions are appropriate.

Examples

In presenting the following results, no attempt will be made to give a complete picture of any compound discussed. The main purpose is to show the type of results generated and some comparative results that are believed to be interesting.

The occlusive study for ^{14}C-phenyl-2-ethyl-6-methyl aniline hydrochloride (MEA) was done to observe the metabolic fate and urine metabolites. Defining a major urinary component would serve as an appropriate measure of exposure to MEA. The major balance information is shown (Table II) with the main dose appearing in the urine after 48 hours.

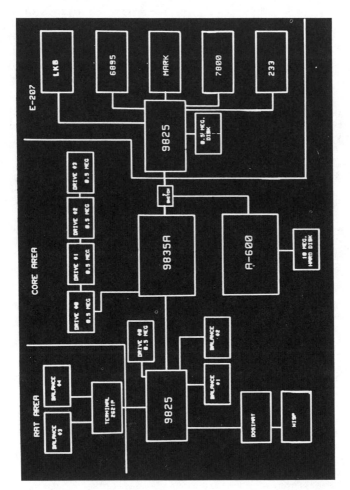

Figure 8.   Schematic of laboratory mini-computer network with
liquid scintillation counters indicated at far
right.

Table II: Occlusive Dermal Absorption in the Rats of
2-ethyl-6-methyl aniline

(Dose - 0.1 mg/kg; Time - 48 hrs.)	
Fraction	% of Radioactive Dose
Urine	78.4
Feces	2.3
CO_2	1.3
Skin	2.0
Foil	4.2
Adhesive	6.0
Carcass	3.1
Cage Wash	0.7

Some of the dose does remain on the foil and adhesive. The main (60% of dose) urinary component was identified as the sulfate ester conjugate of 2-ethyl-4-hydroxy-6-methylaniline. In another occlusive study, CGA-73102, ^{14}C-phenyl-(O-n-butyl-O'-(2,2-dimethyl-2,3-dihydrobenzofurane-7-yl)-N,N'-dimethyl-N,N'-thiodicarbamate) was done to include results on tissue retention 72 hours after dosing (Table III).

Table III: Occlusive Dermal Absorption in Rats of CGA-73102
After 72 Hours

Fraction	% of Radioactive Dose	
	Male (0.42 mg/kg)	Female (0.46 mg/kg)
Urine	51.4	44.2
Feces	2.2	1.5
CO_2	0.2	0.2
Skin	7.3	4.3
Skin wipe	9.4	7.3
Foil	13.6	6.7
Adhesive	1.5	19.5
Carcass	5.3	5.3
Cage Wash	1.4	0.6
	PPM	
Liver	0.006	0.004
Kidney	0.021	0.004
Other tissues	0.002	0.002

The major balance information is shown with the majority of dose appearing in urine. Again, part of the dose appears on the foil and adhesive. Based on the skin, foil and adhesive values, this compound appears to be absorbed slower than 2-ethyl-6-methylaniline.

For non-occlusive studies of methidathion, $2-^{14}C$-thiadiazole-(S-[(5-Methoxy-2-oxo-1,3,4,-thiadiazole-3(2H)-yl)methyl]O,O-dimethyl phosphorodithioate), the rat vs. mouse results show the mouse to absorb methidathion more rapidly than the rat for either male or female with little differences between sexes (Table IV).

Table IV: Non-Occlusive Dermal Absorption of Methidathion in Rat vs. Mouse (72 hrs.)

| Fraction | Rate to Absorb Half the Dose (Hours) | | | |
| | Males (12 mg/kg) | | Females (12 mg/kg) | |
	Acetone	Formulated*	Acetone	Formulated*
Rat	16.9	15.9	17.2	17.4
Mouse	9.1	10.4	10.5	10.9

% of Radioactive Dose				
Rat				
Urine	34.1	32.7	48.9	36.9
Feces	3.3	4.0	3.3	3.0
Volatiles	0.1	.1	0	.1
CO_2	26.6	16.3	21.8	18.3
Skin	.3	9.9	2.0	4.5
Tissues	1.3	3.0	1.7	3.6
Cage wash	1.7	3.4	2.5	3.9
Mouse				
Urine	14.6	23.5	14.5	16.2
Feces	3.4	4.4	4.4	3.6
Volatiles	1.1	.3	.3	.2
CO_2	64.1	50.9	61.4	55.6
Skin	0.5	0.4	0.7	1.3
Tissues	0.7	0.3	0.4	0.4
Cage wash	5.9	2.0	1.9	3.0

*Petroleum ether plus emulsifier.

Interestingly, the formulated compound is absorbed at essentially the same rate even with petroleum ether and emulsifier present. The distribution information shows only modest differences between sexes or active ingredient alone vs. formulation. The mouse does significantly produce more CO_2, reflected in lower urine values. Also, the low cage wash values indicate minimal cage contamination for either rat or mouse.

Tetrahydrofuran (THF) may be used as a general solvent because of its broad solvent abilities. It has been compared with other commonly used solvents. For methidathion, whether acetone or THF are used, the results are very similar in major balance values and tissues (Table V).

Table V: Comparison of THF vs. Acetone at 72 Hour After
Methidathion Non-Occlusive Dosage

(Male Rats - 12 mg/kg)		
	Tissue Levels μg/gm	
Fraction	Acetone	THF
Plasma	.26	.41
RBC	.31	.45
Muscle	.25	.36
Kidney	.29	.50
Liver	.39	.71
	% of Radioactive Dose	
Urine	34.1	36.4
Feces	3.3	7.4
Volatiles	.1	.7
CO_2	26.6	31.0
Skin	.3	2.9
Cage wash	1.7	3.5

For atrazine, ^{14}C-triazine-(6-chloro-N-ethyl-N'-(1-methyl-ethyl)-1,3,5-triazine-2,4-diamine), ethanol required warming to dissolve atrazine in sufficient concentration to apply a 2.5 mg/kg dermal dose (Table VI).

Table VI: Comparison of THF vs. Ethanol at 72 Hours After
Atrazine Non-Occlusive Dosage

(Male rats - 2.5 mg/kg)		
	Tissue Levels μg/gm	
Fraction	Ethanol	THF
Plasma	.06	.06
RBC	.75	.75
Muscle	.10	.11
Kidney	.49	.47
Liver	.72	.65
	% of Radioactive Dose	
Urine	41.2	35.1
Feces	11.1	9.6
Skin	12.8	40.9
Cage wash	15.9	2.1

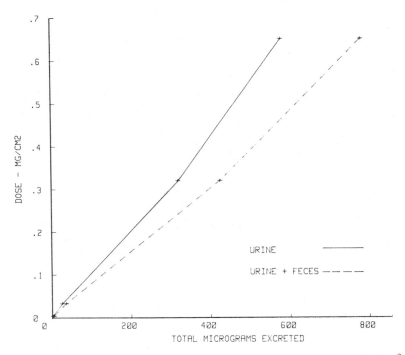

Figure 9.   Relationship of atrazine dermal exposure (mg/cm^2) and amount (micrograms) excreted by the rat.

In fact, flaking was observed on the skin treated with
ethanol as the solvent. THF solved this with a deposition of a
very fine powder adhering to the skin. These observations are
reflected in the skin and cage wash values noted. In most
studies, the cage wash is rarely above 5% of dose. Yet, the
tissue values are not appreciably altered nor are the excretion
values. The atrazine undoubtedly flaked-off onto the cage walls
for the ethanol treatment and not for the THF. Since THF
resolved the treatment problem, yet provided similar results in
tissues in these and other comparisons, it is the solvent that is
often used at present.
      The skin absorption half-life of atrazine at 0.25 mg/kg dose
was 39 hours for males and 43 hours for females. Another value of
interest for monitoring worker dermal exposure is the urinary
excretion half-life (See Table VII).

Table VII: Urine Excretion Half-Lives of Atrazine in the Male Rat

Dermal Dose (mg/kg)	Half-Life (Hours)
0.025	127
0.25	85
2.5	44
5.0	36

      (The term "half-life" as used in our present studies refers
to the length of time required for 50% of the dose to be either
absorbed or excreted based upon fitting the data by a least
squares best fit approach to a variety of models. The computer
selected best fit may not necessarily follow a first-order
equation.)
      At the 0.25 mg/kg level, the half-life for excretion is about
double the half-life for absorption. Of interest, is the significantly more rapid excretion rate with increase of dose. Finally,
when the urine from this multidose study is analyzed by a method
that converts all the excreted metabolites to one entity, in this
case cyanuric acid, a proportional relationship is observed
between dermal exposure (mg/cm^2) and the microgram amount of
excreted atrazine metabolites 144 hours after dosing (Figure 9).
This would indicate the cyanuric acid total method to be an
appropriate one for monitoring worker exposure to atrazine.
      In our studies to date, the compounds in which oral and
dermal studies were done have shown qualitative similarities in
urine metabolic patterns. This was noted in the methyl ethyl
aniline, CGA-73102, methidathion and atrazine studies discussed in
this paper. Thus, based upon our experience, there is no reason
to believe that major metabolic differences occur due to oral vs.
dermal treatment routes. As noted by Pannatier et al (6), specific
examples of skin metabolism are scarce, except for steroid
hormones.

At the present stage of rodent dermal studies, there does not appear to be a set protocol that is the clearly preferred choice. Our experiences to date indicate that the data usage would establish whether the occlusive or non-occlusive approach should be used. We feel that our present multi-tiered strategy for dermal studies will provide a cost and time effective approach which will provide flexibility and allow judgement to be used depending on the objective of the studies. This study design is being used with on-going studies.

Nontechnical Summary

Since one of the measures used in assessing chemical risk and worker exposure is the amount of chemical absorbed through the skin, a method, not using humans, is desirable. These studies describe the use of rodents, preferably the rat, in obtaining such dermal exposure information. The experimental strategy described depends upon a four step procedure using the generated information to move through the steps. Thus, judgement and flexibility are incorporated in designing studies to provide the proper information at reasonable cost. The radioactive chemical treated skin area may be covered (occlusive) or exposed to air (non-occlusive) depending upon the real world situation to be simulated. Both procedures are described in this paper. A unique new technique for performing the non-covered studies is to place jewelry chain shackles on the rear legs preventing disturbance of the dosed skin area. In order to facilitate data handling, several mini-computers were interconnected and the system directly connected to balances and apparatus for counting radioactivity. By use of the occlusive method, an organic base and a thiocarbamate insecticide were shown to be absorbed and excreted readily. Very little material was retained in the tissues of the rats. By use of the non-occlusive method, the insecticide, methidathion, was shown to be absorbed about 3 times faster than the herbicide, atrazine. Also, the mouse absorbed the insecticide faster than the rat. In the case of atrazine, use of four different treatment amounts showed a direct relationship between the amount placed on the skin and the amount found in the urine. This shows that urine analyses for atrazine residues would measure the amount of skin exposure. It is assumed that a similar relationship applies to man and could be used to estimate worker exposure.

This paper presents an organized approach to the use of rodents as a model to estimate the rate of skin absorption of a chemical in man.

Literature Cited

1. Bartek, M. S.; LaBudde, J. A.; Maibach, H. I., J. Invest. Dermat., 1972, 58, 114-123.
2. Hunziker, N.; Feldmann, R. J.; Maibach, H., Dermatologcca, 1978, 156, 79-88.
3. Wester, R. C.; Maibach, H. I., Drug Metab. Rev., 1983, 14 (2), 169-205.
4. Knaak, J. B.; Schlocker, P.; Ackerman, C. R.; Seiber, J. N., Bull. Environm. Contam. Toxicol., 1980, 24, 796-804.
5. Fischer, W. C.; Marco, G. J., Chemtech, 1981, 11, 658-663.
6. Pannatier, A.; Jenner, P.; Testa, B.; Etter, J. C., Drug Metab. Rev., 1978, 8 (2), 319-343.

RECEIVED November 15, 1984

Dermal Dose–Cholinesterase Response and Percutaneous Absorption Studies with Several Cholinesterase Inhibitors

JAMES B. KNAAK[1] and BARRY W. WILSON[2]

[1]Worker Health and Safety Unit, California Department of Food and Agriculture, Sacramento, CA 95814
[2]Department of Avian Sciences, University of California, Davis, CA 95616

Dermal dose–ChE response and percutaneous absorption studies were conducted with parathion, carbaryl, and thiodicarb in the rat. Parathion and thiodicarb inhibited 50% of the red cell cholinesterase activity at dose levels of 3.2 and 33 mg/kg of bw. Carbaryl at the highest dose level tested (417 mg/kg of bw) produced no detectable red cell cholinesterase inhibition. Finite, nonoccluded doses (600 ug) of [^{14}C]labeled parathion and carbaryl were absorbed through the back skin of adult males at the rate of 0.33 and 0.18 ug hr^{-1} cm^{-2} of skin. This rate was sufficient to absorb 57% of the applied dose of parathion and carbaryl over a period of 168 hr. A computer program, Nonlin, was used to calculate the plasma rate constants for simultaneous absorption-elimination. A finite, nonoccluded dose (570 ug) of [^{14}C]thiodicarb was slowly absorbed (0.042 to 0.27 ug hr^{-1} cm^{-2} of skin) and acted as if it were an infinite dose applied to the skin. Approximately 22% of the applied dose was absorbed over a period of 168 hr.

Cholinesterase (ChE) inhibiting organophosphate and carbamate insecticides are used extensively in California agriculture. Workers are exposed to these insecticides during mixing/loading and application and by contacting foliar residues during harvest operations (1,2,3). Exposure to spray and foliar residues often results in the inhibition of red blood cell cholinesterase activity and reported illnesses among farm workers (4). The relationship, in workers, between exposure to pesticides, the rate they are absorbed, and cholinesterase inhibition is not well known. Field monitoring studies indicate that prolonged exposure to moderately toxic organophosphates (OP's) produce the same amount of ChE inhibition (5) as short exposures to highly toxic OP's (3).

The California Department of Food and Agriculture recently established toxicologically safe levels for total residues of parathion [0,0-diethyl 0-(4-nitrophenyl) phosphorothioate],

0097–6156/85/0273–0063$06.00/0
© 1985 American Chemical Society

azinphosmethyl   [O,O-dimethyl   S-[(4-oxo-1,2,3-benzotriazin-3(4H)-yl)
methyl]   phosphorodithioate],   and   methidathion   [S-[(5-methoxy-2-oxo-
1,3,4-thiadiazol-3   (2H)-yl)methyl]   O,O-dimethyl   phosphorodithioate]
and their toxic alteration products on tree foliage (6) using dermal
dose-ChE response data.   This procedure was also used to establish
reentry   times   for   chlorthiophos   [O-[2,5-dichloro-4-(methylthio)-
phenyl] O,O-diethyl phosphorothioate] and carbosulfan [dihydro-2,2-
dimethyl-7-benzo-furanyl   [(di-n-butylamino)thio]   methylcarbamate]
(7,8).

    The differences observed between chlorthiophos, carbosulfan,
and other pesticides that have been examined appear to be largely
due to their rate of absorption, and anti-ChE activity.   These
relationships were recently examined for carbaryl [1-naphthyl
methylcarbamate],   parathion   (9) and   thiodicarb   [dimethyl   N,N'
[thiobis[(methylimido)carbonyloxy]]   bis   [ethanimidothioate]]   (10)
in the Sprague-Dawley rat and are reviewed in this paper.

Methods

Dermal Dose-ChE Response Studies.   A   procedure   developed   by   Knaak
et al. (11) using 220-240 g male Sprague-Dawley rats was used to
determine the relationship between the applied dose and red cell ChE
inhibition.   Four rats per dose level and four or five dosage levels
were used.   In each study, baseline or control ChE activity was
determined using nontreated animals.   The pesticides (carbaryl,
parathion and thiodicarb) were individually applied in 1.0 ml of
acetone to the clipped backs, 25 cm^2, of the rat using a digital
microliter pipet.   Animals treated with parathion were killed 72 hr
after the application of the dose, while animals treated with carbamates; carbaryl, and thiodicarb were killed 24 hr after the dose was
applied.   The log-probit procedure of Finney (12) for determining
LD_{50} values was modified to compute the inhibition ED_{50} for cholinesterase activity (11) using treatment and control means.   The
program computed the slope of the line, the ED_{50} and the confidence
limits for the curves.

Percutaneous Absorption Studies.   The   percutaneous   absorption   of
[ring-U- 14 C]   parathion   (specific   activity,   1.8   mCi/mmole),   [ring-
U-$_{14}$C]carbaryl (specific activity, 1.46 mCi/mmole) (9) and [acetyl-
1-^{14}C] thiodicarb (specific activity 2.19 mCi/mmole) (10) were
studied using the procedures of Knaak et al. (13) for triadimefon.
Adult male and female Sprague-Dawley rats were used in the studies
with parathion, adult males with carbaryl, and adult females with
thiodicarb.   Rats were prepared for dosing, one day prior to treatment, by removing the hair on their backs with an animal clipper.
Templates, cut from neoprene rubber sheeting, were glued to the backs
of the animals using a cyanoacrylate glue.   The treatment areas (A =
9.64 weight $^{0.66}$), comprising 3% of the body surface, were determined
using the body weight to surface area data of Brodie et al. (14).
Queen Anne collars made of polyethylene sheeting were used to prevent
the animals from reaching the treated areas.   In each study, 36 rats
(12 groups of 3 rats per group) were used.   The dose (600 ug of
parathion or carbaryl; 570 ug of thiodicarb), in 0.2 ml of acetone,
was evenly distributed over a 11.9 to 13.8 cm^2 area using a digital
microliter pipet to give approximately 43.5 to 48 ug/cm^2.   The

animals were placed into individual metabolism cages for the complete
and separate collection of urine and feces. Three animals were
killed at 0.5, 1, 4, 8, 12, 24, 48, 72, 96, 120, 144, and 168 hr
after the administration of the dose. Plasma, treated skin, acetone
washings from treated skin, heart, liver, kidney, and the carcass
from each animal were collected at sacrifice. Urine and fecal
samples were collected every 24 hr during the study. Penetrated
skin residues were extracted using methanol followed by acetone.
Unextracted residues were considered to be bound to tissue. Liquid
samples were analyzed by direct scintillation counting methods and
tissue/fecal samples by combusting procedures (13).

Calculations. The count data from the percutaneous absorption
studies were analyzed by the procedures of Knaak et al., (13) utilizing a collection of computer programs: a conversion program, dpm
to ug of pesticide or pesticide equivalents; exponential and linear
regression programs of Heilborn (15). The blood plasma data was
analyzed using the two compartment model of Metzler et al. (16),
where k_{12} and k_{20} are the first order rate constants for absorption into and elimination from plasma. The entry compartment, A,
is represented by skin while the main compartment, B, is represented
by plasma as shown in Figure 1. The dose, topically applied, is
absorbed (penetrates) by the skin (entry compartment). The rate of
absorption (penetration) was obtained indirectly by measuring the
rate the dose is lost from skin (surface, penetrated and bound
residues) or eliminated from plasma (13). The skin absorption rates
were calculated using a modification of the procedure of Marzulli et
al. (17).

Results

Dermal Dose-Response Studies. The dermal dose red cell ChE-response
curves for parathion and thiodicarb are given in Figure 2. Parathion, the most toxic pesticide used, inhibited 50% of the red cell
ChE activity at a dose level of 31 ug/cm^2 (3.2 mg/kg) of treated
skin in 72 hr, while 322 ug/cm^2 of thiodicarb (33.3 mg/kg) gave 50%
ChE inhibition in 24 hr. Carbaryl at dose levels up to 4,000 ug/cm^2
of treated skin (417 mg/kg) did not produce detectable ChE inhibition
24 hr after application of the dose. Thiodicarb was dermally more
toxic than carbaryl, but substantially less toxic (1/10) than parathion.
      A dose of 800 ug of thiodicarb per cm^2 of skin produced the
same amount of inhibition as a dose of 400 ug/cm^2. Doses of parathion above 80 ug/cm^2 inhibited 70 to 100 % of red cell cholinesterase activity and produced mortality in test animals. No deaths
occurred using doses of 800 ug of thiodicarb per cm^2 of skin.

Recovery Studies. The time-course recoveries of [^{14}C]labeled
parathion, carbaryl, and thiodicarb in adult rats are given in Figure
3. The recovery data in this Figure are given in percentage of the
applied dose, except for urine and feces which are expressed in
cumulative percentage of dose. Total recovery is a summation of the
percentages obtained for feces, urine, carcass, and skin. Parathion
was excreted in urine (47, 49%) and in feces (5.3, 3.7%) by males and
females. Recovery procedures accounted for 61% of the dose for adult

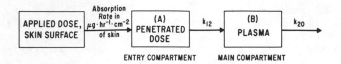

Figure 1. Two compartment model with a central compartment (B) and an entry compartment (A) which takes up the topically applied dose.

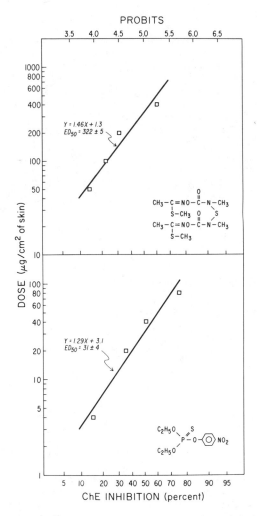

Figure 2. Dermal dose-ChE response curves for thiodicarb (top) and parathion (bottom). Male Sprague-Dawley rats weighing 220-240 g were used. A 25 cm^2 area of skin was treated.

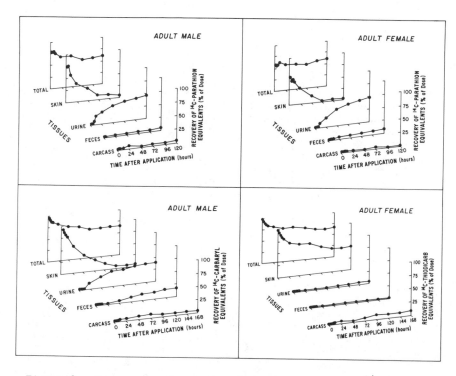

Figure 3.   Time-course recovery of dermally applied [^{14}C] labeled parathion, carbaryl, and thiodicarb equivalents in percentage of dose in feces, urine, carcasses, and skin (surface and penetrated residues) after application. (Reproduced with permission from Ref. 9. Copyright 1984, Academic Press.)

males and females at the end of the study. Carbaryl equivalents were largely excreted in urine (39%) with lesser amounts in feces (15%). Thiodicarb was not absorbed to any extent. Approximately 4.4% was found in urine, 2.5% in feces, 8.8% in the carcass, and 6.6% (estimated) in respiratory air as CO_2 and acetonitrile. The largest percentage of the dose was found on the surface of the skin. Evaporative losses are believed to be responsible for the incomplete recovery of the applied dose in these studies.

Loss From Skin. The dissipation of topically applied [^{14}C]parathion and [^{14}C]carbaryl from skin is given in Figure 4, while Figure 5 gives the dissipation of [^{14}C]thiodicarb. The half-lives for the dissipation of parathion from the skin of adult females and males were 24.3 and 28.6 hr, respectively, while the dissipation half-life for carbaryl from the skin of adult males was 40.6 hr. Thiodicarb dissipated at an initial rate (0-24 hr; t 1/2, α phase) of 40 hr from the skin of adult females and at a final rate (24-168 hr; t 1/2, β phase) of 254 hr.

Surface, Penetrated, and Bound Residues. The time-course recoveries of [^{14}C]labeled parathion, carbaryl, and thiodicarb from skin (surface, penetrated, and bound residues) of adult rats expressed in percentage of residual pesticide are given in Table I. During the first 24 hr following topical application, 94 to 98% of the applied parathion remained on the surface of the skin. Small quantities of parathion penetrated the skin (1.6 to 5.6%) and were available for absorption into blood. Less than 0.3% of the parathion in the skin was present as bound residues. In the case of carbaryl, 74 to 94% of the topically applied dose was found on the surface of the skin over a period of 72 hr. The percentage of penetrated [^{14}C]increased with time along with the percentage of bound residues. Topically applied thiodicarb largely remained on the surface of the skin during the study. A small percentage (3.0 to 10%) of thiodicarb penetrated the skin. Bound residues varied between 0.4 and 3.1% of residual [^{14}C]thiodicarb equivalents.
      The total amount of [^{14}C]labeled parathion, carbaryl, and thiodicarb equivalents present in ug and percentage of dose is given in Table II. Carbaryl, parathion, and thiodicarb reached plateau values of 35, 17, and 7 ug,respectively, per treated area of skin.

Absorption vs Dissipation. The relationship between the loss of the topically applied dose of parathion, carbaryl, and thiodicarb and the absorbed dose is given in Figures 6 and 7. The regression lines showed that the absorbed dose was considerably less than the dose lost from skin. The skin loss data correlated well with the absorption data.

Simultaneous Absorption and Elimination in Plasma. The time-concentration curves for the absorption and elimination of [^{14}C]labeled parathion, carbaryl, and thiodicarb equivalents in plasma of adult rats are given in Figure 8 and the pharmacokinetic constants in Table III. The [^{14}C]equivalents were found in blood shortly after the application of the dose and reached maximum concentrations in plasma in 2.5 to 12 hr. Carbaryl and parathion [^{14}C]equivalents were eliminated during the study, while [^{14}C]thiodicarb equivalents

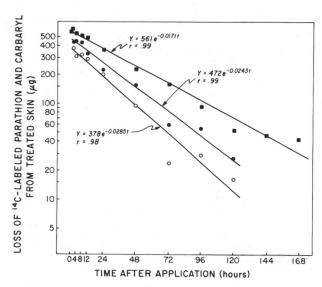

Figure 4. Loss of surface and penetrated [^{14}C] labeled parathion and carbaryl equivalents from skin of adult rats. Key: ■, carbaryl, adult male; ●, parathion, adult male; O, parathion, adult female. (Reproduced with permission from Ref. 9. Copyright 1984, Academic Press.)

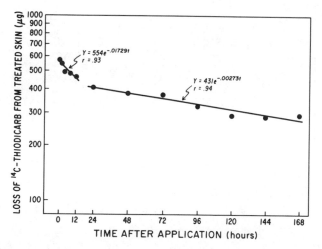

Figure 5. Loss of surface and penetrated [^{14}C] thiodicarb equivalents from skin of adult female rats.

TABLE I. Time-Course Recovery of [14C]Labeled Parathion, Carbaryl, and Thiodicarb Equivalents From Skin of Adult Male and Female Rats

Percentage of Residual [14C]Equivalents[a]

Sacrifice Time in Hours	Washings From Intact Skin[b]			Washings From Ground Skin[c]			Combusted Skin[d]		
	P	C	T	P	C	T	P	C	T
0.5	98.2	94.1	97.0	1.6	4.8	2.6	0.2	1.1	0.4
1	96.0	94.4	93.6	3.8	4.8	5.5	0.2	0.9	0.9
4	–	93.2	94.8	–	5.2	4.5	–	1.6	0.7
8	96.0	92.8	91.4	3.9	5.5	7.5	0.1	1.7	1.1
12	–	91.8	92.2	–	6.6	6.3	–	1.6	1.5
24	94.1	87.6	92.1	5.6	9.6	5.8	0.3	2.8	2.1
48		81.8	92.5		12.0	5.7		6.2	1.8
72		73.9	90.4		19.4	7.2		6.6	2.4
96		62.8	91.2		23.7	6.7		13.5	2.1
120		38.8	89.6		38.6	7.6		22.6	2.8
144		25.4	90.0		31.4	6.9		43.1	3.1
168		29.3	91.0		41.9	6.5		28.8	2.5

a See Figure 2. P, Parathion; C, Carbaryl; T, Thiodicarb.

b Surface residue.

c Penetrated residue.

d Bound residue.

Source: Adapted from Ref. 9, 10.

TABLE II. [^{14}C]Labeled Parathion, Carbaryl, and Thiodicarb Equivalents in Treated Skin in ug and % of Dose[a]

Study	Units	Hours After Application											
		0.5	1	4	8	12	24	48	72	96	120	144	168
Parathion, Males[b]	ug	8.2	17.5	–	17.3	–	13.0	–	–	–	–	–	–
	% of Dose	1.4	2.9	–	2.9	–	2.2	–	–	–	–	–	–
Carbaryl, Males[c]	ug	34.6	33.5	36.5	36.6	39.8	45.6	41.9	41.8	35.2	33.1	35.6	31.1
	% of Dose	5.8	5.6	6.1	6.1	6.1	7.6	7.0	7.0	5.9	5.5	5.9	5.2
Thiodicarb, Females[d]	ug	2.40	5.0	3.67	5.3	6.9	8.4	6.6	9.0	6.6	8.1	9.0	7.2
	% of Dose	0.42	0.88	0.6	0.9	1.2	1.4	1.1	1.6	1.2	1.4	1.6	1.3

a Penetrated and bound residues.
b,c 600 ug applied to skin in acetone.
d 570 ug applied to skin in acetone.

Source: Adapted from Ref. 9, 10.

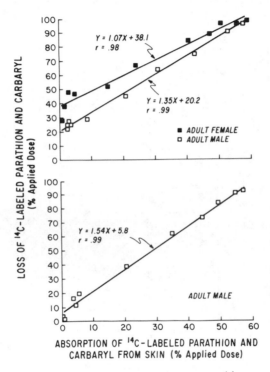

Figure 6. Relationship between the loss of $[^{14}C]$ labeled parathion (top) and carbaryl (bottom) from skin surface (Figure 3) and absorbed $[^{14}C]$ equivalents. (Reproduced with permission from Ref. 9. Copyright 1984, Academic Press.)

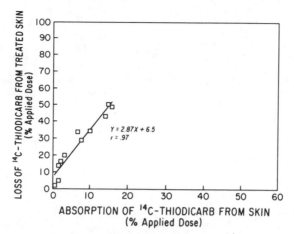

Figure 7.   Relationship between the loss of [^{14}C] thiodicarb from the skin of adult female rats (Figure 4) and absorbed [^{14}C] equivalents.

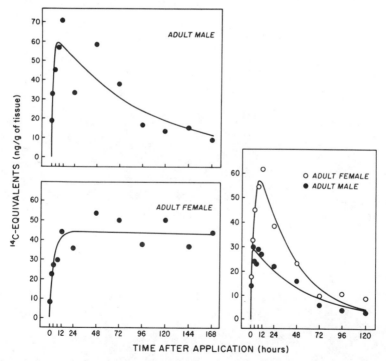

Figure 8. Time–concentration curves for the simultaneous absorption and elimination of [^{14}C] labeled carbaryl (top left), thiodicarb (bottom left), and parathion (right) equivalents in plasma. (Reproduced with permission from Ref. 9. Copyright 1984, Academic Press.)

TABLE III. Pharmacokinetic Constants For the Simultaneous
Absorption and Elimination of $[^{14}C]$Labeled Parathion, Carbaryl
and Thiodicarb Equivalents in Plasma

Constants	Male/ Female	Parathion	Carbaryl	Thiodicarb	Units
Theoretical Initial	M	30_a	64^g		ng/ml
Concentration	F	70^b		44^j	
Absorption Constant	M	1.84^c	0.549^h		h^{-1}
	F	0.326^d		0.241^k	
Corresponding t 1/2	M	0.38	1.26		h
	F	2.1		2.87	
Elimination Constant	M	0.0175^e	0.0103^i		h^{-1}
	F	0.0242^f		–	
Corresponding t 1/2	M	39.5	67.0		h
	F	28.6		–	
Position of Peak					
Time	M	2.5	7.4		h
	F	8.6		12	
Height	M	28.7	59.3		ng/ml
	F	57		44	
R-Squared	M	0.90	0.75		
	F	0.95		0.77	
Absorption-Elimination	M	1:104	1:53		
Ratio k_{12} : k_{20}	F	1:13			

a ± 2	e ± 0.0034	i ± 0.0028
b ± 6	f ± 0.0039	j ± 5
c ± 0.542	g ± 8	k ± 0.089
d $\pm .0701$	h ± 0.256	

Source: Adapted from Ref. 9, 10.

reached a plateau value of 44 ng/ml and remained at this level. The elimination constant for thiodicarb could not be determined under steady state conditions.

Absorption Rates. The skin absorption rates for [^{14}C]labeled parathion, carbaryl, thiodicarb in adult rats are given in Table IV. Female rats absorbed parathion faster than males as indicated in this Table when either the t 1/2 for plasma elimination or for skin loss was used. In males and females, the t 1/2 for skin loss gave higher absorption rates than the t 1/2 for elimination from plasma. This difference is believed to be produced by evaporative losses of parathion from skin. Carbaryl was absorbed at a slower rate than parathion in males when the t 1/2 for plasma elimination or the t 1/2 for skin loss was used.   Differences in the absorption rate for carbaryl (0.18 vs 0.44 ug hr^{-1} cm^{-2}) maybe caused by evaporation. In the case of thiodicarb, t 1/2 for skin loss (α and β phase) was used to determine the rate of absorption because steady state plasma concentrations prevented the calculation of the t 1/2 for elimination of thiodicarb from plasma.

Discussion

Dermal dose–ChE response studies in animal models are valuable in assessing the dermal toxicity of organophosphate and carbamate pesticides to workers. The behavior of the pesticide in the body, however, cannot be determined from dose–response data. Percutaneous absorption studies utilizing [^{14}C]labeled pesticides are required. According to percutaneous absorption studies (17) the amount of pesticide absorbed is a function of the total skin area (cm^2), the concentration of the pesticide on skin (ug/cm^2), and the length of exposure (hr).

The rapid inhibition of red cell cholinesterase in workers dermally exposed to parathion suggested that parathion was rapidly absorbed from skin. In the rat dermal dose response study (9) a period of 72 hr was required for a single topical dose of parathion (32 mg/kg) to inhibit 50% of the red cell cholinesterase activity. Studies by Fredriksson (18) in the cat showed that parathion was absorbed slowly (0.35 ug hr^{-1} cm^{-2}) and that parathion was unsuitable as a model substance for studying percutaneous absorption. The rate of absorption was determined by serial skin stipping and by measuring the disappearance of parathion over a period of 5 hr using a GM tube.

Maibach et al., (19) studied the percutaneous absorption of parathion in man. A period of 5 days was required to completely absorb and eliminate the pesticide in urine. These findings are consistent with the present work of Knaak et al. (9) in the rat where a 5 day period was required to absorb and eliminate a topically applied dose of 600 ug (44 to 48 ug/cm^2). The rate of absorption was determined to be 0.33 to 0.58 ug hr^{-1} cm^{-2} of skin.

Knaak et al. (9) detected parathion equivalents in low concentrations in blood soon after topical application. The parathion equivalents reached a maximum concentration within 12 hr as shown by the blood plasma absorption–elimination curve. These blood levels most likely occur in workers exposed to foliar residues of parathion and are responsible for illnesses reported in workers several hr

TABLE IV. Absorption of $[^{14}C]$Labeled Parathion,
Carbaryl, and Thiodicarb Through Rat Skin In Vivo

Pesticide Age/Sex of Animals	Skin Absorption Rate, r, ug hr^{-1} cm^{-2}	
	1	2
Parathion[a]		
Adult Males	0.33	0.45
Adult Females	0.49	0.58
Carbaryl[a]		
Adult Males	0.18	0.31
Thiodicarb[b]		
Adult Females	0.27[c]	0.042[d]

[a] $r = \dfrac{1/2 \text{ absorbed dose (ug)}}{t\ 1/2\ (hr)} \times \dfrac{1}{\text{area treated in } cm^2}$.
1, t 1/2 for plasma elimination.
2, t 1/2 for loss from skin.

[b] $r = \dfrac{\text{absorbed dose (ug)}}{t\ 1/2\ (hr: \alpha, \beta)} \times \dfrac{1}{\text{area treated in } cm^2}$.

Absorbed dose: 6.6% of dose estimated to be absorbed and
eliminated as CO_2 and acetonitrile; 6.9%
absorbed and eliminated in urine and feces;
8.8% of dose found in carcass. Dose was
absorbed over one half-life.

[c] α phase, t 1/2 for loss of dose from skin.
[d] β phase, t 1/2 for loss of dose from skin.

Source: Adapted from Ref. 9, 10.

after they reenter orchards. Pesticide residues on skin are normally removed by washing at the end of the work day. Such practices, however, do not remove the penetrated dose or the dose absorbed into blood and other body tissues. Several days are normally required to eliminate a dose after the skin has been thoroughly washed. Workers coming in contact with pesticides on a daily basis are exposed to repeated doses of the pesticide. This periodic process may be sufficient to maintain pesticide levels in skin and blood over extended periods of time. In the case of irreversible inhibitors like parathion, ChE activity may be reduced to the same extent by large single or small multiple doses. Immunochemical tests are available to determine the total amount of phosphorylated and non-phosphorylated enzyme (20) in plasma. Tests to distinguish between these forms are presently being developed.

The use of carbaryl has not resulted in illnesses among workers mixing-loading or applying the pesticide and no reentry interval has been established for this pesticide in California. Cholinesterase inhibition is considered to be the major toxic effect of carbaryl. Carbaryl (500 mg/kg) topically applied to the back of the rabbit inhibited 50% of the red cell ChE activity 24 hr after application and activity returned to pretreatment values after 72 hr (21). In the rat study reviewed in this paper, a topical dose of 417 mg/kg did not produce ChE inhibition 24 hr after application indicating that the rate of absorption was low or carbaryl was metabolized in the skin to non-ChE inhibiting products.

Maibach et al., (19) conducted percutaneous absorption studies in man and Shah et al. (22) in the mouse. Carbaryl was absorbed more readily than parathion in these studies. The relationship between the dose and the adverse health effect (ChE inhibition) was not examined. According to the skin loss and plasma elimination data of Knaak et al. (9) reviewed in this paper, carbaryl was not absorbed more rapidly than parathion in the adult male rat. More carbaryl residues were found in skin (penetrated) than were found in the case of parathion. The difference (2X) may be related to the ability of the rat skin to metabolize these pesticides prior to their absorption into blood. Fredriksson (23) showed that parathion was not metabolized to any extent in rat skin. Studies by Chin et al. (24) suggest that carbaryl may be partially metabolized in skin to water soluble products prior to their absorption into blood.

Thiodicarb is a new insecticide being marketed by Union Carbide as Larvin for the control of insects on cotton. Thiodicarb is metabolized in the rat to acetamide, acetonitrile, CO_2, methomyl, and methomyl metabolites. No illnesses have been reported among applicators or field workers coming in contact with this carbamate insecticide. Thiodicarb is somewhat more persistent on crops than methomyl and is less toxic dermally in rabbit studies. The dermal dose–ChE response study showed that a dose of 33 mg/kg produced 50% ChE inhibition 24 hr. after the application of the dose, while a dose of 87 mg/kg of thiodicarb did not produce more inhibition than a dose of 44 mg/kg. The poor solubility of this carbamate in water/lipid most likely prevented the absorption of additional quantities of thiodicarb, thereby reducing its toxicity. Thiodicarb was found in lower concentrations in skin than either parathion or carbaryl during the percutaneous absorption studies. The concentrations in plasma,

however, were similar for parathion, carbaryl, and thiodicarb (57,
59, and 44 ng/ml,respectively).

Thiodicarb was initially lost from skin at a rate similar to
that of parathion and carbaryl. After 24 hr, the rate of loss
decreased by a factor of 1/6. The initial loss of thiodicarb appears
to be due to a combination of events which may include evaporative or
other losses, the initial penetration of the dose into skin and rapid
distribution to blood and other tissues. Absorption was slow after
24 hr as indicated by the t 1/2 for skin loss of 254 hr. Parathion
and carbaryl, on the other hand, penetrated the skin and were
absorbed at a more uniform rate after 24 hr according to the skin
loss data. The plasma absorption-elimination curve for thiodicarb
plateaued after 24 hr. The dose remaining on the surface of the skin
acted as an infinite dose supplying the rat with a low but uniform
amount of thiodicarb.

Pharmacokinetic data may be used for comparing the behavior of a
dermally delivered dose (tissue levels) to one delivered by another
route (i.e., oral and inhalation). Evaluations of this nature are
vitally needed because most data on adverse health effects such as
cholinesterase inhibition, neurotoxicity, teratogenicity and reproductive effects are generated using the oral route and use of this
data may lead to wrong conclusions (25) concerning "safe" working
conditions.

Nontechnical Summary

The effect of a topically applied dose of parathion, carbaryl, and
thiodicarb on red blood cell cholinesterase activity in the rat was
reviewed along with pharmacokinectic data developed on their percutaneous absorption. Parathion and thiodicarb inhibited 50% of the
red cell cholinesterase activity at dose levels of 3.2 and 33 mg/kg
of bw, while no inhibition was detected with carbaryl at dose levels
as high as 417 mg/kg of bw. Parathion and carbaryl were absorbed at
0.33 and 0.18 ug/hr/cm^2, while thiodicarb was absorbed at rates
varying from 0.27 to 0.042 ug/hr/cm^2 of skin. Skin loss and plasma
elimination data were used to calculate the values. The topically
applied pesticides slowly penetrated skin and were available for
absorption into blood and redistribution to other tissues. Recovery
data suggested that evaporative losses occurred during the course of
the 5-day study. The pesticides may be removed from skin by washing,
thus reducing the amount available for absorption.

Acknowledgments

The authors wish to thank Karin Yee and Craig Ackerman for their
assistance in these studies and Union Carbide Agricultural Products
Company, Inc., for support and [^{14}C]labeled carbaryl and
thiodicarb.

Literature Cited

  1. Knaak, J. B.; Jackson, T.; Fredrickson, A. S ; Maddy, K. T.;
      Akesson, N. B. Arch. Environm. Contam. Toxicol. 1976, 9,
      217-229.

2. Knaak, J. B.; Jackson, T.; Fredrickson, A. S.; Rivera, L.;
    Maddy, K. T.; Akesson, N. B. Arch. Environ. Contam. Toxicol.
    1980, 9, 231-245.
3. Spear, R. C.; Popendorf, W. J.; Leffingwell, J. T.; Milby, T. M;
    Davies, J. E.; Spencer, W.T. J. Occup. Med. 1977, 19, 406-410.
4. Maddy, K. T., Peoples, S. A.; Edmiston, S. C. "Pesticide Related
    Human Illnesses in Callifornia" Vol. VII, Jan-Dec 1981, Cali-
    fornia Department of Food and Agriculture, Sacramento, CA.
5. Knaak, J. B. 1980, Unpublished report.
6. Knaak, J. B.; Iwata, Y. In "Pesticide Residue and Exposure";
    Plimmer, J. R., Ed.; ACS SYMPOSIUM SERIES No. 182, American
    Chemical Society, Washington, D.C., 1982; pp. 23-39.
7. Iwata, Y.; Knaak, J. B.; Carmen, G. E.; Dusch, M. E.;
    Gunther, F. A. J. Agric. Food Chem. 1982, 30, 215-222.
8. Iwata, Y.; Knaak, J. B.; Carman, G. E.; Dusch, M. E.;
    O'Neal, J. R.; Pappas, J. L. J. Agric. Food Chem. 1983, 31,
    1131-1136.
9. Knaak, J. B.; Yee, K.; Ackerman, C. R.; Zweig. G.; Fry, D. M.;
    Wilson, B. W. Toxicol. Appl. Pharmacol. (submitted 12/83).
10. Knaak, J. B.; Ackerman, C. R.; Wilson, B. W. 1984, Unpublished
    report.
11. Knaak, J. B.; Schlocker, P.; Ackerman, C. R.; Seiber, J. N.
    Bull. Environ. Contam. Toxicol. 1980, 24, 796-804.
12. Finney, D. J. "Probit Analysis": 3rd. ed; Cambridge University
    Press; New York, 1972.
13. Knaak, J. B.; Yee, K.; Ackerman, C. A.; Zweig, G.; Wilson, B. W.
    Toxicol. Appl. Pharmacol. 1984, 72, 406-416.
14. Brodie, S.; Comfort, J. E.; Matthews, J. C. Missouri Agr. Expt.
    Sta. Bull. 1928, 15.
15. Heilborn, T. "Science and Engineering Programs Apple II
    Edition"; Osborn/McGraw-Hill, Berkeley, California.
16. Metzler, C. M.; Elfring, G. L.; McEwen, A. I. Biometrics 1974,
    30, 562-563.
17. Marzulli, F. N.; Brown, W. C.; Maibach, H. I. Toxicol. Appl.
    Pharmacol. 1969, Supplement No. 3, 76-83.
18. Fredriksson, T. Acta Dermato-Venerologica 1961, 41, 353-362.
19. Maibach, H. I.; Feldmann, R. J.; Milby, T. H.; Serat, W. F.
    Arch. Environ. Health 1971, 23, 208-211.
20. Eckerson, H. W.; Oseroff, A.; Lockridge, O.; LaDu, B. N. Bio-
    Chem. Genet. 1983, 21(1-2), 93-108.
21. Yakim, V.S. Giegieno i Sanitarija 1967, 32(4) 29-33.
22. Shah, P.V.; Monroe, R. J.; Guthrie, F. E. Toxicol. Appl.
    Pharmacol. 1981, 59, 414-423.
23. Fredriksson, T. Acta Dermato-Venereological 1961, 41, 335-343.
24. Chin, B. H.; Sullivan, L. T.; Eldridge, J. N.; Tallant, M. J.
    Clin. Toxicol. 1979, 14(5), 489-498.
25. Knaak, J.B.; Peoples, S.A.; Jackson, T.; Fredrickson, A.S.;
    Enos, R.; Maddy, K. T.; Bailey, J. Blair; Dusch, M. E.; Gunther,
    F. A.; Winterlin, W. L. Arch. Environm. Contam. Toxicol. 1978,
    7, 456-481.

RECEIVED September 14, 1984

The Use of Monkey Percutaneous Absorption Studies

ROBERT B. L. VAN LIER

Toxicology Division, Lilly Research Laboratories, Greenfield, IN 46140

The assessment of percutaneous absorption for pesticides has played an increasingly important role in risk evalua- tions for users of these products. Wester and Maibach (1-10) showed in a series of papers that the rhesus monkey was an appropriate model to predict the percutane- ous absorption of pesticides in man. A similar technique in which radiolabeled pesticide is given in two sequen- tial studies has been employed in this laboratory. The disposition of an intravenous dose is determined by assaying plasma, urine and feces until at least 90% of the dose is recovered. Following a wash-out period of at least 5 half-lives, an equal dose is applied to the fore- arm of the same monkeys. Each monkey is placed in a metabolism chair for 24 hours to prevent removal of the dose from the application site. Thereafter, the site is thoroughly washed and the monkeys returned to metabolism cages. Plasma and excreta are collected, assayed and the extent of absorption is assessed by comparing the area under the plasma level-time curve (AUC) to that from the intravenous dose. Additionally, comparison of the amount excreted in urine and feces is used as another measure of absorption. For a study with oryzalin, these procedures yielded dermal absorption values of 1.64 and 1.89 percent of the applied dose, respectively.

The increasing production of new chemicals and pesticides by industry has prompted significant growth and awareness in the field of toxicology. The decade of the 1970's witnessed a heightened concern about new technology and the long-term impact the use of new chemicals may have on the environment and human health.

As industry sought to develop new, safer and more specific pesticides for agricultural use, toxicology studies became more elaborate, sophisticated and more sensitive. Toxicokinetic prin- ciples were used too infrequently in setting doses for subchronic and chronic studies. Maximum tolerated doses used in these tests may have well exceeded the metabolic capacity of the test animal.

0097–6156/85/0273–0081$06.00/0

Nevertheless, the toxicologist, by regulatory mandate, is forced to increase the dose in each study to produce some demonstrable adverse effect (11). In the case of some compounds which do not produce acute toxic effects in mammalian species, the dose levels used in subchronic and chronic studies were quite high.

Exposure by workers in the manufacture of agricultural chemical products or by the mixer, loader or applicators who use these products may be considerable. Thus, the risk to these workers may be greater than to the consumer of treated products. The two recognized major routes of exposure are inhalation and topical. However, contrary to what was first believed, topical exposure constitutes the major route and it is for this reason that interest in percutaneous absorption of pesticides has increased to a considerable degree.

In order to assess the risk from topical exposure a number of investigators have sought animal models that could predict percutaneous absorption rates of chemicals in humans. Considerable efforts by Wester and Maibach (2-6) have shown that monkeys and pigs give dermal absorption data most comparable to humans with a range of drugs and pesticides which varied in their physicochemical properties as well as use. A similar rank order for species comparisons has been observed in in vitro (12-14) absorption data which in most cases exceeded the human values (Table I). For this reason, and because of the availability of rhesus monkeys within our facility, dermal absorption studies with rhesus monkeys were considered an appropriate model.

Table I. Ranking of Skin Permeability of Different
Species as Determined in vitro; Listed
in Decreasing Order of Permeability

Tregear (1966)[a]	Marzulli et al. (1969)[b]	McGreesh (1965)[c]
Rabbit	Mouse	Rabbit
Rat	Guinea pig	Rat
Guinea pig	Goat	Guinea pig
Man	Rabbit	Cat
	Horse	Goat
	Cat	Monkey
	Dog	Dog
	Monkey	Pig
	Weanling pig	
	Man	
	Chimpanzee	

[a]Ref. 12.
[b]Ref. 13.
[c]Ref. 14.
Source: Reproduced with permission from Ref. 15. Copyright 1980, Elsevier Biomedical Press.

There are a number of practical limitations that must be considered in conducting dermal absorption studies.

1. Much of the work described in the literature using monkeys has used a 6 cm² site on the ventral forearm.(8,9) This is a practical surface area and one which does not overly stress the animal. Other workers have suggested using as much as 16 percent of the body surface.(15,16) For a mature 4 kg rhesus monkey, the body surface area has been estimated to be 2900 cm² and 16 percent represents 475 cm², or about a 9" x 9" square! Such a large area could not be practically covered even on the back of a monkey.

2. Specific activity of available radiolabeled compound is often more of a problem than might be realized from the literature. Topical doses often cited range from 2 to 100 µg/cm² with 4 µg/cm² used quite often. If one assumes that a safe but lower limit of radioactivity would be approximately 10 µCi/animal, the specific activity would have to be at least 400 µCi/mg or, for a compound of 200 molecular weight, about 80 mCi/mmol. Such high activity for ^{14}C custom synthesized compounds is most often not available. In fact, if synthesized at this specific activity, many compounds undergo self-radiolysis, a process by which the emitted beta energy from ^{14}C is absorbed by the molecule itself producing decomposition. With custom synthesized radiochemicals, where little is known about their stability, compounds are rarely synthesized with specific activities in excess of 7.5 mCi/mmol. Thus, it is rarely possible to conduct studies at the 4 µg/cm² dose level with many experimental pesticides using carbon 14 radiotracer.

3. Radiocarbon counting statistics also are a major consideration in the conduct of dermal absorption studies. Since rhesus monkeys can produce from 1 to 2 liters of urine per day, counting a 1 ml aliquot of urine entails the use of a very large multiplication factor to express the amount excreted in the urine. Furthermore, since the concentration is generally low, the sample count will not be sufficiently accurate unless a considerable period of counting time is allotted. This is less true for plasma or fecal homogenates, but these too must be counted for long times to get meaningful quantification of their content. On the other hand, if the overall experimental error is 5 percent, less precise counting of samples from later time points will not significantly alter the results.

4. Another important limitation for risk assessment to mixers, loaders or applicators is the manner in which these workers are likely to be exposed to the chemical. Marketed pesticides are available in a variety of concentrated product forms ranging from dry pellets or powders to solutions in organic solvents and surfactants such as emulsifiable concentrates. Most of these products are mixed with water and applied in some way to soil or a food crop. The mixers and loaders may be exposed to concentrates which have a greater potential of being absorbed, while the applicator is exposed to a less absorbable form but over a potentially greater surface area.

In the case of overhead orchard spraying the exposure may be considerable; however, the vehicle (essentially water) is less likely to promote absorption. Field studies indicate that the arms, hands, and face receive the highest rate of exposure.(17) The amount absorbed can vary depending upon exposure site. Thus, a small deposit on a readily penetrable site can lead to just as much absorbed as a large deposit over a less penetrable area. In the case of organophosphates and carbamates, vapor exposure may be considerable and this, too, must be taken into account in the design of an absorption study. Thus, care must be exercised in planning and interpretation of the percutaneous absorption studies when the data are to be applied to a specific group of workers exposed to a given pesticide.

In the conduct of a monkey dermal absorption study, four mature rhesus monkeys are used in each experiment. These monkeys are obtained from the Charles River Breeding Laboratories. All monkeys have been acclimated to the facility for at least 1½ years and are accustomed to the use of metabolism cages and chairs.
The study is divided into two phases. If nothing is known about the disposition of the compound, it is preferable to conduct the intravenous phase first. However, if the time course of excretion can be predicted, it is quicker to conduct the topical study first. Levels are usually lower and background counting rates are more quickly reached, permitting the intravenous phase to be started sooner.
One day prior to starting the topical study, the monkeys are anesthetized with 10 mg/kg ketamine and 0.04 mg/kg atropine. The ventral forearm is shaved with electric clippers taking care not to abrade the skin. The following day, the animals are reanesthetized and, using a template, a 2 x 3 cm. rectangle is drawn on the skin. The dose is applied carefully using a hair dryer to evaporate the solvent. The site is covered using a neoprene rectangle with a stainless steel wire cloth (Ludlow and Saylor, St. Louis, MO) and adhesive tape attached. The square steel screen is from 20-60 mesh and is affixed to the neoprene with cyanoacrylate glue (Figure 1).
The monkeys are placed in plexiglass restraining chairs (Plas-Labs, Lansing, MI) where they have access to food and water. The arm on which the compound has been applied is restrained; however, the other is permitted to remain free. A midline barrier keeps the animal from reaching over and removing the protective cover and freeing the treated arm. Urine and feces are collected in a plastic tray at the base of the chair. During this period, the animals void only small quantities of urine.
After 24 hours, the arm is washed with soapy water followed with a swab soaked in acetone. Wash water and swab are saved and the latter extracted with solvent. The protective screens are also collected and washed with soap and water. The extracts and all the washes are assayed for radiocarbon content to determine the percent of dose recovered from the application site. The animals are returned to metabolism cages and daily urine, feces and plasma samples are collected.

The disposition of radiocarbon should be followed to permit a reasonable estimate of absorption to be made. For some herbicides, 7 days was sufficient; however, for organophosphates or carbamates, the time course of absorption and excretion would be much faster, and collection times and termination of the study should be adjusted accordingly.

After radiocarbon levels have returned to background, the second phase can be initiated. The dose given should be the same as that used previously and it is important that a soluble form of the compound be given. Water or saline are preferable vehicles, but rarely seem possible. Ethanol is most often used. Less polar organic solvents should be avoided. The dose is given in the saphenous vein, and the disposition similarly determined. Two-three ml heparinized blood are usually collected prior to dosing, at 15 and 30 minutes and again at 1, 2, 4, 6 and 24 hours. Daily samples are taken thereafter until a good profile of plasma radiocarbon disappearance can be determined.

Figure 2 illustrates the plasma disappearance of oryzalin, a dinitroaniline herbicide (3,5-dinitro-N^4,N^4-dipropylsulfanilamide) from a monkey given an intravenous dose of 2.0 mg/kg. Both alpha and beta half-lives were determined assuming a two-compartment open model. Values of 2.5 and 93 hours, respectively, for each phase were determined by a non-linear least square regression analysis of the model equation using MLAB ([18]). The volume of distribution obtained suggests significant plasma protein binding which has been confirmed by in vitro studies with purified protein fractions. The area under the plasma level time curve was obtained by summing trapezoidal areas between each time point.

Data from three topical studies with oryzalin are shown in Figure 3. The first experiment shows the plasma level data for the usual system of 2.0 mg/kg applied to 6 cm^2 equivalent to 1300 µg/cm^2. The second curve is the same dose applied to twice the surface area (660 µg/cm^2). The third curve is for 0.1 mg/kg applied to 6 cm^2. This latter experiment was made possible with the availability of a high specific activity lot and is equivalent to 67 µg/cm^2. The nondescending curves probably reflect the longer absorptive phase from topical application or a very slow diffusion rate through the skin. This rate appears similar in all three experiments, and may account for the fact that not all the dose is recovered during the one-week study.

Recoveries from the application site are shown in Table II.

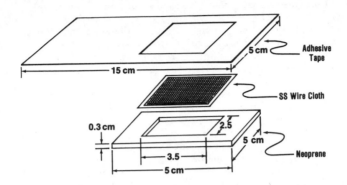

Figure 1.   A 5 x 5 cm protective patch made of neoprene and
stainless steel woven cloth.

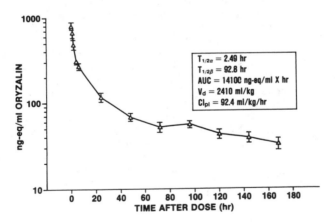

Figure 2.   Plasma disappearance of radiocarbon from monkeys.
Oryzalin (2.0 mg/kg) given in ethanol intravenously.   N=4.

Table II. Recovery of Applied Dose of [14]C Oryzalin in
Ethanol from Application Site

	Study 1[a]	Study 2[b]	Study 3[c]
	Percent of Applied Dose		
Rinse water	42.2±11.5	66.7±2.1	55.2±6.7
Swab	1.6±0.31	2.9±0.44	1.5±0.15
Screen	-	6.4±0.60	9.8±1.7
Dressing	29.1±6.7	-	-

a. 2.0 mg/kg - 6 cm^2
b. 0.1 mg/kg - 6 cm^2
c. 2.0 mg/kg - 12 cm^2

The first experiment utilized a gauze dressing to protect the site.
The later two studies utilized the neoprene screen patch. Total
recoveries from the site were only 66 to 76 percent. This is
typical and has also been seen in published studies with mosquito
repellents by Reifenrath, et al.(19)
     Urinary and fecal excretion for each of the three experiments
is shown in Figure 4. The amounts excreted are very small and a
descending excretion rate is observed in each case. Apparent
differences may not be real, considering the small quantities which
are being measured.
     Table III illustrates the two methods which are used to
estimate dermal absorption.(20,21)

Table III. Estimation of Dermal Absorption for
2.0 mg/kg Oryzalin

I. $\dfrac{\text{AUC (topical)}}{\text{AUC (intravenous)}} = \dfrac{231}{14,100} \times 100 = 1.64\%$

II. $\dfrac{\Sigma \text{ Excretion (topical)}}{\Sigma \text{ Excretion (intravenous)}} = \dfrac{1.59}{84.0} \times 100 = 1.89\%$

The first compares the ratio of the two areas under the curve (AUC)
for topical versus intravenous dosing. The area estimates are from
zero to 168 hours and do not use extrapolated areas beyond this
time. This gave a value of 1.64 percent. For the 12 cm^2 exposure
experiment, the value was 1.85 percent. A second comparison is
obtained by comparing total excretion for each experiment, topical
versus intravenous. This gave an absorption estimate of 1.89
percent for the first experiment, 4.0 percent for the second
experiment, and 1.78 percent for the third experiment (0.1 mg/kg).
These data demonstrate that no significant change in absorption
estimates occurred when the application area was doubled or when
the surface dose was reduced 20-fold. This is in contrast to what
is usually expected in percutaneous absorption studies,(22) but was
also observed by Reifenrath, et al. for mosquito repellents as seen
in Table IV.

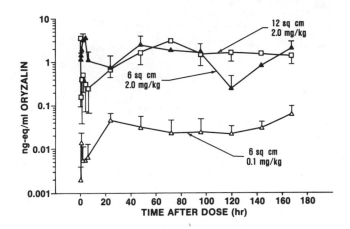

Figure 3.   Plasma disappearance of radiocarbon from monkeys.
Oryzalin given in ethanol topically.   N=4.

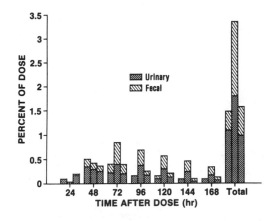

Figure 4.   Mean urinary and fecal excretion of radiocarbon from
monkeys receiving oryzalin topically. Experiment 1 (right-most
bar), 2.0 mg/kg applied to 6 cm^2; experiment 2 (middle bar),
2.0 mg/kg applied to 12 cm^2; experiment 3 (left-most bar),
0.1 mg/kg applied to 6 cm^2.

Table IV. Percutaneous Penetration and Total Absorption of
Repellents in Relation to the Dose of the
Chemical Applied to the Hairless Dog

Compound	Topical Dose ($\mu g/cm^2$)	Penetration (% of Applied Dose*)	Mean Total Absorbed ($\mu g/cm^2$)
Ethylhexanediol	4	8.8±2.0	0.35
	320	10.3±1.9	33.0
m-Deet	4	12.8±4.6	0.51
	320	9.4±3.6	30.1
Sulphonamide**	100	9.1±3.6	9.1
	320	7.5±2.2	24.0
	1000	5.4±2.2	54.0

*Values (means ± 1 SD) are corrected for incompleteness of urinary excretion.
**n-Butanesulphonamide cyclohexamethylene.
Source: Reproduced with permission from Ref. 19. Copyright 1981.
Pergamon Press, Ltd.

This author studied the percutaneous penetration of ethylhexanediol, N,N-diethyl-m-toluamide (m-Deet) and n-butanesulphonamide
cyclohexamethylene in the hairless dog. Decreasing penetration
with increasing dose was noted with m-Deet and the sulphonamide but
not with ethylhexanediol. None of the differences were significant
at the 95 percent confidence level. These compounds, like
oryzalin, were absorbed at 10 to 12 percent or less, so that the
assumed relationship between surface dose and penetration may not
be too significant for compounds which are poorly absorbed.
    Several problems exist in conducting percutaneous absorption
studies in rhesus monkeys.

1. As demonstrated, often only one or two doses are feasible.
    These may well exceed exposure rates; however, application
    rates similar to what is seen in field studies are likely to
    yield non-detectable levels.

2. Although studies could be done using arms and legs versus
    chest, back or forehead, the amount of time all such studies
    would take would be prohibitive and not likely to produce
    radically different results. Significant differences in
    penetration rates for different skin sites have been observed
    with some pharmaceuticals and pesticides indicating that
    axilla and scrotal skin were more readily penetrated(10,23);
    however, it is hoped that these areas will not be exposed to
    pesticides during normal use.

3. Since monkeys are expensive and special facilities are neces-
    sary to house and maintain them while using radiolabeled
    substances, only a limited number are likely to be utilized in
    these types of studies.

4. Without direct assay of the skin at the site of application,
    it is not likely that recovery of the entire dose will ever be
    complete.

5. When the excretion rate as estimated by the intravenous study
    is faster than the percutaneous absorption rate, plasma levels
    are likely to be very low and difficult to measure. The
    length of time in which percutaneous absorption is allowed to
    occur may not reflect the field situation. This would be the
    case for pesticides with low penetration potential more than
    rapidly absorbed pesticides which may be entirely absorbed
    within a few hours. A worker may or may not wash the affected
    area, depending upon his personal hygiene habits.

Percutaneous absorption studies utilizing rhesus monkeys have
one important single advantage. That is, their skin type and
absorption characteristics seem to be similar to humans. This is
of utmost concern since the purpose of this study is to simulate
the human case. This is not a toxicology study, and it should not
be the purpose of this study to estimate a worst case scenario as
in a hazard identification study. Thus, in spite of the many
shortcomings of the described procedures, monkey percutaneous
absorption studies could play an important role in pesticide risk
assessments.

Nontechnical Summary   In this paper, the process of risk assessment with compounds which exhibit chronic but not acute toxicity is
first reviewed. The remainder of the paper is spent on reviewing
the procedure for quantifying absorption through the skin. The
test animal used is the rhesus monkey since previously published
work has shown this animal to yield data most similar to man. Data
are presented on oryzalin for which dermal absorption was less than
2 percent of the applied dose. The problems and shortcomings of
the procedure as well as its advantage (similarity to man) are also
discussed.

Acknowledgments   Gratitude is expressed to James White and W. Dean
Johnson for their cooperation in conducting these studies and to
Michael K. Scott and Allen Johnson, Linda D. Cherry, Mark D. Gunnoe
and Dix E. Weaver for their technical assistance.

Literature Cited

1. Wester, R. C.; Maibach, H. I.   Toxicol. Appl. Pharm. 1975, 32,
    394-398.
2. Wester, R. C.; Maibach, H. I.   In "Cutaneous Toxicity"; Ed.
    Drill, V.; Lazar, P. Academic Press, New York, 1977, 111-126.
3. Wester, R. C.; Maibach, H. I.   In "Animal Models in Derma-
    tology"; Ed. Maibach, H. I., Churchill Livingstone, New York,
    1975, 133-137.
4. Wester, R. C.; Maibach, H. I.   J. Invest. Dermatol. 1976, 67,
    518-520.
5. Wester, R. C.; Noonan, P. K.; Maibach, H. I.   J. Soc. Cosmet.
    Chem. 1979, 30, 297-307.

6. Feldmann, R. J.; Maibach, H. I.   J. Invest. Dermatol. 1970,
    54, 339-404.
7. Feldmann, R. J.; Maibach, H. I.   J. Invest. Dermatol. 1969,
    52, 89-94.
8. Wester, R. C.; Maibach, H. I.   J. Invest. Dermatol. 1976, 67,
    518-520.
9. Wester, R. C.; Maibach, H. I.   Tox. Appl. Pharm. 1975, 32,
    394-398.
10. Maibach, H. I.; Feldmann, R. J.; Milby, T. H.; Sevat, W. F.
    Pestic. Arch. Environ. Health 1971, 23, 208-211.
11. "Pesticide Assessment Guidelines Subdivision F", U.S. Environ-
    mental Protection Agency, 1983.
12. Tregear, R. T.   "Physical Function of Skin", Academic Press:
    New York, 1966.
13. Marzulli, F. W.; Brown, D.W.C.; Maibach, H. I.   Tox. Appl.
    Pharm. Suppl. 3, 1969, 76-83.
14. McGreesh, A. H.   Tox. Appl. Pharm. Suppl. 2, 1965, 20-26.
15. Wester, R. C.; Noonan, P. K.   Int. J. of Pharmac. 1980, 7,
    99-110.
16. Zenzian, R., USEPA, personal communication.
17. Shah, P. V.; Moore, R. J.; Guthrie, F. E.   Tox. Appl. Pharm.
    1981, 59, 414-423.
18. Day, E. W. (1984), personal communication.
19. Knott, G. P.   MLAB, an on-line modeling laboratory. Nat.
    Inst. Health, Washington, D.C., 1979.
20. Reifenrath, W. G.; Robinson, P. B.; Bolton, V. D.; Alitt, R.
    E. Food Cosmet. Toxicol. 1981, 19, 195-199.
21. Wester, R. C.; Noonan, P. K.   J. Invest. Derm. 1978, 70,
    92-94.
22. Wester, R. C.; Noonan, P. K.; Smeach, S.; Kosobud, L.
    J. Pharm. Sci. 1983, 72, 745-748.
23. Feldmann, R. J.; Maibach, H. I.   J. Invest. Dermatol. 1967,
    48, 181-183.

RECEIVED November 15, 1984

FIELD STUDIES: METHODOLOGY

Field Studies: Methods Overview

H. N. NIGG and J. H. STAMPER

Citrus Research and Education Center, University of Florida, Lake Alfred, FL 33850

Assessment of worker exposure to pesticides through
field studies requires collection devices placed on or
near the worker, extraction techniques, quantification
of the chemical, and statistical analysis. We present
an overview of these methods with specific attention
given to dermal absorption pads, their proper placement
at various body locations, and the statistical
variability in pad contamination which commonly
results. Use of personal air samplers is reviewed.
Sampling of worker urine is discussed, together with
correlations between pad and urine contamination.
Field studies involving pesticide applicators or
mixer-loaders are contrasted with those involving
harvesters. The effect of worker methods or work rate
on exposure is mentioned. The influence of the
extraction method on the calculated dissipation rate of
pesticides from foliar surfaces is discussed. Finally,
biological monitoring and statistical problems are
outlined.

Many of the methods reviewed here have been previously reviewed by
Davis (1). It is our purpose to update that review and to relate
our personal experiences with existing devices for monitoring worker
exposure in order to assist other prospective researchers with the
experimental design of field experiments.

Initiating a Field Study

The goals of a field study help dictate the methods as well as the
subsequent difficulties encountered in the field portion of the
study. For instance, a study to determine the penetration of
pesticides through fabrics might require that collection devices be
placed under the worker's suit and on the surface. To determine the
actual protection provided by the suit might require that urine
samples be collected each day. While 24-hr. urine samples are
preferable for applicator/mixer-loader studies, daily timed urine

samples may suffice for a harvester experiment. Depending on urine
excretion kinetics for the compound used, the suit might be worn on
alternate days or on alternate weeks. Field methods will also be
influenced by the extraction and analytical techniques employed.
The length and complexity of any individual design will depend on
the variation among replications reported by previous researchers in
the literature. Exposure experiments are very expensive and time
consuming; no researcher wants to discover belatedly that only a few
more samples collected and a little more effort expended would have
salvaged a statistically unanalyzable experiment.

Respiratory Exposure

Several questions should be answered prior to any experiment
designed to measure respiratory exposure. Does the application
method provide droplet sizes that are 'breathable'? Is the chemical
volatile under the conditions of use? Are respiratory data required
at all for registration?

   Several approaches to the measurement of respiratory exposure
are available. The first was developed by Durham and Wolfe (2) and
employs a respirator with the collection pads protected by cones
from direct spray. The second common method uses the personal air
sampler with a pump carried by the worker and a collection device in
the general breathing zone. The third method involves a more
careful experimental design. In this case, the worker wears a
pesticide respirator for a certain period of time with the
respirator removed for an equal amount of time. Twenty-four hour
urine samples are collected each day, with any observed increase in
urinary metabolites indicating the degree of respiratory exposure.
It is best to ask the worker to wear extensive protective gear
throughout. Care must be taken with this type design. Since the
goal is to identify an increase which may be small, any extraneous
exposure may obscure this difference and lead to a tenuous result.

   In his review, Davis (1) argued in several ways that the first
two methods suffer from the lack of efficacy data. That is, the
trapping efficiency of a respirator or personal air sampler is
seldom checked for the collection of both aerosols and vaporized
materials. We agree with this assessment. Even when the collection
efficacy is checked, the pesticide may have been applied in a
solvent, and air subsequently drawn through the device. This is
imprecise at best. Collection techniques which include both
aerosols and vapor are more accurate and would better reflect actual
field situations.

   The experimental design for respiratory exposure necessarily
depends on several assumptions and disparate pieces of available
data. The excretion kinetics of the pesticide employed must be
known. If the total dose is excreted by small animals in 24-48 hr.,
the same may also be true of humans, and a simple experimental
design may suffice. If the dose is excreted over a period of a
week, a simple design correlating dose with the immediate effect on
urine will not correctly assess respiratory exposure. The
difficulty with longer sampling periods, occasioned by longer
excretion kinetics, derives from the variation normally observed in
the urinary exposure estimation for field experiments. It is not

unusual to see a 100% coefficient of variation among urinary
excretion samples. As a consequence, the change in urinary levels
comparing respirator vs. no respirator must be very high in order to
validate significance. Part of this variation results from reckless
work practices. Workers spill concentrate. They service
contaminated machinery with bare hands. In one experiment, we
observed a worker remove his gloves, roll up his protective suit,
and retrieve a crescent wrench from the tank. These kinds of
activities obviously decrease the statistical significance of any
observed difference in urinary metabolites when comparing those
wearing protective gear to those not.

The prior knowledge of the excretion kinetics is a key piece of
data. Unfortunately, many pesticides in common use are not excreted
in urine in proportion to dose. This behavior is common for
organochlorines. An example of current interest is dicofol. With
multiple doses this organochlorine rapidly reaches a plateau in
urine, while excretion levels steadily increase in the feces (3).
However, the excretion kinetics available for most compounds have
resulted from studies using only one or a very few oral doses.
Dicofol is an exception.

There are kinetic models which could represent pesticides
recycled into the bile (4). However, laboratory excretion models
generally do not account for the differences in the route of the
dose for workers and subsequent excretion differences.

There are obvious paths toward a solution to this difficulty.
A small animal excretion study with multiple doses could be done.
However, which dosing method should be used? Should the dose be
dermal, as the fieldworker has mostly dermal exposure, or should a
mixture of oral, dermal, and respiratory dosing be used? What if
the compound has associated data suggesting skin penetration is low?
Would then respiratory exposure be the route to investigate? Since
humans will be involved in the fieldwork and subsequently in
regulations, relevance and accuracy in the preliminary small animal
studies are extremely important.

Another possibility is to perform an actual human excretion
study. At the end of the spray season, and with the workers removed
from further exposure, a series of 24-hr. urine samples might yield
the necessary kinetic data. We suggest splitting the daily sampling
periods into two 12-hr. or four 6-hr. segments. For compounds which
are very rapidly excreted, this division into timed segments will
help to obtain the necessary data points. Removal of workers from
exposure is paramount even if the experimenter must wash the
workers' clothing and closely monitor their work activities over
this period. We have discovered, to our surprise, that workers have
interpreted 'removal from exposure' as 'stop spraying,' and then
proceeded to clean and maintain heavily contaminated equipment over
our sampling period. Even if all of these factors are controlled,
the chemical type, its metabolism, and/or variability among subjects
may prohibit the drawing of statistically valid inferences.

Some of the other factors which can (and have) invalidate(d) a
respiratory exposure experiment are loosely fitting respirators,
workers with highly variable hand exposure, varying wind speed and
direction, and spraying when the wind velocity exceeds approximately
10 mph.

From our perspective, a tightly fitting respirator with
collection devices, or an experiment with 24-hr. urine collection
and alternating respirator-no respirator periods, constitute
adequate designs. Of these two, the respirator with a collection
device is the least expensive and easiest to conduct in the field.
The respirator has the advantage of not needing calibration. The
actual material inhaled is measured. It is convenient to wear,
whereas the personal air sampler may be refused by the worker
because of discomfort or inconvenience, particularly in harvester
experiments.

Dermal Exposure Pads

Dermal exposure pads have been constructed of α-cellulose, cloth,
polyurethane foam, and combinations of these materials. They are
generally designed to collect spray materials and have been used for
emulsifiable concentrates and wettable powders mixed with water.
They appear to work well. However, almost never are these
collection devices assessed for pesticide loss. That is, if the pad
is left on the worker for 6 hr., how much material evaporated or
degraded in those 6 hr.? There would appear to be two ways to
assess this loss. Davis (1) reviewed the practice of fortifying
pads with the same pesticide-water mixture as in the field
experiment. Alternatively, unfortified pads could be applied to the
worker, with some left for 1 hr. and then removed, some left for 2
hr. and removed, and so forth. This latter test assumes that the
exposure to the pads is equal for all exposure periods and ignores
temperature effects. Fortified pads placed in an out-of-doors
holding device appears to be the better approach. By removing and
analyzing these pads at intervals, the approximate length of time a
pad should be worn by a worker in the field can be determined. This
is an important consideration for 'unquestionable' worker data,
i.e., the ability to account for the behavior of the pesticide on
the pad during the experiment.
       Once the time of exposure and laboratory recovery studies are
completed, storage stability should be determined. Although a
separate experiment is possible, the simple expedient of storing one
or two fortified pads with each worker's pad set will determine
storage stability as extraction and analyses proceed. The resulting
recoveries also serve as a check on the accuracy of laboratory
technical help. The required number of these fortified pads depends
on the size of the experiment. The criterion is to allow for enough
measurements to statistically validate the quality of both storage
and extraction. We use a minimum of three fortified pads per
exposure day.
       Placement of the pads on the body of the subject has many
ramifications. If a total body exposure estimate is to be made, the
calculation method should be considered. Davis (1) and Popendorf
(5) are good sources for these methods. Pads will then be placed so
as to optimize the total body estimate. Obviously, if the
calculation requires a leg value, accuracy would dictate placing a
pad on the leg. For areas where pads are inconveniently worn, such
as the face, combinations of shoulder and upper body pad residues
may be used as approximations. However, there is at least one

published study in which face exposure itself was significant (6).
Development of methods for measuring face exposure and for measuring
exposure to other body areas where pads are not normally placed
would be helpful to this research area.

The location of pads on the subjects should not be decided upon
hastily. A consensus among regulatory agencies appears to be
forming in favor of protective suit design. For those areas of the
U.S. where temperatures can be very warm and/or humid during a spray
season, data on where the greatest exposure occurs to the worker's
body would be very helpful. That is because these data might allow
development of protective suit designs which do not attempt total
coverage and might prove more comfortable. For instance, the
exposure of an applicator or mixer-loader on the backs of the arms
and legs is not known. It should be known. Whether the lower arms
receive more exposure than the upper arms is seldom monitored. In
many of our measurements, the lower arms received significantly more
exposure than the upper arms, but the generality of this result is
unconfirmed. If these data were available, comfortable protective
suits utilizing relatively open mesh areas might be certifiably
protective at this time. And, actual exposure estimates might, in
fact, be reduced through their use. Certainly, taking these
additional data adds extra work and expense to a study, but the
long-term benefits might be substantial.

Mixer-Loaders and Applicators vs. Harvesters

Applicators and mixer-loaders certainly receive different
levels and types of exposure than do harvesters. The mixer-loaders
have an opportunity for concentrate as well as drift exposure. The
applicator is primarily exposed to drift and the tank mixed
material. The harvester is exposed to a presumably homogeneous
application of pesticide on fruit, leaf, and soil surfaces. Both
groups may also be exposed by working on or around contaminated
machinery and in or around contaminated loading areas.

For applicator, loader-mixer groups we previously discussed
sources of experimental variation. For harvesters, different
sources of variation exist, but these may not be extreme.
Theoretically, harvesters are exposed only to the residues remaining
in the field. They are exposed most heavily when working in that
field. The experiment appears simple. Pads are placed on the body
of the harvester at various locations, the residues on leaves, fruit
and soil are measured, and the appropriate correlations are made.

For the experimenter, however, there are all sorts of possible
constructions. Where should the pads be located? Should they be
placed inside or outside the clothing? Will clothing chosen by the
worker suffice or should standard clothing be issued? Was the field
sprayed during 1 hr., 1 day, or 3 days? If the spraying took longer
than one day, where should the workers start working? Will they
overlap sprayed sections as the work progresses? How many daily
residue samples should be taken as a consequence? Should pads with
a surgical gauze front be used or would polyurethane foam be
satisfactory? How should these pads be assessed for residue loss?
How long should the worker wear the pads? Is the pesticide
converted in the field into a toxicologically important metabolite?

Can it be extracted and analyzed? How should the urine be
collected: 24-hr. urines or a timed grab sample? And finally, how
many sampling periods (days) should the experiment entail in order
to make statistically significant results likely?

These suggestions are offered: The pads should be placed
inside the clothing for lower and upper arm, chest, back, shoulders
and shin exposure. For the upper body, the pads can be conveniently
pinned inside an issued shirt. They can also be pinned inside the
pants, but it should be noted whether the worker wears the same
pants each day. Intuition is a fine tool here, especially as
enhanced by experience, but at least for the first experiment we
recommend the above placement of pads. For later experiments, a
reduction in the number of pads may be possible. It is, however, a
mistake to simply observe a harvest operation and decide a priori
that only leg patches are necessary.

At what time the pesticide application was made is important
for several reasons. If the purpose of the experiment is to
correlate field residues with worker exposure, knowing the pesticide
used and its application date can be crucial. An experiment of this
type should begin at the legal reentry time and extend through at
least two pesticide 'half-lives.' This insures the validity of the
correlation of residues with exposure because a broad range of both
has been utilized. This sampling time may last one week or longer.
The area to be sprayed may be large. We have, for instance, used
three spray machines simultaneously in order to assure a one day
application. All harvesters are then exposed to the same daily
residue over the sampling period.

When a 'blind' harvester experiment is conducted and the
application is made over a few days, the number of residue samples
per substrate should be doubled and taken from where the harvesters
are working that particular day. This will help with the overlap
problem. Even if the experiment is only a one or two day
experiment, reentry should commence as soon as possible after
application. This assures some results at least, from an analytical
standpoint, that may fit an existing model. If the workers reenter
a field after 10 days and the analytical chemist detects no residues
because of low levels, little has been accomplished except the
expense of time and money.

The most commonly used exposure pad for worker reentry
experiments is faced with surgical gauze, backed with α-cellulose
and glassine weighing paper. This pad has proven uncomfortable for
the worker, difficult to attach, and takes time to prepare. We know
of one instance where polyurethane foam pads were used (7). They
are very convenient and may be efficient. However, there is no good
method for assessing the residue collecting efficiency of these
devices for a harvester exposure experiment. In spite of years of
research in this area, the transfer process of field surface
residues to the body of the harvester is not known with certainty.
Probably foliar and field dust are primarily involved. How then is
the efficiency of a collection device for a harvesting operation
measured? The experimenter is presently confined to the application
of pesticide-laden dust or a pesticide solution to the exposure pad,
followed by a disappearance study. Although the disappearance study
may indicate a 50% loss from a pad in, say, 2 hr., the pads may have

to be worn longer. The reason is simple: exposure for a harvester
is generally low and enough residue must be collected for analyses.
We attach the pads just before workers enter the field in the
morning and remove them 4-5 hr. later at the noon break. The amount
detected on the pads can be corrected according to the disappearance
experiment, but this correction is not entirely reliable since the
pesticide may disappear at a different rate when attached to dust,
as may have been the case in the field.

The production of a toxic metabolite on foliage or in soil and
the possible consequence to harvesters have been reviewed (8, 9).
We mention this consideration because of its importance to
harvesters and because the urine analyses may have to account for
the excretion products of these metabolites. Urine collection from
harvesters is not difficult, but consistently reliable urine
sampling is another matter. We have attempted to collect 24-hr.
urine samples, but this did not work well. Harvesters in Florida
are more mobile, appear for work erratically, and are less likely to
understand instructions than the applicator, mixer-loader group.
However, a timed grab sample from the start of work until the noon
break has provided excellent correlations between residue levels on
foliage and urinary metabolites in harvesters (10). We attribute
this to the greater opportunity for significant contamination
incidents of applicator, mixer-loaders over harvesters.

Worker Methods and Work Rates

For the applicator, mixer-loader group the type of equipment used,
the number of tanks applied per unit time, the concentration of the
tank mix, and the loading method all affect the exposure process.
This has been known for years and is described in many published
reports (1, 10).

For harvesters, there are only a few field experiments
described in the literature. The harvesting method and crop have
been studied and some reports exist which can be compared. What
seems apparent from these reports is that the exposure process is
the same for the harvesting of such tree fruits as citrus and
apples. At least, the proportion of harvester exposure to pesticide
on the leaf surface is the same. For other types of crops this
proportion may be different.

Regardless of crop type, the work rate appears to be related to
exposure. This means that the number of boxes picked, crates
loaded, tassels removed, etc., is confounded with residue levels in
affecting exposure. The worker's production delimits the contact
with the plant, a subject which has been studied using movies and
time analysis (11), and estimated with surveys (12). Therefore,
work rate data should be gathered for each subject; it may explain
variation in urinary or dermal exposure unaccounted for by field
residues.

Extraction Methods--Rates of Disappearance

There has been some concern over the method of pesticide extraction,
particularly for harvester exposure residues. For applicators and
mixer-loaders, methods can be developed as needed with defined

substrates. For the extraction of leaf, fruit, and soil surface
residues, peculiar to harvester exposure studies, a standard
methodology has been adopted by many researchers (13, 14). Fruit
and leaf surface residues are recovered with organic solvents from a
mild soap solution in which they have been shaken. Soil surface
residues are recovered by vacuuming surface soil through a 100-mesh
screen. However, at least for foliar residues, some experimenters
shake leaves in organic solvents (15, 16). These organic solvent
residue data are generally higher and usually lead to slower
calculated rates of disappearance, making it appear that the worker
is exposed to higher residues of longer duration.

      Should these differences in extraction methods really be a
concern? Regardless of the volume of research on the harvester
exposure process, i.e., the transport mechanism from foliage or soil
to the worker, it is not precisely understood now, nor is this
understanding likely to arise in the near future. Nor are there
enough researchers or funds available to investigate every exposure
situtation. But models of worker exposure as a function of foliar
residues recovered by the dislodgeable method (non-solvent) have
been and are being produced. A model developed for one chemical is
then used for another. Solvent residue data for a chemical could be
alternatively used in these models once the relationship between the
solvent and dislodgeable methods is understood and quantified. For
now, differences in extraction methods are of concern, but once the
quantitative relationship between the two methods is understood,
this will no longer be true.

      The dislodgeable method washes the leaf surface with a dilute
soap solution and the solution is extracted with the appropriate
solvent. Details on this method may be found in Iwata (13). The
efficacy of the dislodgeable method is commonly assessed by
fortifying leaf washes with the pesticide, allowing this mixture to
equilibrate for the same time as the experimental leaves will be
washed (about 20 min), and extracting. This method is simple and
relatively easy to master. It has been used as the basis for models
of harvester exposure and should be the method of choice for
experimenters.

Biological Monitoring

One of the first applicator studies was undertaken by Quinby et al.
(17). Cholinesterase activity was measured in aerial applicators
together with residues on worker clothing and in respirator pads.
Two features of this study should be emphasized: 1. In spite of
physical complaints by pilots exposed to organophosphate, either
normal or only slightly depressed cholinesterase values were
reported, and 2. Cholinesterase values were compared with the
'normal' range for the U.S. population rather than the pilots' own
individual 'normal' values. In 1952, Kay et al. (18) measured
cholinesterase levels in orchard parathion applicators. These were
compared with cholinesterase levels taken from the same workers
during non-spray periods. Plasma cholinesterase for workers
reporting physical symptoms was 16% lower during the spray period.
The corresponding reduction for symptomless workers was about 13%.
Erythrocyte cholinesterase was depressed 27% for the symptom group

vs. 17% for the non-symptom group, but these means were not
statistically different. Roan et al. (19) measured plasma and
erythrocyte cholinesterase and serum levels of ethyl and methyl
parathion in aerial applicators. Serum levels of the parathions
could not be correlated with cholinesterase levels. However, serum
levels did correlate with the urine concentration of p-nitrophenol.
Drevenkar et al. (20) measured plasma and erythrocyte cholinesterase
levels and urine concentrations of organophosphate and carbamate
pesticides in formulating plant workers. No correlation existed
between urinary metabolites and cholinesterase depression. Bradway
et al. (21) studied cholinesterase, blood residues, and urinary
metabolites in rats. Even under controlled conditions and known
doses, correlations of cholinesterase activity with blood residues
and urine metabolite levels were poor. Eight organophosphates were
included in the Bradway et al. (21) experiment. The overriding
general conclusion from the above is that cholinesterase inhibition
as an exposure indicator contains too many variables, known and
unknown, to be of use (except in a very general sense).

Urinary metabolites of pesticides have been used for a variety
of experimental goals. Swan (22) measured paraquat in the urine of
spraymen, Gollop and Glass (23) and Wagner and Weswig (24) measured
arsenic in timber applicators, Lieben et al. (25) measured
paranitrophenol in urine after parathion exposure as did Durham et
al. (26). Cholrobenzilate metabolite (presumably dichlorobenzilic
acid) was detected in citrus workers (27), phenoxy acid herbicide
metabolites in farmers (28), and organophosphate metabolites in the
urine of ordinary citizens exposed to mosquito treatments (29).
Davies et al. (30) used urinary metabolites of organophosphates and
carbamates to confirm poisoning cases. These studies document
exposure, but no estimate of exposure can be made from urinary
metabolite levels alone. Other studies have used air sampling and
monitored hand exposure in combination with urine levels (31), and
air sampling plus cholinesterase inhibition plus urine levels (32).

The exposure pad method, combined with measurement of urinary
metabolites, has been used to compare worker exposure for different
pesticide application methods (33, 34) as well as to monitor
formulating plant worker exposure (35) and homeowner exposure (36).

Several studies have used the exposure pad method to estimate
total dermal exposure, attempting to correlate urine levels with the
estimate (6, 33, 37–40). Lavy et al. (39, 40) found no such
correlation with 2,4-D or 2,4,5-T. Wojeck et al. (33) found no
paraquat in urine and consequently no relationship between dose and
urine levels. However, the group daily mean concentration of
urinary metabolites of ethion and the group mean total dermal
exposure to ethion on that day correlated positively, with
significance at the 96.6% confidence level (38). For arsenic, the
cumulative total exposure and daily urinary arsenic concentration
correlated positively, with significance at the 99% confidence level
(37). Franklin et al. (6) found a positive correlation between
48-hr. excretion of azinphosmethyl metabolites and the amount of
active ingredient sprayed. A significant correlation could not be
made, however, between 48-hr. excretion and an exposure estimate.
In the Franklin et al. (6) experiment, a fluorescent tracer had been
added to the spray mixture. Qualitatively, unpatched areas (face,

hands, neck) also received significant exposure, perhaps leading to
a weak correlation between the patch estimate and urinary
metabolites. Winterlin et al. (41) monitored the dermal exposure of
applicators, mixer-loaders, and strawberry harvesters to captan
using exposure pads. Although the applicator, mixer-loader group
showed higher dermal exposure, no metabolite was detected in their
urine while harvester urine had detectable levels.

We return, consequently, to the problem of the excretion
kinetics of pesticides, the complexity of which may render useless
any search for a simple linear correlation between dose and urinary
metabolites. Some experimenters have attempted to investigate this
area. Drevenkar et al. (20) studied the excretion of phosalone
metabolites in one volunteer. Excretion reached a peak in 4-5 hr.,
but was not complete in 24 hr. Funckes et al. (42) exposed the hand
and forearm of human volunteers to 2% parathion dust. During
exposure, the volunteers breathed pure air and placed their forearm
and hand into a plastic bag which contained the parathion. This
exposure lasted 2 hr. and was conducted at various temperatures.
There was an increased excretion of paranitrophenol with increasing
exposure temperature. More importantly, paranitrophenol could still
be detected in the urine 40 hr. post exposure. In another human
experiment, Kolmodin-Hedman et al. (43) applied methychlorophenoxy
acetic acid (MCPA) to the thigh. Plasma MCPA reached a maximum in
12 hr. and MCPA appeared in the urine for 5 days with a maximum
after about 48 hr. Given orally, urinary MCPA peaked in 1 hr. with
about 40% of the dose excreted in 24 hr. In a rat experiment, seven
different organophosphates at two different doses were fed to two
rats per compound (21). The rats were removed from exposure after
the third day and blood and urine collected for the next 10 days.
The percents of the total dose excreted in urine over the 10 days
averaged (high and low dose): dimethoate, 12%; dichlorvos, 10%;
ronnel, 11%; dichlofenthion, 57%; carbophenothion, 66%; parathion,
40%; and leptophos, 50%. Very little of this excretion occurred
beyond the third day post exposure. Intact residues of ronnel,
dichlofenthion, carbophenothion, and leptophos were found in fat on
day 3 and day 8 post exposure. In another rat experiment, animals
were dosed once dermally and intramuscularly with azinphosmethyl
(44). About 78% of the dermal dose had been excreted in urine in 24
hr. Its rate of excretion peaked in 8-16 hr., continued at about
the same rate for another 16 hr., and declined to a steady level 16
hr. thereafter. There was a linear relationship between dermal dose
and urinary excretion. The intramuscular dose was excreted much
more rapidly than the dermal dose. No apparent relationship existed
between the intramuscular dose and urinary excretion.

Because these experiments illustrate the excretion differences
between dermal, intramuscular, and oral dose excretion, the
excretion differences between compounds, and also problems about
which urinary metabolite to monitor (see 44), a very comprehensive
experimental design would be necessary to correctly model dermal
exposure, absorption, and urinary metabolite levels. Statistical
problems, centering around replicate variation and the resulting
necessity for abnormally large numbers of replications, could drive
the costs of such an experiment in small animals, and certainly in
humans, to prohibitively high levels.

Replications, Statistical Considerations

Here, we discuss in greater detail some of the statistical considerations inherent in experimental design and return, by way of example, to the assessment in the field of the efficacy of protective clothing in reducing dermal pesticide exposure. Data analysis for such experiments usually necessitates comparing two mean values, each deriving from about the same number of replications. Let us say that one of the means represents exposure to a pad placed outside the clothing while the other represents exposure to a pad placed inside. The number of replications per mean is typically the product of the number of sampling periods (sampling days) and the number of participating subjects, but this is contingent upon validation, by an analysis of variance of the obtained data, that exposure levels do not vary significantly day-to-day or subject-to-subject. This is usually the case if all subjects performed the same tasks each day.

The question must be addressed of how many replicates per pad (subjects X days) will be necessary to validate that an observed difference in means is statistically significant. Two parameters must be estimated preliminarily. First, what difference in means is expected to arise from the data? Second, what variation among replicates is expected? A large estimate for the first expectation or a small estimate for the second expectation would reduce the number of replicates necessary per mean. These two estimates can be made with some reliability, prior to the experiment, only from past experience. Our experience has shown, e.g., that protective clothing reduces mean pad exposure by about 90% (45). Similarly, the use of gloves reduces handwash residues by about 85%, according to a recent study of dicofol by Nigg et al., now being prepared for publication. As for variation among replicates, the coefficient of variation is typically about 100% for exposure pad and handwash residues (10, 45).

Standard statistical procedures then show (46) that, on the basis of the above estimates, two exposure pad means may be judged significantly different at the 95% confidence level by taking at least ten replications per mean. The (approximate) calculation is $n > 8 \ (100\% \div 90\%)^2$ or $n > 10$ replications. For gloves, the corresponding calculation would be $n > (100\% \div 85\%)^2$ or $n > 11$ replications. These numbers represent an absolute minimum based on the above two expected values. An increase in n of 50% to provide some margin for error, in the above cases to $n > 15$ and $n > 17$, is certainly warranted in view of the unavoidable preliminary guesswork involved about sample means and variences.

If more than two means are to be compared concurrently, as with comparing residues at various body locations, the situation becomes somewhat more complicated. While it is now harder to generalize, the optimum number of replications per mean can be roughly adduced by the same calculation, with the final result that the means are grouped into significantly different categories, at some confidence level.

Whether to utilize, e.g., three subjects for six sampling periods each, or six subjects for three sampling periods each, to obtain, say, 18 replications is usually dictated by factors other

than statistical ones. A good rule to follow is not to overload the
design too heavily in favor of either variable. If, e.g., many
subjects are used for a very few sampling days, and the data
indicate large differences from subject to subject (admittedly, an
unlikely result), the available number of replicates now decreases
to the number of sampling days alone. The experiment makes a very
unreliable statement about each of many subjects. No valid overall
conclusion may emerge.

It should be borne in mind that these statistical calculations
have shown significant differences between means, but do not
estimate the difference. Suppose one mean is 90% less than the
other, as above, but that one wishes to validate the claim that 50
of that 90% is statistically significant. The approximate
calculation for the requisite number of replications per mean is now
$n > 8 [100\% \div (90\% - 50\%)]^2 = 50$, or $n > 75$ with the safety factor.

Summary

We present these concluding generalities.

1. The experimenter should always bear in mind those hazards
   to realistic measurements peculiar to field experiments
   which we have emphasized above.

2. Otherwise unexplainable sources of variation within
   replicate samples might become evident if the work
   practices of the subjects are considered. This may require
   a period of careful observation in the field extending over
   a week or longer.

3. The level of and reasons for variation encountered in
   previous published studies can be helpful for experimental
   design. Once this anticipated variation is estimated,
   numbers of replications per sample can be rationally
   established.

4. Frequently, the reason for the failure of a worker exposure
   experiment is the lack of basic information on relevant
   human biochemistry and physiology. A thorough literature
   search for information on the urinary excretion kinetics,
   etc. of the compound under investigation could be a very
   worthwhile prior investment.

Literature Cited

1. Davis, J. E. Residue Rev. 1980, 75, 33-50.
2. Durham, W. F.; Wolfe, H. R. Bull. Wld. Hlth. Org. 1962, 26, 75-91.
3. Brown, J. R.; Hughes, H.; Viriyanondha, S. Toxicol. Appl. Pharmacol. 1969, 15, 30-7.
4. Colburn, W. A. J. Pharm. Sci. 1984, 73, 313-7.
5. Popendorf, W. J.; Leffingwell, J. T. Residue Rev. 1982, 82, 125-201.
6. Franklin, C. A.; Fenske, R. A.; Greenhalgh, R.; Mathieu, L.; Denley, H. V.; Leffingwell, J. T.; Spear, R. C. J. Toxicol. Environ. Hlth. 1981, 7, 715-31.

7. Brady, E. personal communication.
8. Nigg, H. N.; Stamper, J. H.; In "Pesticide Residues and Exposure"; Plimmer, J., Ed.; ACS SYMPOSIUM SERIES 182, 1982.
9. Gunther, F. A.; Iwata, Y.; Carman, G. E.; Smith, C. A. Residue Rev. 1977, 67, 1-139.
10. Nigg, H. N.; Stamper, J. H.; Queen, R. M. Am. Ind. Hyg. Assoc. J. 1984, 45, 182-6.
11. Wicker, G. W.; Guthrie, F. E. Bull. Environ. Contam. Toxicol. 1980, 24, 161-7.
12. Wicker, G. W.; Stinner, R. E.; Reagan, P. E.; Guthrie, F. E. Bull. Entomol. Soc. Amer. 1980, 26, 156-61.
13. Iwata, Y.; Knaak, J. B.; Spear, R. C.; Foster, R. J. Bull. Environ. Contam. Toxicol. 1977, 18, 649-55.
14. Spencer, W. F.; Kilgore, W. W.; Iwata, Y.; Knaak, J. B. Bull. Environ. Contam. Toxicol. 1977, 18, 656-62.
15. Ware, G. W.; Estesen, B.; Cahill, W. P. Bull. Environ. Contam. Toxicol. 1975, 14, 606-9.
16. Ware, G. W.; Estesen, B.; Buck, N. A. Bull. Environ. Contam. Toxicol. 1980, 25, 608-15.
17. Quinby, G. F.; Walker, K. C.; Durham, W. F. J. Econ. Entomol. 1958, 51, 831-8.
18. Kay, K.; Monkman, L.; Windish, J. P.; Doherty, T.; Pare, J.; Raciot, C. Ind. Hyg. Occ. Med. 1952, 6, 252-62.
19. Roan, C. C.; Morgan, D. P.; Cook, N.; Paschal, E. H. Bull. Environ. Contam. Toxicol. 1969, 4, 362-9.
20. Drevenkar, V.; Stengl, B.; Tralcevic, B.; Vasilic, Z. Int. J. Environ. Anal. Chem. 1983, 14, 215-30.
21. Bradway, D. E.; Shafik, T. M.; Loros, E. M. J. Agr. Food Chem. 1977, 25, 1353-8.
22. Swan, A. A. B. Brit. J. Ind. Med. 1969, 26, 322-9.
23. Gollop, B. R.; Glass, W. I. N. Z. Med. J. 1979, 89, 10-11.
24. Wagner, S. L.; Weswig, P. Arch. Environ. Hlth. 1974, 28, 77-9.
25. Lieban, J.; Waldman, R. K.; Krause, L. Ind Hyg. Occ. Med. 1953, 7, 93-8.
26. Durham, W. F.; Wolfe, H. R.; Elliot, J. W. Arch. Environ. Hlth. 1972, 24, 381-7.
27. Levy, K. A.; Brady, S. S.; Pfaffenberger, C. Bull. Environ. Contam Toxicol. 1981, 27, 235-8.
28. Kolmodin-Hedman, B.; Hoglund, S.; Akerblom, M. Arch. Toxicol. 1983, 54, 257-65.
29. Kutz, F. W.; Strassman, S. C. Mos. News 1977, 37, 211-8.
30. Davies, J. E.; Enos, H. F.; Barquet, A; Morgade, C.; Danauskas, J. X. In "Toxicology and Occupational Medicine"; Deichmann, W. B., Ed.; Elsevier, New York, 1979, Vol. IV; pp 369-80.
31. Cohen, B.; Richler, E.; Weisenberg, E.; Schoenberg, J.; Luria, M. Pestic. Monit. J. 1979, 13, 81-6.
32. Hayes, A. L.; Wise, R. A.; Weir, F. W. Am. Ind. Hyg. J. 1980, 41, 568-75.
33. Wojeck, G. A.; Price, J. F.; Nigg, H. N.; Stamper, J. H. Arch. Environ. Contam. Toxicol. 1983, 12, 65-70.
34. Carman, G. E.; Iwata, Y.; Pappas, J. L.; O'Neal, J. R.; Gunther, F. A. Arch. Environ. Contam. Toxicol. 1982, 11, 651-9.

35. Comer, S. W.; Staiff, D. C.; Armstrong, J. F.; Wolfe, H. R.
     Bull. Environ. Contam. Toxicol. 1975, 13, 385-91.
36. Staiff, D. C.; Comer, S. W.; Armstrong, J. F.; Wolfe, H. R.
     Bull. Environ. Contam. Toxicol. 1975, 14, 334-40.
37. Wojeck, G. A.; Nigg, H. N.; Braman, R. S.; Stamper, J. H.;
     Rouseff, R. L. Arch. Environ. Contom. Toxicol. 1982, 11,
     661-7.
38. Wojeck, G. A.; Nigg, H. N.; Stamper, J. H.; Bradway, D. E.
     Arch. Environ. Contam. Toxicol. 1981, 10, 725-35.
39. Lavy, T. L.; Shepard, J. S.; Mattice, J. D. J. Agr. Food Chem.
     1980, 28, 626-30.
40. Lavy, T. L.; Walstad, J. D.; Flynn, R. R.; Mattice, J. D. J.
     Agr. Food Chem. 1982, 30, 375-81.
41. Winterlin, W. L.; Kilgore, W. W.; Mourer, C. R.; Schoen,
     S. R. J. Agr. Food Chem. 1984, 32, 664-72.
42. Funckes, A. J.; Hayes, G. R.; Hartwell, W. V. J. Agr. Food
     Chem. 1963, 11, 455-7.
43. Kolmodin-Hedman, B.; Hoglund, S.; Swenson, A.; Akerblom, M.
     Arch. Toxicol. 1983, 54, 267-73.
44. Franklin, C. A.; Greenholgh, R.; Maibach, H. I. In "Human
     Welfare and the Environment"; Miyamoto, J., Ed.; Pergamon
     Press: New York, 1983; pp 221-6.
45. Nigg, H. N.; Stamper, J. H. Arch. Environ. Contam. Toxicol.
     1983, 12, 477-82.
46. Dowdy, S.; Weardon, S. In "Statistics for Research"; Wiley,
     New York, 1983; p 196.

RECEIVED November 8, 1984

Exposure of Applicators to Monosodium Methanearsonate and Cacodylic Acid in Forestry

L. A. NORRIS

Department of Forest Science, Oregon State University, Corvallis, OR 97331

Effective worker training and supervision and use of protective gear should minimize exposure of both humans and other animals to MSMA and cacodylic acid, herbicides used in forestry. Arsenic (As) concentration in urine, a useful index to exposure, increased rapidly with an applicator's first exposure, then decreased rapidly when exposure ceased; As concentration reflected the degree of applicator exposure and paralleled levels in small mammals in treated areas. Poor handling and application techniques raised As concentrations in urine as high as 1.8 ppm, corresponding to an exposure of at least 0.036 mg As/kg body weight/day. Proper handling techniques and use of protective gear can reduce exposure to < 0.003 to 0.007 mg As/kg body weight/day, if urine is assumed the sole excretory source.

The organic arsenic-containing herbicides cacodylic acid (dimethylarsinic acid) and MSMA (monosodium methanearsonate) are used to kill selected trees (usually conifers) during precommercial thinning in Pacific Northwest forests. Although felling unwanted trees with saws is an alternative to chemical thinning, it is costly, dangerous to forest workers, increases fire danger because felling concentrates slash on the ground, reduces access of domestic and wild animals to forage, and has an unsightly appearance. Chemically killed trees are left standing; the needles or leaves fall first, then the branches, and eventually the main stem.

Both cacodylic acid and MSMA are registered for this use and are being applied by both private and public forest-management groups in the Pacific Northwest and elsewhere in the United States. Total use figures are difficult to compile, the level varying over time; for example, the USDA Forest Service applied 18,000 lb on 3,558 acres in Fiscal Year 1979 (1), but larger amounts were used in the early 1970's when more funds were being allocated for intensive forest management.

0097–6156/85/0273–0109$06.00/0

Several million acres of young, overstocked stands are at or near the age where precommercial thinning is needed. MSMA in particular, and possibly cacodylic acid, could be important tools for this purpose, but both benefits and risks must be assessed. Particularly at risk are pesticide applicators, who have the greatest, and only substantive, potential for exposure. The purpose of this paper is (1) to review (a) studies of applicator exposure to MSMA and cacodylic acid and (b) strategies for applicator protection and (2) to calculate magnitude of applicator exposure.

Application Methods and Opportunities for Exposure

MSMA and cacodylic acid are injected into the tree cambium by one of three methods:
. Hack and squirt--axe or hatchet used to cut into the stem, usually one cut per inch of diameter, and herbicide applied with a plastic squeeze bottle or pump-type oil can,
. Injection hatchet--specially designed hatchet containing an inertia-driven piston which forces the herbicide concentrate into the cut when the hatchet strikes the tree stem, and
. Injection bar--long tube (containing herbicide) with a narrow bit on the end; the bit is plunged into the cambium at the base of the tree, and a small amount of herbicide enters the cut in the tree through a hole in the bit when the operator opens the valve.

Each method allows opportunity for applicator exposure at three points:
. Transporting and transferring the herbicide concentrate from the manufacturer's container to the application equipment,
. Carrying, using, and repairing the application equipment in the field, and
. Emptying and cleaning application equipment at the end of the work day.

Potential Exposure Indexes

Arsenic (As) has been reported in a variety of tissues, any of which are potentially useful as indexes to exposure. However, the organic pentavalent arsenicals are not accumulated in tissues and are rapidly excreted in urine (2-4). Therefore, urine generally is a particularly valuable index to applicator exposure. Exon et al. (5) reported both urine and feces were important pathways of excretion in rabbits exposed to MSMA in their feed. They found 70% of ingested As had been excreted (54% in urine, 46% in feces) during a 17-week exposure period. Arsenic levels in liver, hair, and urine were the same as in controls after 12 weeks of MSMA exposure followed by 5 weeks of control rations, indicating excretion was ultimately fairly complete.
Hair and blood are possible indexes of applicator exposure. Exon et al. (5) reported As accumulation in hair of rabbits, but about 4 weeks of continuous exposure to MSMA in their feed were required before the concentration was high enough to measure with confidence. Dickinson (6) reported nonsignificant As accumulation

in hair of cattle fed enough MSMA in their diet (10 mg/kg/day for 10 or 12 days) to cause the death of the animals. However, As concentration increased measurably in 10 days in hair of cattle exposed to 10 mg/kg/day of cacodylic acid; the concentration continued to increase with duration of exposure. Arsenic in hair may be a useful index to long-term As exposure, but it does not respond with sufficient speed to be useful in short-term tests or for operational monitoring of workers. Wagner and Weswig (7) found a slight increase in As levels in blood of forest workers applying cacodylic acid, but the increases were quite erratic and were not apparent before the second week of exposure.

Hair is simple to collect and analyze, but arsenic levels in hair do not respond rapidly to exposure. Blood both is difficult to collect and does not give a consistent or rapid enough response to As exposure of an organism. Thus, even with the attendant collection problems, urine is the most practical index to the exposure of forest workers to the organic arsenical herbicides. Unfortunately, the pharmacokinetics of these herbicides have not been fully developed for dermal exposure, and there are indications that urine is not the sole excretory route. Thus, estimates of exposure based only on As excretion in urine may be only 30% of actual exposure levels (5, 8).

Applicator Exposure and Influence of Protective Strategies

The First Study. Forest-applicator exposure to MSMA and cacodylic acid was first studied by Tarrant and Allard (9). They collected individual urine samples on Monday mornings and Friday afternoons for 9 consecutive weeks from five applicators (each using a different combination of application method and chemical) and one control. Workers were supplied with clean clothes daily, including two pair of cotton gloves (to be changed at noon, or earlier if one pair became substantially contaminated with herbicide). Complete data were obtained for weeks 2, 3, 4, 7, and 8 (except for the injection hatchet-cacodylic acid combination, which was not included in the analysis).

Analysis of variance showed that As concentration in urine was significantly higher ($P < 0.05$) than in the control (Table I). Concentration was higher by the end of the first work week, and Friday levels were higher than the succeeding Monday levels, indicating absence from contact over the weekend was sufficient to complete elimination (except in a few cases where Friday levels were substantially higher than average). The Friday concentrations did not increase substantively over the 9 weeks, which also indicates rapid clearance and lack of accumulation. None of the workers experienced illness that seemed associated with the herbicide exposure.

Official standards for As in urine following exposure to these compounds is lacking, other than one manufacturer's recommendation of 0.3 ppm. This standard appears to be based on a study of urinary excretion of arsenic in 163 unexposed individuals, which showed a maximum excretion value of 0.85 mg As/day (10); the 0.3 ppm concentration was selected based on a 3-liter daily void of urine and is therefore quite conservative. In the Tarrant and Allard study (9), 47% of the Friday values were > 0.3 ppm; the maximum value was 2.5 ppm. In contrast, only 4% of the observations (all in the injection hatchet-cacodylic acid treatment group) were > 0.3 ppm on Mondays.

Table I. Mean Concentration (+1 Standard Deviation) of Arsenic in Urine from Forest Workers at 2, 3, 4, 7, and 8 Weeks of a 9-Week Exposure Period (9)

Application Method and Chemical	Total As(mg/1)			
	Monday	% > 0.3 ppm	Friday	% > 0.3 ppm
Control, no exposure	0.04 (+ 0.01)	0	0.07 (+ 0.03)	4
Hack and squirt, MSMA	0.07 (+ 0.01)	0	0.26 (+ 0.05)	32
Hack and squirt, cacodylic acid	0.03 (+ 0.01)	0	0.41 (+ 0.08)	46
Injection hatchet, MSMA	0.10 (+ 0.01)	0	0.50 (+ 0.12)	54
Injection bar, MSMA	0.10 (+ 0.01)	0	0.36 (+ 0.07)	42

Source: Reproduced with permission from Ref. 9. Copyright 1972, American Medical Association.

Follow-up Studies. The results of the Tarrant and Allard study (9), combined with an incident in which several dead snowshoe hares with elevated levels of As (more than 100 ppm in various tissues) were found in a treated area, prompted an intensive effort to further elucidate patterns of applicator exposure and to evaluate means of reducing exposure to humans and other animals.

Investigation of the hare mortality incident revealed that careless handling techniques and poor procedures for disposing of leftover herbicide and clean-up water were the likely sources of As for the hares (the high salt content of the material probably attracted them). In interviews, workers from the Tarrant and Allard study indicated that their cotton gloves in particular and sometimes portions of their clothing became quite wet with herbicide. In addition, their hands contacted the herbicide when the application equipment was being filled with herbicide concentrate or when the application equipment had to be repaired or cleaned. In some cases workers were "splashed" with the herbicide during actual application.

Allard (11) conducted a second round of tests to determine how As levels in urine could be reduced through worker training and improved protection. In this test, applicators wore goggles, used an impervious face cream, and were instructed in better techniques for handling of both herbicide concentrate and application equipment. In addition, two groups used rubber gloves instead of cotton gloves.

Arsenic levels in urine were substantially reduced in all crews but the Kaniksu (Table II). It was concluded from periodic observations and interviews of crew members and foremen that impervious gloves, skin cream, and effective training and supervision were the key factors. The foreman and the trainer of the Colville crew had been particularly effective; As level in urine for that crew, which wore only cotton gloves, was similar to that of one crew wearing rubber gloves, and the number of observations > 0.3 ppm was only 1/3 that of a similar crew in the same area the previous year (Table I).

Table II. Mean Concentration of Arsenic in Urine from Forest Workers Applying MSMA or Cacodylic Acid via the Hack and Squirt Method in Operational Precommercial Tree Thinning (11)

	Total As (ppm)[1]					
	Monday			Friday		
Crew	Mean	Max.	% > 0.3 ppm	Mean	Max.	% > 0.3 ppm
MSMA						
Colville	0.05	0.37	8	0.15	0.46	11
Okanogan	0.07	0.50	9	0.24	1.30	33
Wenatchee	0.03	0.14	0	0.07	0.35	7
Cedar Creek	0.04	0.09	0	0.02	0.03	0
Naselle[2]	0.04	0.20	0	0.14	0.54	14
Cacodylic Acid						
Kaniksu	0.01	0.02	0	0.80	1.80	75

1 Controls averaged 0.02 ppm.
2 Crews used rubber gloves instead of cotton gloves.

Wagner and Weswig (7) implemented the best of all these procedures in monitoring an operational thinning program a year later. The crew consisted of five college students and a full-time supervisor who were carefully trained in proper procedures for handling the herbicide (cacodylic acid) and the hack and squirt method. All were impressed with the importance of minimizing personal exposure and based on their performance, seemed to have approached the study as something of a personal crusade.

Wagner and Weswig collected 24-hour urine samples from each worker beginning late Thursday afternoon and continuing until the end of the work day on Friday, when blood samples were collected and analyzed (Table III). At no time during the exposure period of 7 weeks (5 work days/week) did As concentration in urine exceed 0.2 ppm. Arsenic excretion increased once exposure began, reaching the average level during the second week of exposure, but fell rapidly when exposure ended, reinforcing the results from the animal

Table III. Mean Concentration in Blood and Excretion in Urine of
Arsenic from Five Forest Workers Exposed to Cacodylic Acid and
Five Controls (7)

Week[1]	Workers	
	Exposed	Controls
	Arsenic in blood (ppm)	
1	0.05	0.05
2	0.17	--
3	0.26	--
4	0.19	--
5	0.06	--
6	0.06	0.06
7	0.03	--
8	0.03	--
9	0.04	--
10	0.01	--
11	0.02	0.02
	Arsenic in urine (mg/24 h)	
1	0.038	---
2	0.077	0.073
3	0.141	---
4	0.172	---
5	0.106	---
6	0.103	0.042
7	0.169	---
8	0.204	---
9	0.024	---
10	0.068	---
11	---	0.026

[1] Week 1 was a pre-exposure period; weeks 2 through 8 were full
5-day work weeks, although work records indicate application
accounted for only 23.7 hours of each 40-hour work week, and each
worker applied an average of 817 g dimethylarsinic acid/week; week
9 included only 10 hours of exposure, which occurred during the
first 2 days of the week; weeks 10 and 11 were post-exposure
periods.

Source: Reproduced with permission from Ref. 7. Copyright 1974,
American Medical Association.

feeding studies (5). Though As level in blood initially increased, it decreased to control levels in 4 weeks and correlated poorly (correlation coefficient = 0.14) with As excretion in urine. On the basis of 70 kg body weight and the assumptions that (1) excretion level measured at the end of the week is representative of the daily rate and (2) urine is the principal route of excretion, these workers were exposed to an average of 0.002 mg As/kg body weight/day.

Monitoring Operational Projects

Seven operational application units were monitored on the basis of information from the previous tests in an effort to minimize applicator exposure (11). Operational monitoring involved six individual application crews of from five to ten applicators; one crew treated two units. All crews used the hack and squirt method, but some applied cacodylic acid and others MSMA. The time required to complete a unit varied from 1 to 3 months, but not all crews were involved with chemical thinning each day.

Each crew and foreman were briefed on results of previous studies, and the importance of minimizing personal exposure was emphasized. Guidelines on application equipment, protective gear, and methods of handling and applying the herbicide to minimize exposure were presented. Type and density of vegetation, roughness of terrain, and climatic factors varied such that the method and protective equipment best suited to each circumstance were implemented; no effort to "standardize" was made, emphasizing the operational nature of the tests. Single urine samples were collected from each applicator in each unit near the end of the work day on Friday; a similar sample was collected every third Monday, before the work day began. Of the seven units monitored, five were highly successful (no As levels > 0.3 ppm), one was fairly successful, and one (Kaniksu 1) was a failure (Table IV).

Table IV. Mean Concentration of Arsenic in Urine from Forest Workers in Seven Application Units Thinned with MSMA or Cacodylic Acid by the Hack and Squirt Method (12)

| Application Unit | Total As (ppm) | | | | | |
| | Monday | | | Friday | | |
	Mean	Max.	%> 0.3 ppm	Mean	Max.	% > 0.3 ppm
Colville 1	0.06	0.21	0	0.10	0.34	4
Colville 2	0.04	0.21	0	0.06	0.32	2
Colville 3	0.03	0.11	0	0.05	0.13	0
Siuslaw 1	0.03	0.05	0	0.09	0.19	0
Naselle 1	0.03	0.08	0	0.09	0.49	5
Cedar Creek 1	0.06	0.13	0	0.08	0.52	10
Kaniksu 1	0.26	0.50	33	0.38	1.74	45

The pattern of arsenic in urine from the Kaniksu 1 crew is quite
interesting (Table V). Mean As concentration increased immediately,
the number of observations > 0.3 ppm exceeding 50%. As soon as
these results were available, the crew foreman and supervisor were
notified, and they intensified efforts to reduce exposure. They
were partially successful for about 2 weeks (17% of observations
> 0.3 ppm); then the average and maximum concentrations began to
rise. Late in July, 83% were > 0.3 ppm, and thinning was stopped to
prevent futher applicator exposure. During the next 3 weeks, As
concentration in urine dropped. After 2 succeeding weeks when the
average and maximum concentrations were in the normal range (0.02 to
0.03 ppm), the crew returned to thinning for 5 days. All urine
samples collected at the end of that period exceeded 0.03 ppm As;
they averaged 0.85 ppm, and maximum was 1.74 ppm.

Table V. Mean Concentration of Arsenic in Urine from Kaniksu 1
Application Crew (12)

| Date | Day | Total As (ppm) | | Crew Size | % > 0.3 ppm |
		Mean	Range		
June					
15	Tue.	0.08	0.02-0.20	5	0
18	Fri.	0.31	0.08-0.42	5	60
25	Fri.	0.20	0.04-0.33	5	20
July					
2	Fri.	0.21	0.05-0.33	6	33
6	Tue.	0.17	0.03-0.48	6	17
9	Fri.	0.15	0.07-0.37	6	17
16	Fri.	0.29	0.05-0.68	6	33
23	Fri.	0.72	0.19-1.32	6	67
26	Mon.	0.53	0.11-1.01	6	83
30	Fri.	0.49	0.10-1.38	6	50
August					
2	Chemical thinning suspended				
6	Fri.	0.17	0.13-0.36	6	17
13	Fri.	0.02	0.02-0.03	6	0
20	Fri.	0.02	0.01-0.03	5	0
23	Thinning resumed				
27	Fri.	0.85	0.32-1.74	3	100
	(Last day of thinning)				

The daily diary of the Kaniksu 1 foreman noted numerous
occasions when applicators received considerable exposure as a
result of poor handling practices and use of inappropriate gear.
Coincident with applicator monitoring, however, small mammals
(usually mice) were trapped in these seven units and analyzed for
arsenic. Interestingly (though the details are beyond the scope of

this paper), there was a strong relationship between As concentration in small mammals and that in applicator urine (Table VI)--which leads me to believe that care in application is a predominant factor influencing small animal as well as human exposure. Thus, monitoring applicator urine for As may be useful as an index to both applicator and animal exposure.

As Concentration in Urine Related to 24-Hour Excretion in Urine

Wagner and Weswig (7) recommended 24-hour As excretion in urine as the best measure of applicator exposure. Though useful in experimental work, this measure is impractical as an operational monitoring tool: the likelihood of workers successfully collecting uncontaminated 24-hour urine samples on a routine basis seems low. The best monitoring tool is the one which "will be used" and which gives a reasonably good index to exposure.

Table VI. Mean Concentration of Arsenic in Whole Bodies of Small Mammals and in Urine from Applicators (12)

Arsenic in Applicator Urine		Arsenic in Small-Mammal Whole Bodies			
Application Units[1]	% Friday Observations > 0.03 ppm	% Observations			
		< 0.5 ppm	> 1 ppm	> 3 ppm	> 5 ppm
Colville 1	4	54	9	2	0
Colville 2	2	72	9	0	0
Colville 3	0	38	37	9	0
Siuslaw 1	0	83	0	0	0
Kaniksu 1	45	20	50	25	15

[1] No data for Naselle or Cedar Creek units.

Norris (13) conducted a study to determine the relationship, if any, between As concentration in a single (small) urine sample and As excretion in urine over a 24-hour period. In this study, 17 workers applied MSMA by the hack and squirt method. On the designated collection day, each crew member received one large and one small container; all urine excreted during the 24-hour period was collected in the large container except that excreted at the end of the work day, which was collected in the small container. The paired samples (one large and one small) constituted a sample set. The number of sample sets from any one individual ranged from one to nine (average 3.3); in total, 56 sample sets were collected. The volume of both samples in a set was measured and urine analyzed for total As, creatinine, and osmolality.

Multiple regression analysis of data showed that the independent variables (urine volume, As concentration, mg% creatinine, and osmolality) accounted for 76% of the variation in the dependent variable (ug As excreted in 24 hours). Adding independent variables

stepwise, in order of their importance, showed that:
. Arsenic concentration in the small sample accounted for 73.4%
of the variation,
. Urine volume and As concentration in the small sample
accounted for 75.9% of the variation, and
. The other independent variables did not significantly improve
the model.
Thus, two types of data, easily collected, could be used to predict
applicator exposure with reasonable accuracy in operational
monitoring programs, according to the relationship:

$$Y = 12.88 + 1386 (X_1) + 0.14 (X_2); r^2 = 0.76$$

where:
Y = ug As excreted in 24 hours,
X_1 = ppm As in a single urine sample collected at the end of
the work day, and
X_2 = ml urine in the sample.

In this study, the average As concentration was 0.075 ppm
(maximum 0.28 ppm), and the average amount of As excreted 126 ug/24
hours (maximum 323 ug/24 hours). On the basis of 70 kg body weight,
these workers were exposed to an average of 0.002 (maximum of
0.005) mg As/kg body weight/day. Similar values were reported by
Wagner and Weswig (7).

Calculating Applicator Exposure

With the possible exception of Wagner and Weswig (7) and Norris
(13), none of the studies on applicator exposure gives more than an
index to exposure, based on rising and falling As concentration in
single urine samples. Unfortunately (for this purpose), both Wagner
and Weswig (7) and Norris (13) examined situations where applicator
exposure was quite low. However, exposure can be calculated using
the several other data sets in this paper and the following
assumptions:
. All arsenic absorbed is excreted in urine--The validity of
this assumption needs testing; for instance, possible As
excretion in perspiration has not been addressed. If this
assumption is not valid, calculated exposure levels will be two
to three times lower than actual (5, 8).
. mg As excreted/day = 12.88 + 1386(ppm As in single urine
sample) + 0.14(ml urine in single sample)--The validity of this
assumption depends on the degree to which the Norris (13)
relationship is accurate at higher levels of arsenic exposure.
. The average volume of urine voided in a single sample is
373 ml--based on the average reported by Norris (13).
. The body weight of the average forest worker is 70 kg.
Using the data in Tables I-IV and these assumptions, I have
calculated the mean and maximum applicator exposure for each data
set in this paper (Table VII). The overall average was 0.005 mg
As/kg body weight/day, the highest individual maximum 0.036 mg As/kg
body weight/day. If urine is not the sole excretory source of As,
the overall average could be 0.015 mg As/kg body weight/day and the
highest individual maximum 0.018 mg As/kg body weight/day.

Table VII. Exposure of Forest Workers to MSMA or Cacodylic Acid:
Summary of Data Sets Presented in Prior Tables

Crew[2]	Total As in Urine, Friday (ppm)			Calculated As Exposure (mg/kg/day)[1]	
	Mean	Max.	% > 0.3 ppm	Mean	Max.
Table I					
A	0.26	0.36	32	0.006	0.008
B	0.41	0.51	46	0.009	0.011
C	0.50	0.93	54	0.011	0.019
D	0.36	0.58	42	0.008	0.012
Table II					
E	0.15	0.46	11	0.004	0.010
F	0.24	1.30	33	0.006	0.027
G	0.07	0.35	7	0.002	0.008
H	0.02	0.03	0	0.001	0.001
I	0.14	0.54	14	0.004	0.012
J	0.80	1.80	75	0.017	0.036
Table IV					
K	0.10	0.34	4	0.003	0.008
L	0.06	0.32	2	0.002	0.007
M	0.05	0.13	0	0.002	0.004
N	0.09	0.19	0	0.003	0.005
O	0.09	0.49	5	0.003	0.011
P	0.08	0.52	10	0.003	0.011
Q	0.38	1.74	45	0.008	0.035
			Average	0.005	0.013
			Maximum	0.017	0.036

[1] Based on the four assumptions proposed in the text: (a) all
arsenic excreted in urine; (b) mg As excreted/day = 12.88 + 1386 (ppm
As in urine) + 0.14 (ml urine excreted in one sample), see 13; (c)
373 ml urine excreted in one sample, see 13; (d) 70 kg body weight.
Upper case letters represent entries, in order, from Tables I-IV.

[2] Upper case letters represent entries for exposed workers, in order,
from Tables I, II, and IV.

Conclusions

The concentration of total arsenic in urine increases and
decreases rapidly with initiation and termination of applicator
exposure; levels in urine usually are near normal by the Monday
morning following a full week of chemical thinning. Moreover, As
level of exposed applicators seems to parallel that in small mammals
in treated areas. The use of impervious gloves, long-sleeved
shirts, and silicon face cream, combined with effective training and
supervision, markedly reduces urine arsenic levels. Thus, a urine
monitoring program can give a good index to exposure of humans and
other animals during operational thinning. Even single urine
samples can be used to project daily As excretion, facilitating
monitoring and calculation of applicator exposure.

Several monitoring efforts suggest that forest workers applying
MSMA and cacodylic acid may be exposed to As levels as high as
0.036 mg/kg (average 0.005 mg/kg), although the actual level varies
with the worker and the protective measures employed. However,
these levels likely are underestimates because urine may not be the
only source of excretion.

Nontechnical Summary

MSMA and cacodylic acid herbicides are used to thin overstocked
forest stands. Although these arsenic containing herbicides are
injected into the tree stem, applicators may still be exposed during
the handling, application and clean-up stages of operation. The
amount of arsenic in urine is a good indicator of applicator
exposure. The first tests conducted during operational thinning
programs showed the levels of applicator exposure were higher than
advised, and there appeared to be a correlation between the levels
of arsenic in urine from applicators and the whole body levels of
arsenic in small animals. This suggests that minimizing applicator
exposure will also reduce exposure to small mammals. Later tests
showed effective worker training and supervision, and the use of
protective gear are effective in this regard. Monitoring arsenic in
applicator urine is useful for determining if exposure goals are
being achieved during operational forest thinning with MSMA and
cacodylic acid herbicides.

Acknowledgments

This research is supported in part by USDA Forest Service, Pacific
Northwest Forest and Range Experiment Station, PNW 84-359.

Literature Cited

1. "Pesticide-use Advisory Memorandum 246," USDA Forest Service,
   1980.
2. Schroeder, H. A.; Balassa, J. J. J. Chronic Dis. 1966, 19,
   85-106.
3. Hogan, R. B.; Eagle, H. J. Pharmacol. Exp. Ther. 1944, 80,
   93-113.

4. Frost, D. V. Fed. Proc. Fed. Am. Soc. Exp. Biol. 1967, 26, 194-208.
5. Exon, J. H.; Harr, J. R.; Claeys, R. R. Nutr. Rep. Int. 1974, 9, 351-7.
6. Dickinson, J. O. Am. J. Vet. Res. 1972, 33, 1889-92.
7. Wagner, S. L.; Weswig, P. Arch. Environ. Health 1974, 28, 77-9.
8. Dutkiewicz, T. Environ. Health Persp. 1977, 19, 173-7.
9. Tarrant, R. F.; Allard, J. Arch. Environ. Health 1972; 24, 277-80.
10. Mattice, M. R.; Weisman, D. Amer. J. Med. Sci. 1937; 193, 413-20.
11. Allard, J., In "The Behavior and Impact of Organic Arsenical Herbicides in the Forest: Final Report of Cooperative Studies"; USDA Forest Service, Pacific Northwest Forest and Range Experiment Station, Portland, Oreg., 1974; pp. 4-8.
12. Norris, L. A., In "The Behavior and Impact of Organic Arsenical Herbicides in the Forest: Final Report of Cooperative Studies"; USDA Forest Service, Pacific Northwest Forest and Range Experiment Station, Portland, Oreg., 1974; pp. 75-89.
13. Norris, L.A., In "The Behavior and Impact of Organic Arsenical Herbicides in the Forest: Final Report of Cooperative Studies"; USDA Forest Service, Pacific Northwest Forest and Range Experiment Station, Portland, Oreg., 1974; pp. 10-17.

RECEIVED December 3, 1984

Exposure of Strawberry Harvesters to Carbaryl

GUNTER ZWEIG[1], RU-YU GAO[2], JAMES M. WITT[3], WILLIAM J. POPENDORF[4], and K. T. BOGEN

School of Public Health and Sanitary Engineering Health Research Laboratory, University of California, Berkeley, CA 94720

A group of strawberry harvesters was monitored for dermal exposure to the insecticide carbaryl during finite periods in the morning and afternoon of three consecutive days. Dermal exposures were estimated by the use of cotton gloves and patches for hands and body, respectively. The results from this study showed that dermal exposure in the morning was higher than afternoon; that younger and smaller subjects exhibited lower dermal dose rates, and that most workers showed ambidextrous behavior during picking of fruit. The ratios of dermal exposure rate/dislodgeable foliar residues were similar to those found in studies involving other crops and pesticides.

Background

Dermal exposure to captan and benomyl by strawberry harvesters has been the subject of several previous studies (1,2,3). This field study was designed to test a number of hypotheses and the reproducibility of dermal exposure rate measurements taken under field conditions. Most of our past studies have not been designed for a particular pesticide but were modified to accommodate the pesticide chosen by the grower to control a certain pest. In this case, the pesticide was carbaryl (1-naphthyl N-methylcarbamate) an insecticide used to control the spittlebug and leafroller. Our results could then be compared with those obtained by Maitlen and co-workers (4) who studied workers exposed to carbaryl in an apple orchard. Furthermore, attempts will be made to test possible positive correlations between age and dermal dose rate versus productivity and dermal dose rate versus age of harvesters. Difference of dermal exposure due to age or

[1]Current address: Office of Pesticide Programs, Environmental Protection Agency, Washington, DC 20460
[2]Current address: Nankai University, Tjanjin, People's Republic of China
[3]Current address: Department of Agricultural Chemistry, Oregon State University, Corvallis, OR 97331
[4]Current address: Agricultural Medical Research Facility, University of Iowa, Iowa City, IA 52242

gender will be tested. By measuring dislodgeable carbaryl residues on strawberry foliage, ratios of dermal dose rates and dislodgeable residues could be determined and compared with those from previous studies on other crops and pesticides.

Experimental Details

Description of Field Study. The study was conducted on a privately owned strawberry farm near Corvallis, Oregon during three consecutive days in June, 1982. The field had been sprayed with 2 lbs a.i./A of carbaryl 15 days prior to the first day of the study. Eighteen strawberry harvesters volunteered to participate in the study; their personal characteristics and work efficiency are listed in Table I.

Table I. Physical Characteristics and Productivity of Strawberry Harvesters

ID	Sex	Age	Weight kg	Height cm	Surface Area m^2	Daily Prod. cr/hr
6	F	40	69.5	168	1.77	1.04
7	F	12	42.3	163	1.52	0.68
8	F	18	63.6	175	1.78	0.91
9	F	29	56.7	164	1.58	0.99
10	F	13	43.1	149	1.35	0.78
11	F	32	61.3	175	1.72	1.00
12	F	15	59.0	160	1.62	1.00
13	F	16	50.4	173	1.56	0.72
14	M	13	63.6	178	1.76	0.97
15	M	13	70.4	168	1.78	0.57
17	F	12	45.4	157	1.42	0.74
18	F	12	49.9	163	1.52	0.60
20	M	14	56.7	180	1.70	1.04
21	F	14	54.5	165	1.59	0.60
22	F	37	49.9	152	1.46	0.89
23	F	16	49.9	165	1.53	0.96
25	M	12	45.4	160	1.43	0.70
26	M	15	63.6	183	1.84	0.72
					MEAN	0.83

Source: Reproduced from Ref. 17. Copyright 1983, American Chemical Society.

Dermal exposure rates of carbaryl were measured on the workers by
having them wear light cotton gloves (hand exposure) and cotton patch
monitors fastened to their lower legs and forearms. Details for these
monitoring devices may be found in a recent publication (3). Gloves
were kept on for 1-2 h during the morning observation period and were
exchanged for a new set of gloves in the afternoon. Patches were worn
during the entire daily work period. The procedure for hand
monitoring was changed slightly on Day-2 by placing the gloves on the
workers´ hands about two hours after the morning harvest had begun.
The reasons for this change will be explained in a later section.

Dislodgeable foliar residues from strawberry plants were obtained
by collecting 48 circular leaf punches on a random basis, starting
with the first day post-application of carbaryl, finishing on the
last day of the study (Day-17 post-application). A description of the
mechanical leaf punch and the collection technique may be found
elsewhere (1).

Weather data for the three days of the study were recorded as
shown in Table II.

Sample Extraction. Gloves and cotton patches were surface-extracted
with acetonitrile, and the extracts were filtered through 0.22u
MILLIPORE filters. Appropriate aliquots were directly analyzed by
High Performance Liquid Chromatography (HPLC) without further cleanup
or concentration, as will be described below.

Dislodgeable foliar pesticide residues and leaf dust were
isolated by methods described in the published literature (5,6,7,8).
Basically the method for the extraction of dislodgeable carbaryl

Table II.   Meteorological Data at Corvallis Strawberry Farm During
Carbaryl Monitoring Study

| | Date of Observation | | | | | |
| | June 22, 1982 | | June 23 | | June 24 | |
Type of Measurement	AM	PM	AM	PM	AM	PM
Temperature (°C)	12-21	26	16-22	27	17-26	32
Wind Speed (km/hr)	3.07		3.73		5.76	
Precipitation	0		0		0	
Humidity (%relative)	65-100	50	70	60	90	50

residues involved surface extraction with a dilute aqueous solution
of a surfactant (SURTEN), followed by transfer of the residue into
dichloromethane, and a final solution in acetonitrile. Aliquots of
the final extract were analyzed by HPLC.

Leaf dust was originally washed off during surface-extraction of
leaf disks and remained at the interfacial solvent-water layer in the
separatory funnel during the first water-solvent transfer. This
could be quantitatively transferred to a pre-weighed glass filter.
After drying at 110° overnight, the filter was weighed and the dust
calculated by difference.

Analytical Methods. The analytical method for carbaryl and 1-naphthol
by high performance liquid chromatography (HPLC) was recently
described for aqueous samples (9). Similarly, these two compounds
were analyzed in these studies using a Waters 6000A Solvent Delivery
System, WISP Automatic Sample Processor, Data Module and Automatic
Integrator, and Model 4530 Variable Wave Length Detector, set at 230
nm. A Water uBondapak C_{18} reverse-phase column (25 cm x 2 mm i.d.)
was employed. The following experimental conditions were maintained:

      mobile phase: acetonitrile-water (40:60)
      flow rate: 2 mL/min

Under these conditions, carbaryl and 1-naphthol have retention times
of 4.6 and 5.1 min, respectively. Sensitivity is 2 ng for each
compound.

Recovery studies for patches and SURTEN solutions were carried
out by the addition of known amounts of carbaryl and 1-naphthol and
ranged from 85-107% (see Table III).

For routine analyses, the experimental conditions were modified
as follows:
      mobile phase: acetonitrile-water (50:50)
      flow rate: 1.3 ml/min

Under these conditions, carbaryl and 1-naphthol are not resolved
(retention time 5.85 min; see Figure 1). Henceforth, all results will
be reported as carbaryl concentrations.

Estimation of Dermal Exposure. Hand exposure rates, expressed in
mg/h, were calculated from the concentration of carbaryl found in the
glove monitors, divided by the hours that the gloves were worn. To
calculate daily exposure rates, morning and afternoon values were
time-weighted averages. To determine dermal exposure rates for
anatomical regions other than hands, the concentration found on the
patch monitors was extrapolated by the method of Popendorf and
Leffingwell (10) using the 50-percentile man for body surface and a
nomograph (11) relating body weight and height to surface.

Statistical Analysis. T-tests, Kruskall-Wallis and analyses of
variances were performed using SAS, a statistical computer software
program developed by Statistical Analysis Systems, Inc.

Table III. Recovery Studies for Carbaryl and 1-Naphthol

Compound	Sample No.	Amount added	found	Per cent Recovery
		ug		
Carbaryl	Patch-1	69.0	63.9	92.6
	Patch-2	69.0	64.8	93.9
	Patch-3	172.5	184.2	106.7
	Patch-4	172.5	180.0	104.3
	SURTEN #1	828.0	703.2	84.9
	SURTEN #2	828.0	805.2	97.3
	SURTEN #3	828.0	706.7	85.3
	Leaf punch	0	2.0	n/a
1-Naphthol	Patch-3-1	76.0	77.2	101.5
	Patch-3-2	152.4	153.1	106.5
	Patch-3-3	152.4	150.7	98.9

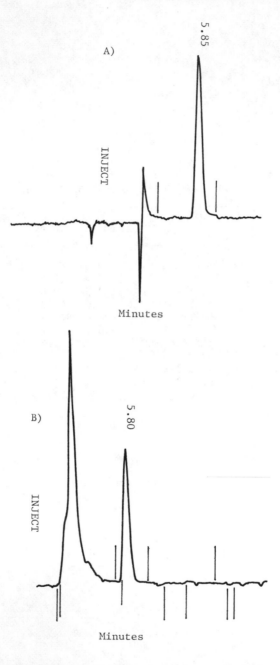

Figure 1.   Analysis of carbaryl by high performance liquid chromatography. (A) standard (137.5 ng of carbaryl); (B) glove extract. Retention time for carbaryl under experimental conditions found in text is 5.80–5.85 min.

Results and Discussion

Dermal Exposure. It has been previously shown that dermal exposure to pesticides by strawberry pickers occurred mainly on hands, forearms and lower legs (1). It was, therefore, decided to monitor these three anatomical regions initially and estimate total dermal exposure. However, in the present study it was discovered that lower leg exposures amounted to less than 4% of total exposure, based on the three anatomical sites. The exception was Worker No. 13 whose lower leg exposure exceeded this value on Day-1 (18%). This high exposure value was discounted as being due to a possible accidental contamination from heavy dew deposits in the early morning hours and Worker No. 13 having come into contact with wet foliage (see discussion on the possible effect of dew on glove monitors). For these reasons alone, exposure values from hands and lower arms were considered.

Table IV is a summary of dermal exposure rates of all workers for three days of observation. The apparently higher exposure rates on the first day are supported by statistics demonstrating that the daily means differ significantly for the three days. It is possible that the heavy dew in the early morning hours of Day-1 (see also Table II for relative humidity) may have affected the absorptivity of gloves used as monitors. Once gloves become wet, they might no longer function as linear monitors over time. Thus, our initial experimental protocol was changed on Day-2 so that gloves were first placed on the subjects 2 h after they entered the field instead of providing them with gloves at the beginning of the morning shift. By that time, most of the dew had dried on the leaves.

Contrary to our expectations about the possible effect of moisture on gloves, Day-1-gloves exhibited higher carbaryl concentrations than on Day-2 and Day-3 (see Table IV). Dose rates for hands on Day-1 and Day-3 were significantly higher in the morning than afternoon. No such differences were observed on Day-2 when gloves worn during the morning and afternoon periods remained relatively dry.

To find an explanation for these results one might reason that wet gloves may possess a larger absorptive capacity for pesticides derived from dislodgeable residues than dry gloves. This might be due to partitioning of pesticides between dislodgeable foliar dust and the aqueous phase of the wet glove. The dew may provide a more efficient contact surface between foliage and glove and create more favorable conditions for the transfer of pesticides. This mechanism differs from that observed in tree crops where dermal body exposure is measured by the use of cotton patches and gloves, and where moisture plays little or no role in monitoring (10).

Recently, two independent studies have indicated that dermal exposure determined from glove monitors may yield higher values than those obtained from hand rinses (12,13). The first investigation (12) was conducted in parallel with the present study and involved three strawberry harvesters exposed to carbaryl. Eliminating the possibility of preferential handedness in harvesting (see below), it was possible to study glove monitors and hand rinses on the same person by monitoring his left and right hands simultaneously. Gloves gave consistently much higher exposure rates if worn for a relatively

Table IV.   Dermal Mean Exposure Rates of Carbaryl of Strawberry
            Harvesters

Anatomical Region	Day of Study			
	Day-1	Day-2	Day-3	Means
	mg/hr			
Both hands, AM	3.01(1.70)	1.23(0.62)	1.47(0.82)	1.90(1.38)
Both hands, PM[1]	1.42(0.80)	1.12(0.73)	0.72(0.38)	1.09(0.71)
Left hand,AM+PM[1]	1.09(0.59)	0.69(0.36)	0.51(0.25)	0.76(0.48)
Right hand,AM+PM[1]	0.90(0.39)	0.51(0.28)	0.51(0.28)	0.64(0.37)
Both hands, AM+PM[1]	1.99(0.92)	1.20(0.54)	1.02(0.47)	1.40(0.78)
Lower arms	0.66(0.41)	0.41(0.27)	0.43(0.30)	0.50(0.35)
Total	2.65(1.14)	1.55(0.61)	1.45(0.69)	1.89(1.00)

( )=standard deviation
[1] Exposure values are time-weighted averages for hours monitored.

Source: Reprinted from Ref. 17.   Copyright 1983, American Chemical
Society.

short time, e.g. less than 1.5 h. When the monitoring time was increased to 3 h, the exposure rates, although still higher , were less divergent than values estimated from hand washes.

In the second study (13), apple thinners were monitored for azinphosmethyl exposure by the use of cotton and nylon gloves or hand rinses with ethanol. Both types of gloves gave higher exposure rates than hand rinses.

Hand rinses will not account for dermal absorption and may thus lead to lower exposure values. On the other hand, glove monitors which have not become moisture-saturated may keep dermal absorption at a minimum by acting as a physical barrier but may still overestimate exposure. Further research is needed to determine which of these monitoring techniques are capable of measuring actual dermal exposure to pesticides.

Comparison of Dermal Exposure With Age and Physical Characteristics. One of the goals of this study was to determine if the age of strawberry harvesters affected dermal exposure to pesticides. The 18 pickers of this study were divided into two groups according to age, youths ($\leq$14 years of age) and adults ($\geq$15 years of age). Other classifications were body weight (< and >50 kg), height (< and >165 cm), and body surface (< and > 1.50 m^2).

Comparing the two age groups, as shown in Table V, right-hand exposure rates of youths was lower than corresponding values for adults. No other significant age related differences were found.

Table V. Dermal Hand Exposure According to Age and Body Weight of Strawberry Harvesters

Variable	Type	N	Exposure mg/h	Kruskall-Wallis x^2	p
Youths	Right hand (means, 3 days)	21	0.54		
				4.94	0.026
Adults		33	0.74		
<50 kg	Left+right,PM (means, 3 days)	21	0.80		
				5.87	0.015
>50 kg		33	1.27		
<50 kg	Left+right,PM	7	0.88	t~3.10	
>50 kg	(Day-1)	11	1.76	df~14.4	
				p= 0.0076	

Source: Reproduced from Ref. 17. Copyright 1983, American Chemical Society.

When the workers were grouped according to physical characteristics, it was found that subjects weighing less than 50 kg showed less hand exposure in the afternoon than adults. No such differences were found when the group was divided according to height and body surface.

Left versus Right-Hand Exposure. Table VI is a detailed compilation of left- and right hand dermal exposure by subject, day, and observation periods. There are six observation periods for each of 18 subjects. In a previous study involving captan and benomyl exposures (3), there were indications that dermal hand exposure measurements might be convenient indicators for assessing left-or right-handed preference by individual strawberry harvesters. The present and more

Table VI. Left- and Right-Hand Exposure Rates of Carbaryl (mg/h)

ID	Day-1 AM		Day-1 PM		Day-2 AM		Day-2 PM		Day 3 AM		Day 3 PM	
	Left	Right	Left	Right	Left	Right	Left	Right	Left	Right	Left	right
6	1.49	0.99	1.01	0.99	0.98	0.83	0.52	0.38	1.09	1.25	0.42	0.59
7	3.82	0.81	0.26	0.48	0.12	0.14	0.09	0.10	0.49	0.69	0.46	0.63
8	1.00	1.22	0.19	0.16	0.21	0.16	0.54	0.42	1.09	1.10	0.39	0.33
9	1.38	1.69	1.52	1.20	0.68	0.82	1.15	1.37	0.16	0.14	0.24	0.25
10	0.39	0.18	0.34	0.51	0.83	0.53	0.65	0.35	1.41	1.15	0.32	0.14
11	0.42	0.60	0.57	0.56	0.19	0.12	0.55	0.86	1.08	0.63	0.29	1.52
12	1.36	0.86	0.59	0.51	1.03	0.78	0.67	0.47	0.71	0.81	0.27	0.27
13	4.12	0.84	1.07	2.10	1.12	0.54	0.97	0.53	0.45	0.20	0.39	0.26
14	0.99	0.83	0.58	1.08	1.07	0.74	1.30	0.13	0.80	0.59	0.33	0.74
15	2.35	1.91	1.37	0.56	0.69	0.78	0.10	0.08	0.29	0.56	0.20	0.18
17	0.76	1.50	0.71	0.57	0.74	0.80	0.16	0.14	0.28	0.59	0.20	0.27
18	0.36	0.44	0.05	0.27	0.47	0.23	0.27	0.51	0.81	0.30	0.11	0.14
20	0.81	1.09	0.46	0.49	1.96	0.29	0.27	1.83	0.56	0.59	0.26	0.28
21	1.74	2.18	1.15	1.25	0.37	0.61	0.27	0.00	2.03	0.21	0.20	0.80
22	3.80	3.20	0.60	0.50	0.20	0.15	0.98	0.91	1.22	1.88	0.70	0.20
23	2.36	2.52	0.33	0.32	0.84	0.89	0.10	0.13	0.46	1.86	0.19	0.22
25	1.57	0.69	0.89	0.34	1.26	0.12	1.78	0.38	0.24	0.16	0.30	0.10
26	2.26	1.61	0.75	1.18	0.57	0.34	0.77	0.48	0.47	0.15	0.36	0.35

detailed study made it possible to apply paired Student t-Test to the data in Table VI. This analysis revealed that only Worker #25 appeared to have a left-handed preference during picking (p< 0.05), while the dermal hand exposure for the rest of the group was not different for either hand. During a pre-study interview of the subjects, Workers #17 and 18 were the only ones who expressed a left-handed preference for manual activities. More detailed studies are required to verify if the technique of dermal hand exposure is suitable for making anthropometric determinations of work habits of fruit harvesters.

A curious correlation between left arm dermal exposure rates and body height was observed (r=-0.404; N=53; p<0.01). The significance of this finding is outside the scope of this study.

Worker Exposure Variability. One of the objectives of this study was to examine the variability of dermal exposure rates and the effects, if any, of external factors on these rates. To determine the significance of individually consistent behavioral patterns having a possible influence on individual exposures, an analysis of variance (ANOVA) was performed on the data in Table VI and the results are shown in Table VII. It is apparent from this analysis that the day

Table VII. Analysis of Variance of Dermal Exposure Incorporating "Day" and "Individual" as Categorical Predictors

Variables	F Value	Degrees of Freedom	p
		"Day"	
Hands (AM)	12.70	2,51	0.0001
Hands (PM)	5.06	2,51	0.01
Hands (all day)	10.60	2,51	0.0001
Total dermal exposure	10.88	2,50	0.0001
		"Individual"	
Hands (AM)	0.922	17,34	>0.05
Hands (PM)	1.415	17,34	>0.05
Hands (all day)	0.802	17,34	>0.05
Total dermal exposure	0.805	17,33	>0.05

and time periods of observation are highly significant predictors for exposure variables, and that factors associated with individual identity do not significantly influence dermal hand exposure rates. Thus, there seems to be greater variability between days and time of day for any individual than between individuals on any given day. These results support the hypothesis that moisture arising from morning dew appears to have an effect on the absorptivity of gloves used as hand monitors.

Productivity Correlations. Productivity expressed as crates harvested/h of each worker (see Table I) for day and time are not significantly different over the three-day course of the study (Kruskall-Wallis X^2=0.63-4.18; df=2; p>0.10). When examining youths and adults (see definition above), it could be shown that the daily productivity of youths was lower than that of the adult group (0.72 cr/h versus 0.89 cr/h) (F=11.56; df=1,48; p=0.0014). This is in

agreement with the finding that workers' daily productivity was
correlated with age (r=0.5; N=51; p=0.0007). Age did not correlate
with AM- or PM-productivity. No significant correlation between
productivity and dermal exposure rates at p<0.01 was found. In an
earlier study involving benomyl exposure by strawberry harvesters,
this correlation was found (3).

Dislodgeable Foliar Residues and Dermal Exposure. Dislodgeable
foliar residues were determined on days 1,3,7,14,15,16, and 17 after
carbaryl had been applied to the strawberry fields at the rate of 2
lb/A. Results of these analyses are found in Figure 2 and Table VIII.
The decline of foliar residues appears to follow first-order
kinetics, and carbaryl has a half-life of approximately 4.1 days. The
three last sampling dates are identical with the study dates. From
these data and exposure rates of corresponding days (Table V), a
ratio can be calculated by the following equation:

$$k_d=(\text{dose rate})/(\text{dislodgeable foliar residue}) \tag{1}$$

This ratio might be considered to represent the ideal area of
foliage contacted by the worker if the residue were quantitatively
transferred from foliage to the skin. In reality, much less than
quantitative transfer is effected. For example, it was shown that
during harvesting of citrus, approximately one-half of parathion and
paraoxon residues was removed during harvesting activity (14).
Furthermore, in tree crops it is unlikely that all of the dry residue
removed from foliage will be adsorbed onto the person, independent of
dermal absorption. Thus, the value of k_d is expected to be smaller
than the actual foliage contacted or disturbed.

The k_d values obtained in this study are shown in Table IX and
are similar to values obtained from studies involving other
pesticides applied on different crops. This is even more surprising
given the range of chemicals and crops studied and considering that
the distribution of doses to the body and presumably the exposure
mechanisms might be quite different.

There are, however, several apparent discrepancies. The first is
the ratio calculated from literature values dealing with carbaryl
exposure to pesticide applicators and fruit thinners in an apple
orchard (4) This ratio (about 0.6×10^3 cm^{2}h^{-1}) was considerably lower
than the range seen in Table IX. The difference may be due to the
fact that Maitlen et al. (4) measured total and not dislodgeable
foliar residues, thus leading to lower values than those obtained by
us and others.

Recent observations (15) on the exposure to the fungicide
vinclozolin by the same group of strawberry harvesters exposed to
carbaryl, reported in these studies, revealed k_d values much larger
than those reported for carbaryl (about 40×10^3). One explanation for
this discrepancy might lie in the nature of vinclozolin residues
resulting from an application which took place over 40 days prior to
the study dates. One might speculate, therefore, that "new" and "old"
residues behave differently in their ability to transfer from foliage
to skin.

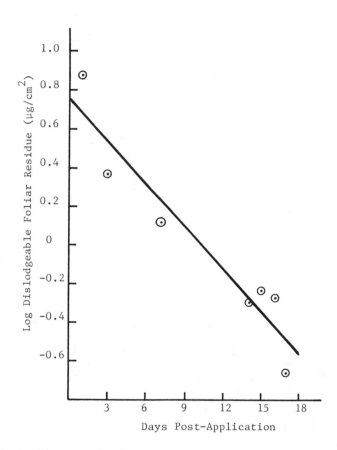

Figure 2. Decline of dislodgeable foliar residue of carbaryl from strawberry leaves; log dislodgeable residues vs. time in days; points are means of values in Table VIII. y=-0.073x + 0.756; r=-0.92. (Reproduced from Ref. 17. Copyright 1983, American Chemical Society.)

Table VIII.   Dislodgeable Foliar Residues of Carbaryl on Strawberry
                              Leaves

Sample ID	Days Post-Harvest	Dislodgeable Residues ug/cm²	PPM(dust) x10³
1.1	1	7.74	50.46
1.2	1	8.41	65.09
3.1	3	3.36	57.10
3.2	3	2.98	56.53
3.3	3	1.35	16.45
7.1	7	1.32	22.55
14.1	14	0.56	8.30
14.2	14	0.51	12.43
15.1	15	0.77	16.06
15.2	15	0.45	6.53
16.1	16	0.41	9.42
16.2	16	0.69	14.57
17.1	17	0.32	2.92
17.2	17	0.15	1.67

Pesticide Treatment: 2 lbs carbaryl/A (SEVIN 4F) on June 7, 1982.

Source: Reproduced from Ref. 17. Copyright 1983, American Chemical
Society.

Table IX. Ratios of Dermal Exposure and Dislodgeable Foliar
                      Residues for Fruit Harvesters

Pesticide	Crop	$k_d \times 10^3$	Literature Cited
Carbaryl (Day-1)	Strawberries	4.34	This study
Carbaryl (Day-2)	Strawberries	2.82	This study
Carbaryl (Day-3)	Strawberries	6.17	This study
Captan	Strawberries	8.57	[3]
Captan	Strawberries	2.90	[1]
Captan	Strawberries	8.00	[1]
Captan	Strawberries	2.62	[1]
Captan	Strawberries	5.97	[1]
Captan	Strawberries	4.73	[1]
Benomyl	Strawberries	7.19	[3]
Chlorobenzilate	Citrus	5.33[1]	[15]
OP Compounds	Citrus	5.1*	[10]

*   geometric mean from 14 observations
** geometric mean from 9 observations

[1] corrected for one side of leaf surface

Source: Reproduced from Ref. 17. Copyright 1983, American
Chemical Society.

Nontechnical Summary

Dermal exposure to the insecticide carbaryl was measured on a group of eighteen strawberry harvesters during three consecutive workdays. Additional analyses were performed on strawberry leaves to determine the concentration of so-called dislodgeable foliar residues. Several significant findings were made in this study: As was already shown in previous studies with different chemicals, the major targets in dermal exposure of strawberry harvesters working in fields which have been sprayed with pesticides prior to harvest, are hands and lower arms. Other parts of the body receive very low or nondetectable amounts of carbaryl. Some problems have been encountered with cotton gloves used as hand monitors, in that dermal exposure obtained by this technique might be overstated. Younger and/or smaller workers (by weight) appear to receive less exposure (mg/h) to carbaryl. Left- and right hand exposure to carbaryl by most workers was indistinguishable. The day and time period of observation have a greater influence on the mean exposure rate than the identity (e.g. work habits) of the individual worker. The ratio of dermal exposure rates to dislodgeable foliar residues, termed "transfer coefficient", has been found to be very similar to ratios obtained from studies involving other crops and chemicals.

Acknowledgments

This study was funded by the US. Environmental Protection Agency through a Cooperative Agreement (CR80-9343-01-0) with the University of California, Berkeley. This paper has not been peer-reviewed by the Agency and, therefore, the contents and conclusions do not necessarily reflect the views of the Agency, and no official endorsement should be inferred. An abbreviated report on this work will appear elsewhere (17).

Literature Cited

1. Popendorf, W.J.; Leffingwell, J.T.; McLean H.R.; Zweig, G.; Witt, J.M. "Youth in Agriculture. Pesticide Exposure to Strawberry Pickers -- 1981 Studies", Final Report, 2nd Draft, U.S. Environmental Protection Agency, Office of Pesticide Programs, Washington, D.C. 20460, Sept. 1982.
2. Everhart, L.P.; Holt, R.F. *J. Agric. Food Chem.* 1982, 30, 222-227
3. Zweig, Gunter; Gao, Ru-yu; Popendorf, W.J. *J. Agric. Food Chem.* 1983, 31, 1109-1113.
4. Maitlen, J.C.; Sell, R.C.; McDonough, L.M.; Fertig, S.N. In "Pesticide Residues and Exposure";Plimmer, J.R., Ed.; ACS SYMPOSIUM SERIES No. 182, American Chemical Society; Washington, D.C., 1982; pp. 83-103.
5. Gunther, F.A.; Westlake, W.E.; Barkley, J.H.; Winterlin, W.; Langbehn, L. *Bull. Environm. Contam. Toxicol.* 1973, 9, 243-249.
6. Gunther, F.A.; Barkley, J.H.; Westlake, W.E. *Bull. Environm. Toxicol.* 1974, 12, 641-644.
7. Iwata, Y.; Spear, R.C.; Knaak, J.B. Foster, R.J. *Bull. Environm. Contam. Toxicol.* 1977, 18, 649-653.

8. Popendorf, W.J.; Leffingwell, J.T. Bull. Environm. Contam.
    Toxicol. 1977, 18, 787-788.
9. Jones, A.S.; Jones, L.A.; Hastings, F.L. J. Agric. Food Chem.
    1982, 30, 997-999.
10. Popendorf, W.J.; Leffingwell, J.T. Residue Reviews 1982, 82, 125-
    201.
11. Sendroy, J.Jr.; Cecchini, L.P. J. Appl. Physiol. 1954, 7, 1-12.
12. Noel, M.E.; Zweig, Gunter; Popendorf, W.J. Abstracts of Papers,
    185th National Meeting of the American Chemical Society,
    March 1983, CHAS 27.
13. Davis, J.E.; Stevens, E.R.; Staiff, D.C. Bull. Environm. Contam.
    Toxicol. 1983, 31, 631-638.
14. Spear, R.C.; Popendorf, W.J.; Spencer, W.F.;Milby, T.H. J. Occup.
    Med. 1977, 191, 411-414.
15. Nigg, H.N.; Stamper, J.H.; Queen, R.M. Amer. Ind. Hyg. Assoc. J.
    1984, 45,182-186.
16. Zweig, Gunter; Leffingwell, J.T., unpublished data.
17. Zweig, G.; Gao, Ru-yu; Witt, J.M.; Popendorf, Wm.; Bogen, K.J.
    Agric. Food Chem. In Press.

RECEIVED August 28, 1984

Application Exposure to the Home Gardener

DAVID A. KURTZ and WILLIAM M. BODE

Department of Entomology, Pennsylvania State University, University Park, PA 16802

Exposure to the home gardener applying pesticides was measured using carbaryl as a model pesticide. In 15 minutes, volunteers applied 10 grams active ingredient in dusts and 2-3 grams in wettable powders or aqueous suspensions used to make pressurized spray mixtures. Exposures received from application to corn and beans plants were similar. Slightly higher exposures were received by dusting than in the use of wettable powder and aqueous suspension formulations from pressurized sprayers. Exposure data were calculated using 6 clothing regimens. The use of long sleeves produced exposures of 0.7-0.9, 0.2-0.3, and 0.2 mg carbaryl/15 min. for the three formulations, respectively. Exposures with short sleeves were an order higher. Highest exposures were at the shoe and cuff sample pad locations. When corn was sprayed, thigh pads received exposures similar to the shoe pads. With beans, thigh pad exposure was similar to upper body pad exposure. Inhalation exposure was found to be significantly less than covered-body dermal exposures.

Pesticide products are widely used not only in commercial applications but also in and around homes in the United States. In a 1971 survey of suburban residents of Philadelphia, PA; Dallas, TX; and Lansing, MI (1), 92.5% of the 525 respondents reported using pesticides. Vegetable gardens, an important home activity, are frequently treated with insecticides to prevent damage to garden crops.

Outside of professional worker applications, there are few published reports of studies conducted to measure the exposure of humans to insecticides. These studies have pertained to workers in manufacturing plants (2), people spraying agricultural crops (3), and persons involved in urban pest control (4). Such studies usually consisted of individual non-replicated observations.

0097–6156/85/0273–0139$06.50/0
© 1985 American Chemical Society

Information regarding the quantities and kinds of insecticides used on non-commercial vegetable gardens is not readily available. Likewise, there is a paucity of reports of scientific studies of the amounts of insecticides to which persons might be exposed during application in the home garden (4). Even though most available insecticides are not highly toxic, it is apparent that many users are lax in protecting themselves from exposure to these potentially harmful materials.

This paper presents a study of exposure for people applying an insecticide in a home garden situation. Measurements will be taken primarily of dermal exposure since it has been found to be the major exposure pathway in prior studies (2-5). Assuming the protective effect of clothing worn during application, estimations will be made of exposures under various clothing regimens. Inhalation exposure will also be estimated. The insecticide carbaryl was chosen for this study because it is commonly used by home gardeners, it has a relatively low mammalian toxicity, and residues can be quantified with a rapid and inexpensive method. An estimated 3.5 million pounds of carbaryl active ingredient were used in homes and gardens in 1972 (1). The production of carbaryl for all domestic users was estimated for 1978 to be 15-25 million pounds (4).

Materials and Methods

Field Application.   The compound carbaryl (1-naphthol methylcarbamate) was used as a model insecticide in this study. Three formulations were utilized to determine exposure differences between formulations; these were dust, wettable powder, and aqueous suspension. These are summarized in Table I.

Two kinds of vegetables, sweet corn and bush green beans, were treated to determine differences in the application exposure. The corn plants were 1.0 to 1.3 m high when treated and the bean plants were 0.2-0.3 m high. Drought conditions led to lower than expected plant height and row density. A sufficient number of each vegetable was planted to provide untreated rows for each trial.

Volunteers were recruited from the community to make the carbaryl applications. No special attempts were made to influence

Table I.   Application Variables Used in the Study: Formulations, Description and Source, and Mechanical Applicators

General Type	Active Ingredient	Formulation	Mechanical Applicator
Dust	5%	Agway 5% Dust	Shaker (n=2) Dust pump (n=22)
Wettable Powder	50%	Union Carbide 50WP	Hand held pressurized tank
Aqueous Suspension	43%	Union Carbide XLR	Hand held pressurized tank

how the applications were made other than to use the instructions on the manufacturer's label. Each volunteer on a given day applied all three formulations to either corn or beans. One set of 12 persons treated corn and another set of 12 treated beans (some of these were the same people).

Insecticide deposits on each person were sampled with 10 cm square gauze pads attached with masking tape to selected locations on white Tyvek (spunbonded olefin) coveralls and/or directly on the bodies of the applicators. The locations of the pads are listed in Table II. Another residue sample was taken from the dust/pollen mask worn over the nose and mouth of each applicator. A gauze pad covered by a square of denim or blue jean material and attached at the calf area of the coverall served to indicate the protection provided by typical leg covering. A new coverall with attached set of clean pads was worn for each trial. See Figure 1 for pad placement.

The 5% dust was applied either from the shaker can as purchased or by a mechanical duster. The shaker can was used in two instances, once on corn and once on beans. Thus, most of the dust applications were done with a pump-type device. Applicator exposure included filling the device prior to and emptying it following application.

The wettable powder and the aqueous suspension were mixed with one gallon of water in a 3-gallon compressed air sprayer. Exposure included measuring and adding the formulation to the sprayer as well as emptying the sprayer after the plants were sprayed. The volunteers were told to use 1 tablespoon of formulation with a gallon of water, as per label instructions, and they were offered the choice of a measuring tablespoon or a common kitchen tablespoon.

Each volunteer was given a 15 minute period for the field application to the vegetable crop. Our observer kept track of time

Table II. Body Area Representation by Pads (a)

Body Part Description	Area, cm^2	Pad Location		Pad Area, cm^2	
Face, neck front, lungs	740	face mask		120	
Shoulder, upper arms	1250	shoulder tops		50	
Back (whole torso)	3515	upper back		25	
Chest (whole torso)	1850 (b)	upper chest,	R,L	25	
Forearm (with wrists)	625	forearm,mid,	R,L	25	
Hand	820	hand	R,L	820	(c)
Thigh (knee-hip)	1757	thigh, mid,	R,L	25	
Lower leg	1187	cuff	R,L	25	
Ankle	50	shoe vamp	R,L	2.5	(d)
Foot	585	foot top,out	R,L	25	

(a) Largely from Davis (10), modified by others (11-13). Foot areas and confirmation of others from our own measurements.
(b) Area for either R, right, or L, left, side
(c) Whole hands to wrists were washed
(d) Exposed area for ankle calculation; hidden area was about 22.5

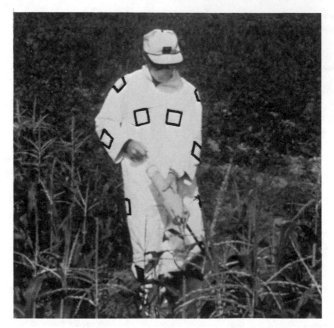

Figure 1. Application to corn by a volunteer with a pump duster.

and row length and recorded actions that might affect the treatment
of the data later. Data on weather conditions were also recorded.
     Following each application the volunteer's hands were
individually rinsed with 200 ml ethanol containing 0.03% NaOH. Each
hand was put into a plastic bag containing the solution and shaken 20
times. A 20 ml aliquot of the extraction mixture was then
transferred from the bag to a glass sample tube, which was capped,
and placed into a cooled, light-excluding container.
     Individual gauze pads were then removed from the coveralls and
the volunteer with freshly cleaned forceps. After all pads were
removed, a 5x5 cm square was cut with scissors from the center of
each and placed also in a glass sample tube.
     Before and after each application of a spray, a 20 ml aliquot
was obtained from the sprayer through the wand for later analysis.
The analysis data of these samples were used to confirm the amounts
of the active ingredient originally measured out by the volunteer.
See Table III.

Sample Analysis.   All samples were analyzed by the method of Chiba
(7). The pads were first extracted by dipping 5 times into 20 ml
of methanol containing 0.03% NaOH. Excess methanol was squeezed from
the pads which were then removed from the tube. The solution was
then treated the same way as published.
     All samples were analyzed within 6 hours after field work since
degradation can occur and a rigorous time schedule was required to
insure proper analytical results. Recoveries from 10 and 50 µg of
field applied carbaryl standard solutions onto gauze pads were 101

and 98%, respectively (n=6). Field applied XLR aqueous suspension solution was similarly recovered at 98 and 101%, respectively (n=5).

Because of the methanol toxicity to humans, the handwashes were done by shaking the hands with ethanol instead of methanol. However, the colorimetric reaction when done in ethanol is not the same as with methanol. The color reaction is only about 1/5 as sensitive, and, further, decomposition occurs somewhere in the process. For these reasons considerable care was taken to keep the ethanol solutions of carbaryl in the dark and cooled with ice. They were also analyzed as quickly as possible after the field work. Recoveries from 50 and 200 μg of field applied carbaryl standards solutions into ethanol solutions were 144 and 189%, respectively. Field applied XLR aqueous suspension solutions were similarly recovered at 90 and 45%, respectively (n=3).

The calibration graphs for the calculation of concentrations of carbaryl in the solutions were determined by regression of the log-transformed data (8).

Exposure Determinations.   Six clothing regimens were devised that covered the full range of potential body coverings that people would wear when spraying in their home gardens. These were no clothes, shorts only, shorts with tank top, short sleeved, long sleeved, and maximum clothing. The shorts only and shorts with tank top were calculated as though barefoot. The short sleeve regimen included shoes, shorts, and a short-sleeved shirt. The maximum clothing used not only long sleeved pants and shirt but also gloves and a face mask. These regimens are pictured in Figure 2.

The various pads represented portions of the body where they were placed, as found in Table II. When the pad, mask and hand exposures were multiplied together by the appropriate area factors, also in Table II, and the skin-exposed areas added together, the exposure was found for a given clothing regimen. For the purposes of these calculations clothing worn over a body area provided full protection from the applied pesticide either as a dust or spray. In related data to be published later and in other studies (9) there has been shown at least a 95% protection feature for single layered and even light weight clothing. An accidental spill, of course, would soak through clothing, but we did not see this type of exposure in any of our 72 field trials.

Results

Field Application Information.   Exposure to the gardener depends on several factors, among which the most important are: 1. the time spent in applying a pesticide, 2. the concentration in the formulation, 3. the precision of applying the pesticide, and 4. personal tidiness. The discussion of these follows:

The time spent by our volunteers was made constant at 15 minutes. We chose to set this parameter to a constant value in order to reduce the number of dependent variables in assessing exposure. It was felt that 15 minutes was a good estimate of the time a person would spend in the garden doing this activity at any given time.

Formulation Measurement.   Measurement of pesticidal formulations in the preparation of spray solutions was left to the individual volunteer. Under the general instruction of measuring one

tablespoon into the sprayer, it was found that there was a wide range
in the amount actually used. Table III shows that people measured
more wettable powder and less aqueous suspension than expected. The
overall range for both preparations measured by the volunteers was
1.7 to 20.4 grams. It can be concluded that people measured from a
half to over 4 true tablespoons of the dry powder in their estimate
of a tablespoon. Since our operating premise for these studies was
to get information under realistic conditions, we had provided an
ordinary kitchen tablespoon as well as a measuring tablespoon for
this preparation. Because the former was a shallow spoon, its level
measure was well under a true level tablespoon. This and the fact
that some people do measure shallow could lead to the lower figure
shown in the range. On the other hand people also have the tendency
to call a heaping tablespoon a true tablespoon.

Table III.   Amounts of Formulation Measured by Volunteers for Spray
Suspensions (12 Replications)

Plant Height	Formulation	Laboratory Measured One Tablespoon, g.	Volunteer Measurement, g.	
			Mean (s)	Range
Corn	Wettable Powder	4.34	5.6 (3.0)	1.7-10.6
	Aqueous Suspension	15.9	9.9 (3.5)	4.6-15.0
Beans	Wettable Powder	4.34	7.4 (5.0)	2.0-20.4
	Aqueous Suspension	15.9	9.0 (3.0)	3.2-13.1

Measurement of the liquid formulation, on the other hand, was
more accurately done, as shown in the table. Since the range for the
liquid measure was 3.2 to 15 g, the observation is made that people
measure liquids to a smaller degree than intended.

Formulation Application.   The application of the formulations
in the garden is summarized in Table IV. The amounts of wettable
powder and aqueous suspension solutions applied from a pressurized
hand-held sprayer by the various volunteers was pretty constant over
the 15 minute period. We had, for better or worse, kept the pressure
in the tank at a nearly constant level; the sprayer was usually
pumped up once during the spray period. The mean volume sprayed was
2.8 L for corn and 2.9 L for beans (which is approximately 0.75 of a
gallon). The range of the volumes dispensed was 1.7 to 3.6 L. In
noting the ranges, there was little difference between the two
formulations, as expected. There was also little difference in the
ranges of spray volume dispensed on beans verses corn.

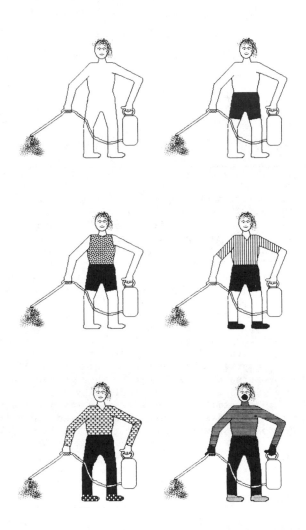

Figure 2. Diagrams depicting the six clothing regimens used in the computation of expected dermal exposure. (a). No clothes. (b). Shorts only. (c). Shorts with tank top. (d). Short-sleeved. (e). Long-sleeved. (f). Maximum clothing protection. Diagrams were prepared on an Apple MacIntosh computer through the courtesy of The Computer Store, State College, PA.

Table IV. Weight of Dust and Volume of Spray Applied by Volunteers
           in 15 Minutes (12 Replications)

Formulation	Corn			Beans		
	Mean	(s)	Range	Mean	(s)	Range
Dust, g	190	(98)	41 -320	220	(210)	23 -680
Wettable Powder, L	2.8	(0.4)	2.2-3.5	2.9	(0.4)	2.2-3.5
Aqueous Suspension, L	2.8	(0.6)	1.7-3.5	2.9	(0.4)	2.2-3.6

     The dust formulation was applied similarly on corn and beans as
shown in the Table. There is not a clear reason why corn should
receive a lower amount unless it is found only in the high
variability of the application. In this case the range of
application on beans was 23 to 680 g, a 30-fold range! On corn it
was better but still very large at 41 to 320 g. This clearly shows
how variable an ordinary gardener's estimate is of how much pesticide
is needed to do the job. Some people just dust a tiny amount on the
leaves while others produce totally white leaves.
     Table V shows the amounts of active ingredient in the amounts of
the formulations applied by volunteers. These data were taken
directly from Table IV and are presented to give the reader some
impression of the amounts of carbaryl used in these trials. The data
can be used when comparing the use of the three formulations
providing the exposures discussed below. They do show that far more
carbaryl was used in 15 minutes when applied as a 5% dust than as
either of the two formulations applied as a sprayed-on suspension.
The higher aqueous suspension dosage is unexpected since its
concentration is only 43% while that of the wettable powder is 50%.

Table V.   Weights of Active Ingredient Applied by Volunteers
           in 15 Minutes (12 Replications)

Formulation	Corn, g			Beans, g		
	Mean	(s)	Range	Mean	(s)	Range
Dust	9.5	(4.9)	2.05-16	11	(10.5)	1.15-34
Wettable Powder	2.1	(1.20)	0.68-4.6	2.8	(1.54)	0.93-5.9
Aqueous Suspension	3.2	(1.36)	1.27-5.6	3.0	(1.07)	1.10-4.6

This difference is overwhelmingly made up by the tendency of
volunteers to overmeasure wettable powders.

Garden Area Covered. The third variable in application is the
precision of the worker, to wit, how much does he put on the plants
and how much on other things including himself. The data in Table VI
give some indication of this variable. It shows the row length
covered by volunteers in 15 minutes. As expected the mean row length
was smaller for corn than for beans since corn was taller. The
difference was small, however. There was up to a ten-fold range in
this data. Some caution must be used in this calculation since at
this particular time there was sparse growth of the vegetables due to
drought conditions. The corn reached only about 2/3 its normal
height and the beans were often only sparsely spaced in the rows.

Table VI. Row Length of Vegetables Treated by Volunteers
in 15 minutes (12 Replications)

Plant Height	Formulation	Row Length, m (a)		
		Mean	(s)	Range
High (Corn)	Dust	140	(70)	34- 270
	Wettable Powder	140	(83)	170- 980
	Aqueous Suspension	160	(130)	170-1800
Low (Beans)	Dust	180	(100)	52- 370
	Wettable Powder	220	(160)	210-2000
	Aqueous Suspension	220	(180)	260-1200

(a) High figures in beans due to sparse growth.

Calculated Exposure According to Various Clothing Regimens. The
estimated dermal exposure of volunteers treating home gardens was
calculated by various clothing regimens using the body areas in Table
II as a guide. Tables VII and VIII give these estimates for
applications made on corn and beans, respectively. There was no
statistically significant difference in the body exposure with a
given clothing regimen either between plant height or between method
of application. The high variation of results from volunteer to
volunteer prevented any possibility of finding differences respecting
these factors. The data suggest that dusting of low vegetables, such
as green beans, results in a larger exposure than does the use of
pressurized water mixtures of other formulations. Results also
suggest that the wettable powder formulation produces the lowest
exposure. When taller plants are to be sprayed, such as corn, the
data suggest that both the dust and the aqueous suspension result in
about equal exposure with the wettable powder still giving the lowest
exposure.

Exposure for all 3 formulations by the no-clothes regimen resulted in 5-10 mg total body exposure to the active ingredient, carbaryl. Persons wearing short-sleeves were exposed to 2.5-5.0 mg. Those wearing long sleeves were exposed to 0.3-0.9 mg; and those wearing a maximum of clothing, 0.15 to 0.5 mg. LD_{50} values for carbaryl are 4000 mg/kg in dermal exposure to rats (6) and 500 mg/kg (acute oral, female rat). For other insecticides that might be used, the toxicity data is 1000 mg/kg (acute oral, female rat) for malathion and 4-13 mg/kg (acute oral, rat) for parathion (14).

In the only other study of urban application of carbaryl by Gold, et al., (4) total dermal exposure (no clothes) was found to be 7.35 mg/15 min. which is similar to our results. This study included 38 persons performing 50 applications from turf to trees and in the home as well as small commercial operations. Garden usage amounted to 24% of the applications in the study. Dusting and aqueous suspension applications were only 6% each, wettable powder, 88%. The study showed a slightly lower exposure when calculated to a long-sleeved regimen, 3.76 mg/15 min. However, their hand exposures were exceptionally high, 2.97 mg/15 min; our hand exposures were only 0.12 mg/15 min. When the hand exposure is subtracted from the long-sleeved regimen, their data is similar to ours, 0.23 to 0.29 mg/15 min for pressurized spraying and 0.68-0.89 mg/15 min for dusting.

In looking at these data by clothing regimen, we see that the exposure is reduced (in various stages) as the clothing cover is increased. We have stated that the skin is protected to a high degree by clothing which is supported in a later section of this paper. If it is assumed that 90-95% protection is afforded even with light weight clothing, and this is not an unreasonable assumption, then the data of Tables VII and VIII are valid.

Application to Corn. Spraying with shorts only or shorts and tank top with bare feet did not reduce exposure a significant amount over the no-clothes regimen. In corn application, Table VII, the

Table VII. Estimated Exposure to Unprotected Body Areas in Home Garden Application of Three Formulations of Carbaryl onto Tall Vegetables (Corn) by Clothing Protection Regimen (12 Replications)

| Clothing Regimen | Dusting | | Pressurized Spraying | | | |
| | | | Wettable Powder | | Aqueous Suspen. | |
	Mean,mg	(s)	Mean,mg	(s)	Mean,mg	(s)
No clothes	9.9	(8.1)	7.7	(6.9)	11.0	(9.7)
Shorts only	7.3	(5.3)	5.0	(4.6)	7.6	(6.6)
Shorts + tank top	5.6	(4.4)	4.3	(4.5)	5.8	(4.5)
Short-sleeved	3.7	(3.7)	2.4	(2.9)	3.8	(3.5)
Long-sleeved	0.89	(0.48)	0.28	(0.16)	0.23	(0.10)
Maximum	0.50	(0.30)	0.18	(0.12)	0.15	(0.09)

Table VIII.   Estimated Exposure to Unprotected Body Areas in Home Garden Application of Three Formulations of Carbaryl onto Low Vegetables (Beans) by Clothing Protection Regimen (12 Replications)

| | Dusting | | Pressurized Spraying | | | |
| | | | Wettable Powder | | Aqueous Suspen. | |
Clothing Regimen	Mean,mg	(s)	Mean,mg	(s)	Mean,mg	(s)
No clothes	10.2	(8.9)	5.4	(3.1)	6.8	(5.4)
Shorts only	9.5	(8.3)	5.2	(3.1)	6.4	(5.0)
Shorts + tank top	8.3	(7.6)	4.8	(3.1)	6.0	(4.8)
Short-sleeved	5.2	(5.8)	3.1	(2.8)	3.7	(3.3)
Long-sleeved	0.68	(0.32)	0.24	(0.10)	0.29	(0.40)
Maximum	0.46	(0.30)	0.19	(0.13)	0.24	(0.40)

exposure was reduced to about 1/3 for each formulation by wearing short-sleeved clothing. The addition of sleeves brought a greater reduction of exposure for the use of the aqueous suspension than for the other formulations. In this case the exposure of 0.23 mg was 1/16 that for the short-sleeved regimen. This is explained in the case of dusting where the hands were proportionately higher in exposure. When wettable powder was used, the added sleeves reduced the exposure from 2.4 to 0.28 mg or about 1/9 the higher level. When dusting was done, the least amount of reduction was observed, from 3.7 to 0.89 mg or about 1/4 the level.

Application to Beans. In application to green beans, Table VIII, we see first that dusting resulted in the highest exposure to carbaryl regardless of the clothing regimen. The use of short sleeved clothing did bring the exposure, when spraying beans, to about half that with no clothes. An order of magnitude improvement-1/10 the level-was obtained, however, when long sleeves were worn. This is significant in that the additional discomfort of the heavier clothing gave such a large increase in protection.

The comparisons by clothing regimen of mean exposures between corn and beans are presented in Figure 3a-c. The figure parts show the comparison using the dusting, wettable powder, and aqueous suspension formulations, respectively,. The variability of the data is shown in Figure 3d. Few statistically significant differences can be drawn from his data because of this high variability.

Comparison with Commercial Application. We found applicator exposure in home gardens to be considerably less than that found in commercial orchard spraying as the 3 studies cited below show. All used air-blast spraying of carbaryl:

In 1962 in Quebec (3), the dermal exposure was found to be 6.3 mg/15 min. as a mean of 7 subjects; the range was 4.6-7.6. The exposure was determined by the adsorption to forehead and wrist pads. This approximated the long-sleeved regimen where our home gardener received a much lower 0.2-0.3 mg/15 min. for high plants!

a)

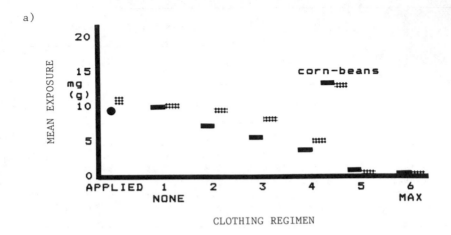

b)

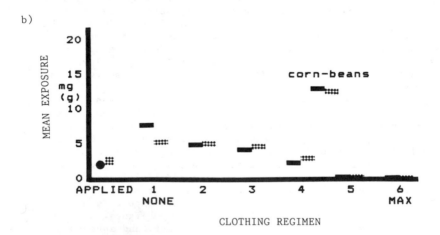

Figures 3a and 3b. Mean exposures for both corn and beans
application calculated for each of the six clothing regimens for
(a) dusting and (b) wettable powder spraying. Applied amount
uses the g unit on vertical axis. Clothing regimens are 1, no
clothes; 2, shorts only; 3, shorts with tank top; 4, short-
sleeved; 5, long-sleeved; and 6, maximum clothing protection.

c)

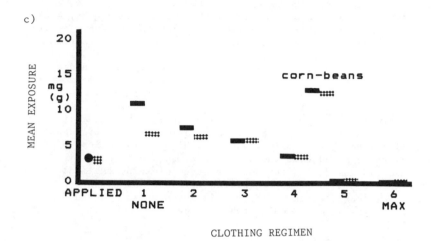

CLOTHING REGIMEN

d)

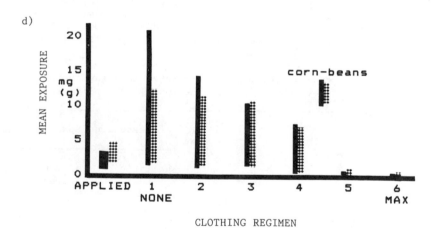

CLOTHING REGIMEN

Figures 3c and 3d. Mean exposures for both corn and beans application calculated for each of the six clothing regimens for (c) aqueous suspension spraying. Clothing regimens are 1, no clothes; 2, shorts only; 3, shorts with tank top; 4, short-sleeved; 5, long-sleeved; and 6, maximum clothing protection. (d) Variance of the exposures for aqueous suspension spraying calculated for the 6 clothing regimens. Each bar is 2 standard deviation units in length pictured +/- about the mean.

In 1961-62 in New South Wales of Australia (16), a study gave
long-sleeve regimen exposure of a slightly lower level, 2.5 mg/kg.
This information is the summary of data found for 8-16 subjects.
Again, this is 10 times the exposure we found.

These data can also be compared with a newer study (2) where
the exposure was calculated for workers wearing short sleeved shirts,
no hat or gloves, and long pants. They found these workers received
a mean of 15 mg/15 min. exposure (range: 0.4-53 mg/15 min.). Again,
this most closely compares with our long-sleeve regimen. Hence the
home gardener is receiving about 1/50 as much exposure as commercial
spraymen for an equivalent time period and clothing worn.

Application Vector to the Person Applying. Calculations were
made to estimate the portion of applied material that actually
reached the skin of the applicator. See Table IX. The high and low
plant applications gave similar results. Higher proportions of the
spray mixtures applied with the pressurized sprayer reached the
worker than did the dust. For short-sleeved clothing regimens, this
amounted to about 0.1% from pressurized sprayers and 0.05% by
dusting. For long-sleeved regimens this amounted to about 0.01% from
pressurized spraying and 0.008% from dusting.

Exposure Profile Verses Height above Ground.   Summary. The data
obtained in this study were configured to show the amounts of
formulation reaching the worker as a function of height above ground.
The data were adjusted to show the quantity found on 25 cm^2 of
surface area at the location of the pad (or hand) placement. Tables
X-XII show the data on this pad collection for dusting, wettable
powder spraying and aqueous suspension spraying, respectively.

Table IX. Mean Percentage of Carbaryl in Spray Reaching the Body
by Plant Height for Two Common Clothing Regimens (12 Replications)

		Dusting	Pressurized Spraying	
			Wettable Powder	Aqueous Suspension
Plant Height	Clothing Regimen	%	%	%
High, Applied amount		9.5 grams	2.1 grams	3.2 grams
	Short-sleeved	0.039	0.11	0.12
	Long-sleeved	0.009	0.013	0.007
Low, Applied amount		11.0 grams	2.8 grams	3.0 grams
	Short-sleeved	0.047	0.11	0.12
	Long-sleeved	0.006	0.009	0.010

Table X. Amount of Carbaryl Active Ingredient Adhering to Individual Pads or Hands as a Function of Body Location and of Plant Height. Dust Formulation (12 Replications)

Location	High Plant Height (Corn)				Low Plant Height (Beans)			
	Right, µg		Left, µg		Right, µg		Left, µg	
	Mean	(s)	Mean	(s)	Mean	(s)	Mean	(s)
	Mean	(s)			Mean	(s)		
Mask (a)	14.9	(8.9)			10.5	(6.9)		
Shoulders (a)	3.3	(2.2)			2.9	(1.6)		
Back	3.2	(1.5)			3.6	(2.7)		
Chest	9.2	(21.) (b)	8.0	(10.3)	5.8	(6.7)	3.9	(3.8)
Forearms	14.2	(39.) (c)	4.4	(8.6) (d)	3.6	(5.0)	5.5	(8.5)
Hand (a)	11.8	(13.)	7.9	(9.9)	3.8	(3.8)	5.3	(5.3)
Thigh	13.2	(19.)	24.	(38.)	4.6	(7.5)	5.6	(5.8)
Cuff	22.	(35.)	25.	(32.)	36.	(52.)	52.	(58.)
Shoe	37.	(35.)	39.	(38.)	53.	(58.)	66.	(50.)

(a) adjusted to 25 cm^2 analysis area.
(b) One high outlier, 74, when removed, changed the mean to 3.3 (4.9)
(c) One high outlier, 139, when removed, changed the mean to 2.9 (2.8)
(d) One high outlier, 32, when removed, changed the mean to 2.0 (0.9)

In all cases the highest concentrations of pesticide were found at the shoe and cuff area. Moving upward, the thigh pad was pivotal in describing exposure differences between spraying our high and low plant vegetables, corn and beans. For corn, the thigh pad had relatively high exposure, but for beans the exposure was significantly lower, approximately 1/10 as much, a finding that was expected. For beans, the levels of carbaryl found on the thigh pad were very similar to other pads located higher on the body all the way to the head. For corn, the drop-off to lower exposure levels occurred higher than the thigh pad, specifically, the hands, forearms and chest. Again, the drop-off from thigh to the higher pads was about 1/10.

The mask pad covering the face, when adjusted to 25 cm^2 area, appears to have heavier exposures than the chest and shoulders for dusting, only slightly heavier exposures for wettable powder spraying, and similar or lighter exposures for aqueous suspension spraying. The higher dust exposure may be from the worker scratching his face and nose in response to the dust irritant which was noted for a fair number of volunteers.

In making comparisons between these pads, care should be taken to compare means having similar variances (standard deviations). Occasional outlying values in the data sets caused standard

Table XI. Amount of Carbaryl Active Ingredient Adhering to Individual
Pads or Hands as a Function of Body Location and of Plant Height.
Wettable Powder Formulation (12 Replications)

Location	High Plant Height (Corn)				Low Plant Height (Beans)			
	Right, μg		Left, μg		Right, μg		Left, μg	
	Mean	(s)	Mean	(s)	Mean	(s)	Mean	(s)
		Mean	(s)				Mean	(s)
Mask (a)		2.8	(1.8)				2.5	(2.4)
Shoulders (a)		1.9	(0.9)				1.0	(0.4)
Back		1.9	(0.6)				1.7	(1.4)
Chest	1.8	(0.7)	3.8	(6.2)	0.9	(0.8)	1.0	(0.8)
Forearms	1.6	(1.1)	5.2	(9.6)	0.7	(0.4)	0.6	(0.4)
Hand (a)	3.0	(2.3)	2.7	(2.8)	2.2	(2.4)	1.3	(1.4)
Thigh	22.	(24.)	17.	(24.)	0.8	(0.7)	2.3	(2.9)
Cuff	12.	(12.)	23.	(32.)	34.	(47.)	28.	(31.)
Shoe	32.	(40.)	40.	(43.)	44.	(48.)	28.	(40.)

(a) adjusted to 25 cm^2 analysis area.

deviations to far exceed the mean values. In cases where the
standard deviation was more than twice the mean, the outliers were
removed and the data set recalculated; such recalculations are noted
in the tables. The data without outliers were used to prepare
figures showing the vertical height profile of exposures. Figures 4
(dusting), 5 (wettable powder), and 6 (aqueous suspension) are shown
with the accompanying table.

Pad Exposures in Clothing-Protected Areas. A previous
suggestion was made that clothing protects the body from dusting and
spraying in the home garden. Information supporting that suggestion
is found in Table XIII. The data presented here are for pads that
were hidden for one reason or another: under-jean pad, inside-arm
pad, and inside-shoe pad. The under-jean pad was taped under the
surface of washed jean material located about the middle of the lower
leg which simulated typical trouser wear. The inside-arm pad was
taped to the person's skin 1-5 inches above the wrist. It was not
fully protected by shirt material since it was placed just next to
the open cuff; the conclusions drawn from the data should take this
in account. Part of the inside-shoe pad was exposed to the spraying
depending on the type of shoe the person was wearing.

The under-jean pad exposure amounted to about 1 μg per pad. It
received less exposure for spraying beans than for spraying corn. It
was about 6% of the thigh pad and less when compared to the cuff pad.

The inside-arm pads, having an approximate exposure of 1.5 to

Table XII.Amount of Carbaryl Active Ingredient Adhering to Individual Pads or Hands as a Function of Body Location and of Plant Height. Aqueous Suspension Formulation (12 Replications)

	High Plant Height (Corn)				Low Plant Height (Beans)			
	Right, μg		Left, μg		Right, μg		Left, μg	
Location	Mean	(s)	Mean	(s)	Mean	(s)	Mean	(s)
	Mean	(s)			Mean	(s)		
Mask (a)	1.9	(1.0)			2.0	(1.4)		
Shoulders (a)	1.4	(0.7)			2.7	(4.3)		
Back	10.6	(27.) (b)			1.7	(0.8)		
Chest	3.9	(8.8) (c)	2.0	(2.3)	0.8	(0.5)	1.4	(2.3)
Forearms	9.1	(22.) (d)	8.7	(19.) (e)	0.8	(0.7)	0.8	(0.6)
Hand (a)	2.2	(1.2)	2.4	(1.8)	1.4	(1.1)	1.5	(1.3)
Thigh	26.	(41.)	22.	(22.)	1.2	(0.9)	5.2	(8.6)
Cuff	39.	(39.)	28.	(37.)	38.	(45.)	34.	(41.)
Shoe	41.	(54.)	41.	(49.)	45.	(47.)	51.	(59.)

(a) adjusted to 25 cm^2 analysis area
(b) One high outlier, 91, when removed, changed the mean to 2.4 (1.5)
(c) One high outlier, 32, when removed, changed the mean to 1.4 (.94)
(d) One high outlier, 77, when removed, changed the mean to 2.9 (4.1)
(e) Two high outliers, 24, 66, removed, changed the mean to 1.5 (.97)

3.0 μg in spraying corn, are compared to the hands (25 cm^2) which received an exposure of about 2.3 μg (aqueous suspension) to 10 μg (dusting). In spraying beans the inside-arm pads received 0.75 to 0.9 μg in compressed air spraying and 2.9 in dusting. This is compared to the hands which received 2.3 μg (aqueous suspension) to 8 μg (dusting). For these protected pads dusting produced the highest exposure and the use of an aqueous suspension the lowest exposure.

The inside-shoe pads ranged in exposure from 1.6 to 3.1 μg in the application to corn. The exposure was 0.9 to 3.3 μg (outliers removed) in compressed gas spraying and 4.0 to 4.9 in dusting when applying to beans. This compares to shoe exposures of 32 to 41 μg for corn and 28 to 66 for beans.

Inhalation Exposure.   Inhalation exposure was not directly measured in this study. We quickly found in pretrials that the volunteers were terribly unhappy wearing a respirator. This would confound the naturalness of the study so much as to adversely affect the operation of the major part of the study. Information can be obtained in this area, however, by comparing the face mask with pads located nearby. Shoulder pad exposures were adjusted to the facial mask area and subtracted from the mask exposure on a case by case

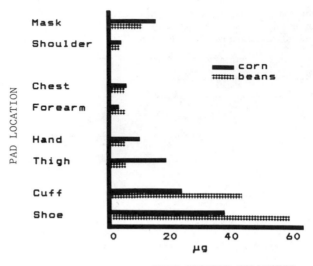

Figure 4. Pad collection profile of mean carbaryl residues for
dusting application as a function of body location. Each location
represents 25 cm² area. Outliers described in Table X have
been removed.

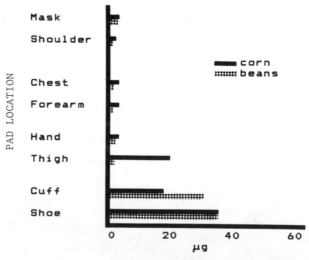

Figure 5. Pad collection profile of mean carbaryl residues for
wettable powder application as a function of body location. Each
location represents 25 cm² area.

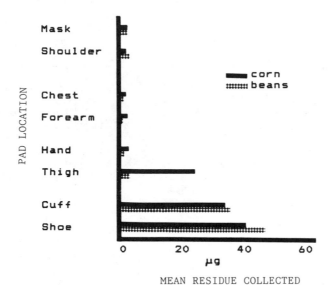

Figure 6. Pad collection profile of mean carbaryl residues for aqueous suspension application as a function of body location. Each location represents 25 cm^2 area. Outliers described in Table XII have been removed.

Table XIII. Amount of Carbaryl Active Ingredient Adhering to "Hidden"
Pads as a function of Body Location and of Plant Height
(12 Replications)

Location	High Plant Height (Corn)				Low Plant Height (Beans)			
	Right, µg		Left, µg		Right, µg		Left, µg	
	Mean	(s)	Mean	(s)	Mean	(s)	Mean	(s)
Dust								
Inside-arm	3.2	(2.3)	3.2	(2.3)	2.9	(2.5)	2.9	(2.5)
Under-jean	0.93	(1.10)	0.95	(0.47)	0.63	(0.60)	0.62	(0.51)
Inside-shoe	3.1	(3.9)	2.3	(3.1)	4.0	(5.4)	4.9	(5.9)
Wettable powder								
Inside-arm	2.0	(2.1)	2.0	(2.1)	0.9	(0.5)	0.9	(0.5)
Under-jean	1.25	(1.83) (a)	1.66	(2.13) (b)	0.94	(2.28) (c)	0.38	(0.30)
Inside-shoe	2.5	(3.2)	2.0	(2.4)	2.4	(2.2)	3.3	(4.1)
Aqueous suspension								
Inside-arm	1.5	(1.5)	1.5	(1.5)	0.75	(0.45)	0.75	(0.45)
Under-jean	0.64	(0.37)	0.70	(0.38)	0.33	(0.31)	2.1	(5.0) (d)
Inside-shoe	2.9	(3.2)	1.63	(1.64)	4.3	(9.1) (e)	4.8	(9.8) (f)

(a) If 2 outliers are rejected, data values become 0.50 (0.39).
(b) If 1 outlier is rejected, data values become 1.01 (0.58).
(c) If 1 outlier is rejected, data values become 0.28 (0.26).
(d) If 1 outlier is rejected, data values become 0.71 (0.62).
(e) If 2 outliers are rejected, data values become 1.03 (0.50).
(f) If 2 outliers are rejected, data values become 0.86 (0.57).

basis. The remaining exposure information is summarized in Table
XIV. The adjusted exposure when spraying corn amounted to 48 µg in
dusting, 5.7 µg in spraying the wettable powder, and 2.1 µg in
spraying the aqueous mixture. The data are similar when beans were
sprayed. The data points where the volunteer was known to have
touched his mask were removed from this calculation, but some of the
points may still have contamination resulting from touching the nose
and face and in adjusting the face mask. These data can be used to
determine if further studies are needed in this area.
    Three published studies show very low inhalation exposure. In a
previous study by Jegier in Quebec (3) workers in orchard air-blast
spraying received only 0.072 mg/15 min. compared to a long-sleeved
dermal exposure of 6.3 mg/15 min. Simpson (5) found in Australia
that the respirator portion of orchard air-blast spraying gave an

Table XIV. Carbaryl Available for Inhalation Exposure. Amount
on Mask Adjusted for Incident Exposure on Shoulder Pad

Application Method	High Plant Height (Corn)		Low Plant Height (Beans)	
	Mean, μg	(s)	Mean, μg	(s)
Dusting	48	(36.)	28	(19.)
Wettable Powder	5.7	(8.0)	6.9	(6.4)
Aqueous Suspension	2.1	(4.9)	3.5	(3.6)

inhalation exposure of 0.12 mg/15 min. His short sleeved-long pants
clothing covering gave a dermal exposure of 2.5 mg/15 min. Gold, et
al., (4) found only 0.014 mg/15 min. inhaled carbaryl in his very
recent urban study. This amount is negligible to the dermal exposure
resulting from the use of limited clothing even if inhaled carbaryl
is taken up much more quickly.

Conclusions

One of the original purposes in the gathering of data for the
operator exposure in home garden spraying was to collect data under
natural conditions. In so doing, we realized we would collect highly
variable data. Consequently, we did not observe statistical
differences in plant height or in formulation effects. We have,
however, learned much by observing both the mean, which is still the
best estimate, and the variance of the collected data.

Only low levels of pesticide reached the user. The mean total
body exposure for all formulations was 10 mg on the tall plant-height
and 7.5 mg for the low plant-height vegetables, a quantity equivalent
to only a light salting of vegetables at the dinner table.

Each mean had a high variance; the ranges were 2 to 33 mg for
corn and 1.7 to 29 mg for beans. While one person received 33 mg
some obtained only 2 mg exposure which was accomplished without any
instruction or elaborate preparations as we observed.

Most exposure occurs at the foot and leg areas of the body even
when spraying plants as high as a meter or so. Hence clothing that
covers all of the lower part of the body gives the greatest clothing
protection. Nearly full protection is gained by the use of shoes,
long trousers, and long-sleeved shirt. To prevent possible
inhalation a disposable paper pollen mask would help to further
reduce inhalation exposure.

Suggestions for Reduction of Personal Exposure. To address the
purpose of eventually reducing exposure to the general public, our
main problem would be to focus on instruction that gives the greatest
reduction first. The following areas as determined from this study
will result in quick and nearly complete reduction of exposure:

First. wettable powders could be prepackaged in tablespoon or

even in teaspoon packets to avoid excessively high concentrations
when used in sprayers. Such packets could allow safe handling
especially if the packet itself would dissolve in the appropriate
volume of water. Overmeasurement was found to exist up to at least 4
times the label-instructed amount. For dusts, a color picture should
be provided on the label showing the approximate density when applied
according to label instructions. We found some applications so heavy
that the plants appeared to have white leaves. Liquids or emulsifiable concentrates are not so much a problem for overmeasurement. To
reduce the spillage of these materials a medicine dropper with a
marked level and attached inside the cap of the concentrated
pesticide could provide the home gardener with an ease of measure but
reduce the chances of spillage from a measuring spoon.
       A second area to vastly reduce exposure is the wearing of a full
cover of clothes as described above. We did not measure the
protection of clothes to any detailed extent, but we did find at
least a 20 to 1 protection ratio under new but laundered jean
material. With this ratio in mind and looking at the larger
proportion of areas covered by just adding long sleeves to short
ones, we calculated a reduction of at least 95% from total body
exposure by the wearing of clothing.
       A third way of reducing the exposure is to suggest that the user
use imagination in the spraying. Imagination can offer ideas to
reduce contact by moving backwards down the rows, moving against the
wind, and planning the direction of travel in the areas to be
sprayed. To do this the label could use small diagrams or pictures
depicting each of these situations. Suggestions could also be made
for the home gardener to perform a dry run over the area...even by
spraying plain water.
       A fourth way of reducing exposure, though not particularly
studied in these experiments, is that the user should thoroughly wash
his hands and equipment after application. The waste water is
allowed to flow preferentially into garden areas or areas that are
not play areas for children or pets. Of course, the clothing worn as
protection should also be washed up directly after use.
       Finally, one additional suggestion is to avoid using dusts where
the particles are dry. The dust is easily transferred from the hands
to the face. In most of the clothing regimens we found higher
exposure results from their use.

Nontechnical Summary

The determination was made as to the amount of pesticide a home
gardener receives when applying in his home garden. The amount of
carbaryl, a model pesticide, reaching the applicator was 8.5 mg,
equivalent in weight to a few grains of table salt. Virtually all of
this covered the feet and lower legs when applying to low-height
vegetables. When applying to tall vegetables, such as corn, the
thigh area also obtained exposures similar to lower legs. The lowest
exposure, when applying to both corn and beans, was obtained by the
use of wettable powder formulation in pressurized sprayers. Somewhat
higher exposures were obtained in the use of aqueous suspensions in
pressurized sprayers and dusts. Because of the protective qualities
of clothing when worn and cleaned afterwards, the wearing of
long-sleeved clothing reduced exposure about 1/20 to 0.4 mg.

Inhalation exposure was negligible. One final finding is that people tend to undermeasure liquids in spoons and drastically overmeasure powders in spoons.

Acknowledgments

The authors wish to acknowledge the helpful role given by the 17 volunteers as well as the following technical help: Michael E. Arner, Robert E. Davis, Andrew G. Fieo, Constance L. Fisher, William C. Erwin, John J. Kmetz, and Barbara Zogren. Special thanks is given for given for leadership, technical help, and aid in the calculation of data to Kathrine Kowalski Giri. This paper is published as Journal Series paper No. 7041 of the Pennsylvania Agricultural Experiment Station. This material is based upon work supported by the U. S. Department of Agriculture under agreement No. 80-CSRS-2-0511.

Literature Cited

1. Von Rumker, R.; Matter, R. M.; Clement, B. P.; Erickson, F. K. "The Use of Pesticides in Suburban Homes and Gardens and their Impact on the Aquatic Environment," Report from the Office of Water Programs, U. S. Environmental Protection Agency, U. S. Government, EP2.25:2, 1972.

2. Comer, S. W.; Staiff, D. C.; Armstrong, J. F.; Wolfe, H. R. Bull. Environ. Contam. Toxicol. 1975, 13(4), 385-391.

3. Jegier, Z. Arch. Environ. Health 1964, 8, 670-674.

4. Gold, R. E.; Leavitt, J. R. C.; Holcslaw, T.; Tupy, D. Arch. Environ. Contam. Toxicol. 1982, 11, 63-67.

5. Simpson, G. R. Arch. Environ. Health 1965, 10, 884-5.

6. Gaines, T. B. Toxicol. Appl. Pharmicol 1960, 2, 88.

7. Chiba, M. J. Agric. Food Chem. 1981, 29, 118-121.

8. Kurtz, D. A. Anal. Chim. Acta 1983, 150, 105-114.

9. Moraski, R. V.; Nielsen, A. P. in THIS BOOK SERIES PUBLICATION.

10. Davis, J. E. Residue Reviews 1980, 75, 33-50.

11. Durham, W. F.; Wolfe, H. R. Bull. World Health Organization 1962, 26, 75-91.

12. Berkow, S. G. Am. J. of Surgery 1931, 11, 315-317.

13. Du Bois, D.; Du Bois, E. F. Arch. Int. Med. 1916, 17, 863-871.

14. "Farm Chemicals Handbook", Meister Publishing Co.: Willoughby, OH, 1984, 70th ed.; pp. C44, C138, C172.

RECEIVED October 31, 1984

Monitoring Field Applicator Exposure to Pesticides

T. L. LAVY and J. D. MATTICE

Altheimer Laboratory, Department of Agronomy, University of Arkansas, Fayetteville, AR 72701

For the past 6 years the research team at the pesticide laboratory of the University of Arkansas has been conducting research
on pesticide applicator exposure studies. During this period we
have analyzed over 9000 samples from nine different studies to
evaluate applicator exposure to 2,4,5-T, 2,4-D, 2,4-DP, paraquat,
EPN, MSMA, picloram, and methyl parathion. During these studies
we have attempted to determine, not only how much exposure applicators receive, but also how large a dose they absorb. We have
attempted to learn how to best collect samples incorporating
quality controls which allow us to best evaluate exposure and
dose measurements. The results of our individual studies have
been published elsewhere (see related literature following the
references). Consequently, the primary purpose here is to present further details and some general conclusions of these studies. In addition, we offer our opinions on how best to design
and conduct exposure studies.

Exposure and Dose

The following three parameters are involved in determining the
potential health effects of pesticides on humans: 1) toxicity of
the compound, 2) absorbed dose, and 3) absorption and excretion
rates.
    It is important to note the difference between exposure and
dose. Exposure to a chemical occurs when a person makes contact
with a chemical. Unless the compound causes damage to the part
of the body it comes into contact with, exposure per se does not
represent a danger. The absorbed dose may be defined as that
amount of the chemical that actually gets inside the body. The
amount that enters the body is related to the amount of exposure
occurring but many factors play a role in determining the fraction of the exposure that is absorbed into the body. Some of
these factors probably controlling the absorption include the
binding properties of the chemical, volatility of the chemical,
resistance to photodecomposition, the moisture and lypophillic

0097-6156/85/0273-0163$06.00/0
© 1985 American Chemical Society

properties of the skin contacted, portion of the body contacted,
and duration of the skin-chemical contact. The retention time in
the body depends upon the rate of absorption and the rate at
which the chemical is excreted from the body. Quantitative
measures of danger to the human are also dependent upon the toxicity of the chemical. Exposure in itself is important from a
health standpoint to the extent it governs the absorbed dose.

Collection of Samples

During most of these studies we have analyzed samples from three
different sources 1) air monitors for determining the concentration of pesticide in the air, 2) patches attached to the
applicators clothing to obtain an estimate of dermal exposure,
and 3) urine to determine the absorbed dose.
     The concentration of pesticide in the air in the worker's
breathing zone was determined by attaching to the worker's belt a
battery-powered pump with a known flow rate. An inlet tube containing the appropriate trapping medium was attached to the pump
with a length of Tygon tubing. The inlet tube was then attached
to the worker's collar. The total time that the pump was on was
recorded. Since the flow rate through the pump was known, the
volume of air drawn through the pump could be calculated. The
amount of pesticide on the trapping medium divided by the volume
of air pulled through the resin gives the concentration of pesticide in the air.
     Analysis of gauze or denim patches of known area attached to
clothing near bare skin areas allowed us to estimate the exposure
per unit area for that skin. Estimates of the area of bare skin
based on photographs of the workers and information from Durham
and Wolfe (1962) enabled us to estimate the amount of pesticide
deposited on the skin.
     In the case of picloram and the phenoxy compounds, analysis
of samples from total urine excreted each 24 h enabled us to
determine the amount of absorbed dose. It has been shown
(Matsumura, 1970; Gehring, 1973; and Sauerhoff, 1977) that both
2,4-D and 2,4,5-T are excreted in the urine almost quantitatively
within 5 days of being orally ingested; therefore, measuring the
total amount of these compounds excreted in the urine over this
time gives a good measurement of absorbed dose.
     It is realized that the pharmacokinetics governing absorption
and excretion rates for many pesticides have not been fully evaluated. This fact should not automatically release the
researcher conducting applicator exposure measurements from any
obligations to attempt to gather information regarding the
absorbed dose. Since analysis of urine sometimes reveals the
presence of a degradation product or the parent pesticide itself,
as in the case of the phenoxy herbicides, a researcher is remiss
if he does not at least attempt to locate a definable urinary
component.
     Air was shown to be a very minor route for internal dose.
Even if all the pesticide that a person breathed in were
absorbed, it would still account for only a fraction of 1% of the
absorbed dose as measured by urine analysis.
     We had hoped that there would be a good correlation between

the exposure as determined by analyzing patches and the total absorbed dose as determined by analysis of urine. If the correlation did exist, future exposure studies would be much easier to perform. They could be accomplished in one day, and there would be no need for collection, storage, and transportation of urine samples over a several day period. However, in studies involving 40 workers applying phenoxy herbicides we found a very poor correlation between the amount deposited on patches and the amount excreted in urine.

Since air was an extremely minor pathway to absorbed dose and since there was a very poor correlation between the amount of pesticide on the patches and the amount of pesticide in the urine, we have chosen in our last phenoxy study to analyze only urine samples since they provide a measurement of the absorbed dose whether its entry into the body is via oral ingestion, inhalation, or dermal absorption.

Overcoming Inconsistencies and Minimizing Errors

We have found that there is consistently a wide variation in exposure from worker to worker performing the same duty and also for the same worker performing the same job at two different times. To help overcome the problem of large, inherent variability, large crew sizes are suggested. In our latest 2,4-D forestry ground applicator study the simultaneous monitoring of 20 workers using the same application method has been employed.

In all of our studies where urine has been analyzed, we have collected one total 24-h sample or two 12-h samples over the 5-day period. To determine the amount of the pesticide absorbed, one needs to know both the volume of urine excreted and the concentration of pesticide in that urine. We have observed more than a 10-fold difference in the volume of urine excreted by two different people doing the same type of work. Consequently, trying to determine dose based upon the concentration of a grab sample and a "typical" or "average" excretion volume is unacceptable. Without the total urine sample, two people who have received the same absorbed dose could show a 10-fold difference in concentration of pesticide in their urine and, consequently, in their absorbed dose simply because of dilution.

Conducting the Field Applicator Exposure Studies

The following describes important considerations that we have found to be essential to a well-designed field applicator exposure to pesticide study. First, a detailed protocol critiqued by several knowledgeable researchers is essential. It is nearly impossible to devise a protocol which has too much detail. One must attempt to plan for all of the possible pitfalls which may occur.

Laboratory Techniques. Prior to initiating a field study, all laboratory components must be ready.
1. One must determine that the technicians and equipment can successfully execute the confirmed method that will be used to analyze the actual field samples.

2. It must be demonstrated that a high and repeatable recovery
    percentage is attainable from all samples at several pesti-
    cide concentration levels.
3. One should know the storage and stability characteristics of
    each sample type or have made provisions to guard against
    degradation prior to analysis.
4. Fortification of several samples, a minimum of 10% of the
    total unknowns should be made and these samples interspersed
    among the actual "unknown" samples. These samples should be
    labelled in such a way that the analyst will not know they
    are fortified samples.
5. A second confirmatory column or a different analytical tech-
    nique should be employed to confirm the identity of the ana-
    lyte.
6. If urine or blood samples are to be used to determine the
    absorbed dose, it is helpful to have pre-study information
    which will give the researcher an opportunity to design his
    sample collection scheme in a manner which will be simplest
    to achieve and which will provide the most quantitative
    information. Much has been written with regard to the excre-
    tion rates, quantitative nature of the excretion, and other
    data on the phenoxy herbicides. For other compounds where
    less is known, if the manufacturer can not provide detailed
    information on the excretion data, the researcher may be
    required to conduct a small controlled study, evaluating
    excretion rate, and other important characteristics of the
    compound prior to conducting a full-scale field study. It is
    necessary to know if one should analyze for the parent com-
    pound or a metabolite. If a metabolite is to be analyzed, it
    is necessary to know if its amount can be related to the dose
    of the parent compound.

Crew Parameters. Much of the accuracy and completeness of sample
collection depends upon the human subjects who are being monitored. If one is interested in measuring the dose of crewmembers
carrying out their normal activities, it is important to communicate with them and try to monitor their activities without
interrupting their normal routines.
1. Selection of crewmembers accustomed to performing the opera-
    tion being monitored is mandatory if the researcher's goal is
    to measure "real-world" exposure levels.
2. Crew motivation is a vital component of any applicator expo-
    sure study. Without the interest, concern, and cooperation
    of the field crew, there is little likelihood of conducting
    a meaningful exposure study. It is important for the prin-
    cipal investigator to go to the field, meet the workers, and
    discuss the protocol with them at least once prior to
    actually beginning the study. The crew must be aware of, and
    involved in, the action. One method we have used to help
    motivate crewmembers is to offer them $100 per week for their
    full cooperation in the study which requires them (to the
    best of their ability) to deliver every drop of their urine
    beginning a day before the application through at least four
    days following application. This request may be annoying but
    it is essential. It may require the worker to carry his

urine container to such places as church, on dates, on trips, etc. In emergencies where some urine was lost and it was possible for the worker to estimate the amount lost, he would record this information. When an excessive number of "emergencies" occurred, the $100 was to be withheld. As an enforcement tool each worker was aware that each of his urine samples was being analyzed for creatinine content. We had indicated to the worker that with this measurement we could tell whether he provided us with all of his urine or only a portion of it. Although analysis of urine samples for creatinine does not always provide as quantitative tool as desired for documenting the completeness of the urine sample, its use was effective in gaining compliance of the workers.

3. It is necessary to be knowledgeable about the applicator history of the crewmembers involved. If they have been applying the pesticide of concern in weeks prior to conducting the test, the workers may enter the test with a positive background level. For that reason it is always essential to take pre-application day urine or blood samples to establish the quantity of absorbed dose more clearly.

4. Crewmembers must be fully informed and knowledgeable concerning how to take the sample, when to begin collection, how to store the sample, the numbering scheme employed and how to deliver the sample to the center for storing and processing.

5. Prior to participating in the study, the workers should sign consent forms, which in writing explains to them the intent of the study, how it is to be carried out, and the fact that they may quit at any time. In no case should the study require the worker to become more heavily exposed to pesticide than he ordinarily does.

On-Site Requirements. In collecting the samples, a well-planned strategy must provide for supplies and equipment as well as storage, handling, and shipping of the samples.

1. The collection site should have adequate cooler space for storing samples. In addition, bench space is necessary for weighing urine samples, taking aliquots for shipment to the analytical laboratory, etc.

2. It is important that one of the field members be in charge of recording starting and stopping times and for calling off the operation if in violation of wind or temperature conditions.

3. Strict adherence should be made to the protocol. When irregularities occur, the study should continue but extensive notes should be made. Our studies have indicated that considerably more exposure occurs to workers when irregularities such as malfunctioning equipment occur.

4. A photo of each field worker in his application attire is a must. These photos are especially helpful in estimating the amount of bare skin exposed, type of shirt, gloves, boots, and other clothing worn.

5. Fortification of samples in the field is as important, or perhaps more so, than those in the laboratory. Field for-

tification of urine samples with known amounts of the pesticide in question provides the researcher with an insurance
policy. If the samples get temporarily lost in transit, get
warmer than the protocol allows, or if excessive time
elapses before analysis, meaningful data can still be
obtained since presumably the fortified samples will have
undergone the same history as the actual field unknowns. The
urine used for fortification should be from a sample that was
collected the day prior to spraying to insure low chemical
background. Labelling of the field fortified samples should
be done in a manner that the chemist in the laboratory can
not differentiate between the unknown and the fortified
sample at the time of analysis.

6.   Use of pre-printed stick-on labels prepared in the laboratory
     but attached to the containers in the field greatly facili-
     tate record keeping and sample collection. Even then some-
     times problems occur.

7.   Extensive notes should be taken in the following areas: wind
     and climatic conditions, duration of study, kind and amounts
     of material used, type of equipment used, all application
     parameters (nozzle size and type, height above canopy if
     aerial) and, as mentioned earlier, all irregularities with
     regard to the application.

Follow-up Responsibilities. Since the field crews play such a
vital role in a successful field applicator exposure study, it is
important that the researcher find the time to share his results
with the field crew. Rapid sample analysis will result in more
accurate analyses and aid in rapid publication of the results.
It is important that the facts derived from study be relayed to
the scientific community through journal publication. The data
should be reported in a clear and uniform manner to allow comparison with other published studies. In addition, the results
should be presented to the worker in the field in a manner he can
understand. Newspapers, television, or farm magazines can be
effectively used.

Observations on Results From Our Studies. (For more complete
data, consult the Related Literature.) In both a 2,4,5-T and a
2,4-D applicator exposure study some of the workers entered the
study with low but positive levels of the phenoxy compound in
their urine. It has been shown that contaminated gloves and
footwear can serve as a continuing exposure source. In surveys
conducted with many forestry applicators it has been revealed
that they routinely shower and change clothes daily after working with herbicides in the forest; however, when asked whether
they used the same boots and gloves, almost invariably the reply
was that they did wear the same boots and sometimes even the same
gloves even when not using chemicals. Other researchers have
found that lower body parts may be exposed to high pesticide
levels. As an example studies by Nigg and Stamper (1983) have
shown that the legs and feet are the most heavily exposed body
parts. Thus, it would not be suprising that boots were heavily
contaminated.

For many crewmembers, in addition to the exposure occurring during normal application duties significant exposure and consequent absorbed dose occurs during equipment repair and cleaning. Evidence for this type of re-exposure becomes evident when one compares the urine excretion pattern from a normal one-time exposure (Figure 1) with that of a crewmember, who presumably received continued re-exposure for several days following herbicide application (Lavy and Mattice, 1984) (Figure 2). Since analysis of our total urine excretion patterns reveals that workers routinely receive inadvertent exposure at times in addition to the application day, it is imperative that total urine be collected if one is interested in obtaining quantitative measurements of the total absorbed dose.

Our results in the 2,4,5-T study have shown that mixers of pesticide concentrates and backpack sprayers who routinely walk through the treated area receive the highest absorbed dose. Flagmen for the helicopter crews and crew supervisors absorbed lower amounts than the mixers and backpack sprayers. Aerial application crews appeared to have lower absorbed doses than backpack or mist blower crews. The absorbed dose for the crewmembers ranged from 0.001 mg/kg for the helicopter flagmen to 0.062 mg/kg for the mixers of the concentrates (Lavy et al., 1980).

Results from our study on helicopter-applied 2,4-D conducted in the Pacific Northwest showed that pilots and batchmen received the highest absorbed dose followed by mechanics, supervisors, and observers. The observers were stationed 200 to 500 feet from the heliport.

Applicators of pesticides do receive an absorbed dose. The important question is whether or not this absorbed dose is dangerous. We have calculated margin of safety (MOS) values for our studies in order to answer the question. We have used worst case data (i.e. worker with the highest absorbed dose); thus, MOS values for the typical worker will probably be greater.

A value of 20 mg/kg 2,4,5-T has been ascribed by EPA, in their Position Document 1 on 2,4,5-T as used in the RPAR process, as the No Observed Effect Level (NOEL). The scientific advisory panel on 2,4-D set a value of 24 mg/kg as NOEL (Hall, 1980). Levels for both of these compounds are for teratogenicity, the most sensitive of the health effect tests in use. By dividing the absorbed dose data (obtained by analyzing the total urine excreted on the day of the application plus the next four days) into the appropriate NOEL, the MOS value is obtained. These values for the workers wearing normal clothing in the 2,4-D study are as follows: pilots and batchmen 1200; mechanics 4400; supervisors 10,000; and observers 49,000. Thus, none of the workers appear to be receiving an absorbed dose even approaching a health threatening level. The observers in the 2,4-D study were purposely added to the study to allow a measurement of the absorbed dose occurring to those nearby but not involved with the spray operation.

Normal clothing afforded a high level of protection to the workers as determined by analyzing patches attached both outside and inside their normal clothing. However, since some compounds

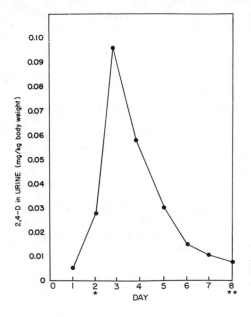

★ Treatment I - Ordinary precautions observed

★★ Treatment 2 - Special precautions observed

Figure 1.   Urinary excretion pattern for a one-time exposure to
2,4-D.

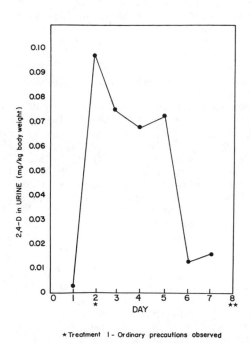

* Treatment I - Ordinary precautions observed

★★Treatment 2 - Special precautions observed

Figure 2. Urinary excretion pattern for a person being re-exposed to 2,4-D after initial exposure.

are considerably more toxic to humans than are the phenoxy herbicides, when applying these compounds protective clothing may be
necessary. Researchers have a responsibility to choose comfortable, inexpensive clothing or devices to protect the worker. If
practical clothing is not provided, more than likely it will not
be worn by the worker unless constant enforcement is made. Some
protective clothing, if worn in the South in the summer, will
cause severe heat problems for the workers.

The use of closed systems is effective in decreasing worker
exposure. Use of closed systems was common for aerial applicators using the more toxic methyl parathion. It was interesting
that hand mixing and application was more common when compounds
with lower toxicity were being used.

A well-designed applicator exposure study can provide information on the extent of the absorbed dose people applying the
pesticide are receiving. Our studies have shown that people
applying pesticides do receive an absorbed dose, and differing
amounts of dose are associated with different application techniques. We have found no case where a worker has received a dose
near a level that causes effects to be observed in laboratory
animals. If an extremely toxic chemical is being used, the
absorbed dose can be reduced by use of protective clothing and
also by the use of closed systems.

Nontechnical Summary

Through these studies we have acquired considerable data on human
exposure as well as experience in designing and conducting research to
monitor real-life exposure of pesticide applicators. Exposure is
relevant to human health only in relation to the dose taken into the
body, its toxicity, and the rate of excretion. In our studies we have
monitored no group nor individual whose dose approaches a level which
could affect human health. Our studies have shown that exposure and
dose are influenced materially by human attire and habits, type and
function of equipment, and safety precautions such as protective
clothing or washing soon after exposure to a concentrate.

Acknowledgments

The authors appreciate the assistance of Martha Davis in
preparing this paper.

Literature Cited

Durham, W.F.; Wolfe, H.R. Bulletin of World Health Organization,
     1962, 26, 75-91.
Matsumura, A. Sangyo Igaku 1970, 12, 446-51.
Gehring, P.J.; Kramer, C.G.; Schwetz, B.A.; Rose, J.Q.; Rowe, V.K.
     Toxicol. and Appl. Pharmacol. 1973, 26, 352-61.
Sauerhoff, M.W.; Braun, W.H.; Blau, G.E.; Gehring, P.J.
     Toxicology 1977, 8, 3-11.
Nigg, H.N.; Stamper, J.H. Chemosphere, 1983, 12(2), 209-215.

Lavy, T.L.; Mattice, J.D. Project Completion Report to United
   States Department of Agriculture on Exposure of Forestry
   Applicators Using Herbicide Formulations Containing 2,4-D,
   2,4-DP (dichlorprop) or Picloram in Non-Aerial Applications,
   Spring and Summer, 1982. 1984, in press.
Lavy, T.L.; Shepard, J.S.; Mattice, J.D. Journal of Agriculture
   and Food Chemistry, 1980, 28, 626-30.
Hall, J.F. letter to the U.S. Environmental Protection Agency
   dated 14 Nov. 1980, p. 6, in Lavy, T.L., "Determination of
   2,4-D Exposure Received by Forestry Applicators," project
   completion report submitted to the National Forest Products
   Association, Washington, D.C., 1980.

Related Literature

Flynn, R.R. Masters Thesis, University of Arkansas, Fayetteville,
   1983.
Forbess, R.C.; Talbert, R.E.; Lavy, T.L.; Morris, J.P.
   "Evaluation of Paraquat Use and Applicator Exposure in Grape
   Vineyards," project completion report to the Southern Region
   Pesticide Impact Assessment Program, Washington, D.C., 1981.
Lavy, T.L. Project Completion Report to Nation Forest Products
   Association on Determination of 2,4-D Exposure Received by
   Forestry Applicators, Spring, 1980.
Lavy, T.L.; Mattice, J.D.; Flynn, R.R. Special Technical Testing
   Publication 795, American Society for Testing and Materials,
   1983, 60-74.
Lavy, T.L.; Mattice, J.D. In "Chemical and Biological Controls in
   Forestry"; Garner, Willa Y.; Harvey, John, Jr., Eds.; 1983,
   319-330.
Lavy, T.L.; Walstad, J.D.; Flynn, R.R.; Mattice, J.D. Journal of
   Agriculture and Food Chemistry, 1982, 30, 375-81.
Leng, M.L.; Lavy, T.L.; Ramsey, J.C.; Braun, W.H. "Review of
   Studies with 2,4,5-T in Humans Including Applicators under
   Field Conditions," Paper presented at the American Chemical
   Society Symposium on Worker Exposure, Washington, D.C., 1981.
Lincoln, C.; Lavy, T. "EPN Usage as a Cotton Insecticide," pro-
   ject completion report to the Southern Region Pesticide
   Impact Assessment Program, Washington, D.C., 1981.
Roeth, F.W.; Lavy, T.L.; Burnside, O.C. Weed Science, 1969, 17,
   202-05.

RECEIVED September 25, 1984

EXPOSURE STUDIES
WITH SPECIFIC CHEMICALS

Methyl Parathion Residue in Contaminated Fabrics after Laundering

JOAN LAUGHLIN, CAROL EASLEY, and ROGER E. GOLD

University of Nebraska, Lincoln, NE 68583-0802

Denim fabrics of cotton and cotton-polyester were contaminated with methyl parathion (MeP) in emulsifiable
concentrate, wettable powder, and encapsulated formulations, and then laundered. After laundering at 60°C,
40°C, and 30°C, the fabrics were analyzed for residue
by gas chromatography. A 1.25% concentration or 54%
a.i. were used to contaminate fabrics. Phosphate,
carbonate, heavy duty liquid, and AATCC Standard 124
detergents were used at 0.3 g/150 ml for powders and
0.4 ml/150 ml for liquids. Emulsifiable concentrate
was most difficult to remove. Statistical homogeneity
was found among the detergents. No differences were
found between 60°C and 49°C water washing, but 30°C
produced lower removal. The undiluted (54% concentrate) was almost impossible to remove by laundering.

Limiting or reducing exposure of agricultural workers during mixing,
handling and application of pesticides has increased in importance
with the recent shifts in pesticide use from organochlorines to higher toxicity organophosphates. Wolfe (1) established that the
principal route of pesticide intake into the human body is dermal
ingestion rather than oral or respiratory ingestion. Thus, attention
has focused on using protective systems or clothing to protect the
skin to minimize dermal absorption. OSHA Standard 1919.267a (2)
suggested that protective clothing include a "washable fabric."
Matthews (3) describes minimum protective clothing as durable cotton
overalls, a long-sleeved shirt, and trousers. The recommendations
for laundering include hot water washing with soap or detergent
(3, 4). The National Institute for Occupational Safety and Health
(5) recommends laundering in a pH 10 solution. Hayes (6) recommends
use of soap, detergent, or washing soda. No research is cited to
support these recommendations.

Refurbishment is an essential and critical part of continued

0097-6156/85/0273-0177$06.00/0
© 1985 American Chemical Society

safety. Completeness of pesticide removal in laundering is essential
if the garment is to be worn again. As the concentration of active
ingredient in the pesticide increases, the success of laundering in
reducing the pesticide residues in the fabric decreases. Multiple
washings help decrease the amount of pesticide residue (7-9). The
Federal Task Group on Occupational Exposure to Pesticides (2) requires that "all protective clothing shall be thoroughly washed after
each day's use.....the clothing shall be adequately cleaned before
it is passed on."

Recent work has shown that, once contaminated, usual textile
items in pesticide applicators' wardrobes are difficult to decontaminate through household laundering procedures currently in use
(10-16). These researchers found that laundering greatly reduces
the amount of pesticide residues present. But Finley and co-workers
found that even three launderings were not effective in removing all
residue. Bioassay has shown that residues remaining after repeated
launderings were biologically active (17). Recommendations have been
made that hot water temperature of at least 60°C be used for laundering pesticide workers' clothing.

Applehans (18) lists several factors that increase the rate of
organophosphate pesticide degradation: temperature of 32°C or more,
a basic pH, organic compounds in the soil, and activity of micro-
organisms. Laundering aids or practices that correspond with these
factors can be established.

The usual processes of soiling and the resultant mechanisms of
soil removal from textile substrates are complicated by the chemical
nature of pesticides as soil. Generally, soiling depends upon the
chemical nature of the textile; the characteristics (geometry) of
the fiber, yarn, and fabric; the chemical treatments of the textile;
and the conditions of textile use (19). Soil can be particulate or
liquid and of an oil base or a water base. The mechanisms of enhanced soiling, and therefore difficulty in soil removal, include
penetration of the soil (dependent upon surface tension of soil and
fiber, viscosity of the soil, and distance between fibers and
interstices between yarns), entrapment in the structure of the fiber
and(or) in spaces of fibers fractured by the mechanical wear of
laundering during use. Raheel (20) photomicrographed the entrapment
of particulate soil in fiber fractures. Obendorf and Klemash (21)
established, through scanning electron micrographs and x-ray diffrac-
tion analysis, the presence of oily soil in the lumen of cotton and
the folds of cotton's convolutions, and in the capillary spaces
between polyester fibers.

Although several studies have examined the pesticide residue in
garment fabric after laundering (7-16, 22-24) few studies have
explored the relationship of soiling mechanisms and textile geometry
to this particular problem (9, 23).

Problem

The purpose of the study was to determine effective laundering procedures for decontaminating work-weight fabrics. The effect of
fiber composition, pesticide formulation, detergent type, wash
temperature, wash cycle procedures, laundry additives, and pesticide
concentration on pesticide residue remaining after laundering were
examined.

Transfer of the pesticide from contaminated fabric to clean cotton fabric through contamination of the washing equipment to subsequent laundry was also determined.

Methods and Materials

Fabrics. Two denim fabrics of 100% cotton and 50/50 cotton-polyester were used. A catalogue survey showed these fiber contents to be common in men's work clothing. Both fabrics were a 2/1 left-hand twill weave. The cotton and cotton-polyester fabrics had a thread count of 60 x 42 and 65 x 47, respectively. Average weight of both fabrics was 321.4 g/m^2.

Chemicals. Three formulations of methyl parathion [0,0-dimethyl 0-p-nitrophenyl phosphorothioate (MeP)] were used to contaminate the fabrics: 1) emulsifiable concentrate (EC); 2) encapsulated (ENC); 3) wettable powder (WP). The active ingredient (a.i.) present in the three formulations was analyzed to insure that actual percent a.i. agreed with label specifications. Analyses of the a.i. in each formulations were 95% to 120% of the labeled amounts (25). Based on these analyses a 1.25% concentration solution of MeP, a common concentration for agricultural application, was prepared from each formulation by adding distilled water. For the work done with full strength pesticide, an emulsifiable concentrate formulation of methyl parathion, 54.0% a.i., was used to contaminate the fabrics.

Contamination of Fabric. Denim fabric swatches were contaminated by pipetting one ml of MeP solution onto the fabric. During the contamination process, a magnetic stirrer provided uniform agitation of the solution. Swatches were supported horizontally during contamination and drying.

Laundry Process. Fabric swatches were individually laundered in stainless steel canisters of an Atlas Launder-Ometer (model B5), using a modified AATCC test method 61-1980 (26). Constant temperature of the Launder-Ometer water bath was maintained. At the end of each cycle, water was decanted from the canisters. Additional water of the specified temperature was then added for the subsequent cycle. Following completion of the laundry process, the fabric swatches were air-dried and then retained in glass for extraction.

Extraction Procedures. To extract the MeP, 150 ml glass-distilled acetone was added to each jar containing a laundered swatch. The jar was shaken for one hour at 170 revolutions per minute, and the acetone extract was decanted and replaced by an additional 150 ml acetone for a second hour of shaking. The fabric swatch was removed at the end of the two-hour period, and the two extracts were combined.

Gas Chromatographic Procedures. Extracts were analyzed by means of a Hewlett-Packard gas chromatograph, model 5850A, with a nitrogen-phosphorus I.D. packed with 3% OV-25 on 100-120 mesh chromosorb W HP. The column temperature was 213°C, that of the inlet was 217°C, and the

detector was 300°C. Nitrogen carrier gas flow was 21.5 cc/minute,
air flow was 50 cc/minute, and hydrogen was 3 cc/minute. Replicated
injections of 1.06 µl were made from each sample solution for
calibration.

Bioassays. Biological assays with Blattella germanica (L) (German
cockroaches) biotype: Orlando normal were performed to assess biological activity. Trials were conducted in environmental chambers
at 30°C and 10-20% R. H. Ten adult males were placed on each of the
treated fabrics, dorsum up. The cockroach mortality was recorded
after 24 and 48 hours.

Statistical Analysis. Differences in the amounts of MeP (ng/cm^2)
between the control and laundered swatches were expressed in percentages of insecticide residue remaining. Statistical differences
were tested with Factorial Experimental ANOVA, Least Significant
Means, and Duncan's Multiple Range Test.

Experimental

The purpose of this study was to determine the effects of fiber
composition, MeP formulations, and selected laundry procedures on
removing MeP residues from contaminated fabrics and to determine
whether residues are transferred in laundry.

Laundry Procedures. Four laundry procedures were examined for MeP
residue remaining after one laundering.

1. Pre-rinse: Each contaminated swatch was pre-rinsed for two
   minutes in warm water at 49°C, then laundered in a 12- minute hot
   water (60°C) phosphate detergent wash, and two warm water rinses
   (49°C), three minutes and five minutes, respectively. The
   phosphate detergent selected was AATCC Standard Detergent 124, a
   12% phosphate detergent used in textile research.
2. Phosphate detergent wash (Det.): Same as described for the pre-
   rinse, with the omission of the pre-rinse cycle.
3. Phosphate detergent wash plus ammonia laundry additive (Det. +
   NH$_3$): Same as the phosphate detergent wash with the addition
   of ammonia laundry additive (3.5%-4% ammonia concentration) in
   the wash cycle.
4. Phosphate detergent wash plus bleach laundry additive (Det. +
   NaOCl): Same as described for the phosphate detergent wash with
   the addition of liquid chlorine bleach (5.25% sodium hypochlor-
   ite) laundry additive in the wash cycle.

Contaminated swatches that were pre-rinsed were placed individually
in 500-ml glass jars with distilled water and agitated on an
Eberbach mechanical shaker to simulate the pre-rinsing cycle of an
automatic washing machine.

Contamination of the Fabric Before and After Laundry. Estimating
the extent to which fabrics had been initially contaminated was
necessary for comparison with post-laundry residue levels (Table 1).
Contaminated (control) fabric swatches for each fabric and formula-

tion were used as an indicator of initial contamination and as a baseline (100%) for percentage residue after laundering calculations.

Transfer of Contamination in Laundry. Sustained transfer occurred when a clean fabric was laundered in equipment that had been used to wash contaminated fabric. The transfer fabric was an all cotton batiste of plain weave construction. These fabric swatches (8 x 8 cm) were subjected to one complete laundering cycle immediately after the contaminated fabrics had been through one wash and two rinse cycles.

That is, following completion of the laundering process, the contaminated denim fabric swatch was removed, the rinse water decanted, and a clean cotton transfer fabric added to each canister along with 150 ml of phosphate detergent solution. Warm water (49°C) was used for the wash and two rinse cycles. After laundering, the transfer fabric was air-dried and retained in glass for solvent extraction.

Biological Assays of Fabric. Blattella germanica (L.) (German cockroaches) biotype: Orlando normal were used to determine if insecticide residues present in the laundered contaminated fabrics and the laundered transfer fabrics were biologically active. All trials were conducted in environmental chambers at 30°C and 10-20% R. H. Cockroaches were anesthetized with CO_2, after which ten adult males were placed on each of the fabrics, dorsum up. Cockroaches recovered within five min and actively sought the confines of the petri dish barrier. The cockroaches were held on the swatches for 24 h and mortalities were recorded.

Detergents and Wash Temperatures. The purpose of this phase of the study was to determine whether commercially available detergents were as effective in pesticide residue removal when used in washing procedures at "hot," "warm," and "cold" water temperatures. The important and unique contribution of this study was the close duplication of in-home laundry procedures, with commerically available detergents and common laundering temperatures. Contaminated swatches were laboratory-laundered in a 60°C (hot) wash/49°C (warm) rinse; 49°C (warm) wash/49°C (warm) rinse; or 30°C (cold) wash/30°C (cold) rinse water temperature using one of four laundry detergents. Three commercially available detergents were selected to represent principal detergent categories: phosphate, carbonate, heavy duty liquid, and a high (12%) phosphate detergent (AATCC 124). The powdered detergents were used at 0.3 g/150 ml, and the heavy duty liquid at 0.4 ml/150 ml.

Pesticide Concentration Levels. The purpose of this experiment was to determine completeness of residue removal during laundering when a range of concentration levels had been used to contaminate denim fabric. Five concentrations of MeP EC were prepared as contaminants: 0.25%, 0.5%, 1%, 2% and 54% (undiluted). Fabric swatches were laundered through one cycle: a 60°C wash and two 49°C rinses. All procedures were as previously described.

Multiple Launderings. Fabric swatches were contaminated with 1.25%

a.i. (field strength) or 54% a.i. (undiluted) MeP EC. Contaminated
swatches were individually laundered one through ten complete laundry
cycles. A 49°C wash and rinse water temperature were used as this
combination was most frequently selected by consumers (27). Other
procedures were as earlier described.

Results and Discussion

Analysis of variance (ANOVA) comparing the degree of contamination
between fabrics and formulations showed no significant difference
(F=1.601, d.f.=5,12), indicating that both fabrics initially retained like amounts of MeP. Comparisons of fabric contamination
after laundry were calculated to ascertain the amounts of MeP remaining after the laundry process.

Residue Remaining After Laundering. The laundry process removed a
mean of 80% to 99% MeP (Table I). Residues were lower for encapsulated (ENC) and wettable powder (WP) formulations, with ranges of
1% to 7% MeP residue. Emulsifiable concentrate (EC) MeP residues
were higher, ranging from 12% to 20%, indicating that EC formulation
apparently was more difficult to remove.

Table I. MeP Residues after Laundering

Treatment	Pre-rinse %	Det. %	Det. + NH_3 %	Det. + NaOCl %
EC-C	12.2	16.5	19.4	11.2
EC-C/P	11.8	15.4	16.3	13.7
ENC-C	2.6	1.9	2.1	2.2
ENC-C/P	2.1	3.2	2.5	2.1
WP-C	0.9	6.7	6.4	6.2
WP-C/P	0.1	4.3	3.7	3.7

Pre-rinsing proved to be effective when fabric and formulation
were considered, that is, percentages of MeP residue were generally
lower than for the other laundry procedures. MeP residue was significantly lower (P $\leq$ 0.05) when the wash cycle was the first aqueous
solution, than when the pre-rinse cycle was the initial aqueous
solution. This significant finding could have resulted from assistance of detergent or detergent plus additive. MeP residue removal
during the washing cycle may be partially attributed to the
alkalinity (pH 9.7) of the phosphate detergent, since MeP is hydro-
lyzed to 4-nitrophenol in an alkaline medium (10).

Differences Attributable to Fabric and Formulation. Although it was
observed that the EC formulation was more difficult to remove from
both fabrics than the ENC or WP formulations, fiber content of
fabrics made no difference in the completeness of MeP residue
removal (Table II). It was initially suspected that since EC formulations are oil-based, there might be an affinity for oleophilic
polyester fibers, although no significant difference between fiber
content was shown based on gas chromatographic analysis.
       Significant differences (P $\leq$ .01) in the MeP residue after
laundering were found among the three formulations; therefore,

Table II. MeP in Contaminated Fabrics Before and after
Laundering and MeP in Transfer Fabrics after Laundering

Treatment	After Laundry X mg/cm^2	Transfer Fabric X ng/cm^2	Treatment	After Laundry X mg/cm^2	Transfer Fabric X ng/cm^2
EC-Cotton			EC-Cotton/Polyester		
Before Laundry (0.62/mg/cm^2)			Before Laundry (0.59 mg/cm^2)		
Pre-rinse	0.08	4.54	Pre-rinse	0.02	4.07
Det.	0.09	4.55	Det.	0.07	5.92
Det. + NH	0.00	5.14	Det. + NH	0.03	5.36
Det. + NaOCl	0.08	4.95	Det. + NaOCl	0.07	3.58
ENC-Cotton			ENC-Cotton/Polyester		
Before Laundry (0.59 mg/cm^2)			Before Laundry (0.59 mg/cm^2)		
Pre-rinse	0.00	5.22	Pre-rinse	0.00	5.31
Det.	0.02	10.64	Det.	0.01	5.44
Det. + NH	0.02	6.24	Det. + NH	0.01	5.44
Det. + NaOCl	0.04	5.81	Det. + NaOCl	0.02	5.85
WP-Cotton/Polyester			WP-Cotton/Polyester		
Before Laundry (0.66 mg/cm^2)			Before Laundry (0.84 mg/cm^2)		
Pre-rinse	0.00	5.24	Pre-rinse	0.01	13.00
Det.	0.05	9.41	Det.	0.08	10.56
Det. + NH	0.05	9.88	Det. + NH	0.06	11.20
Det. + NaOCl	0.04	7.26	Det. + NaOCl	0.06	9.38

statistical partitioning was done to identify where specific differences occurred. Partitioning revealed that the cause of differences
among formulations was the higher percent of EC residue, indicating
difficulty in removal. The ENC formulation was most consistently and
effectively removed. The WP formulation was also easily removed; but
with more variability.

Pesticide Transfer through Laundry. The laboratory laundry equipment
had retained MeP such that the cotton transfer fabric washed through
a full cycle immediately following the laundering of the contaminated
denim fabric retained 3.58 ng/cm^2 to 13.00 ng/cm^2 MeP (Table II).
There was a significant correlation (r=0.63, d.f.=70, p $\leq$ 0.01) between the amount of MeP on the contaminated denim fabric before
laundering and the amount of MeP on the transfer fabric after laundering in contaminated equipment. A negative correlation (r=0.26,
d.f.=70, p $\leq$ 0.05) was found between the amount of MeP on the laundered contaminated denim fabric and the laundered transfer fabric.
Thus, a relationship was observed between the amount of MeP introduced by contaminated denim fabric and the amount of residue in the
transfer fabric. The percentage of MeP retained in the transfer
fabric after laundering ranged from 0.0061 to 0.00181% of contamination. There were no differences attributable to the fiber content
of contaminated denim and in washing the contaminated denim fabric.
Significant differences in the amount of MeP transferred were found
among the three formulations (F=14.46; d.f.=5,65, p $\leq$ 0.01).
Duncan's Multiple Range Test showed ENC and EC were similar, but
different from WP. This high transfer of WP MeP may be attributable
to the particulate nature of the formulation, which may be left

behind in the washing apparatus or lodged in the interstitial spaces
of the fabric or yarn.

Detergents. The four detergents were similar in MeP residue remaining after laundering (F=0.5919; d.f.=3,72, p=0.6263). The MeP
residues after laundering with AATCC 124% detergent were 47.3% of
contamination at 30°C, 26.6% of contamination at 49°C, and 20.6% of
contamination at 60°C. MeP residues after laundering with commercial
phosphate detergent ranged from 51.5% to 24.3% of orginal contamination; for carbonate detergent, residues ranged from 51.1% to 27.9% of
contamination; and for heavy duty liquid, residues ranged from 50.1%
to 14.9%. Although statistical homogeneity was found among the four
detergents, a definite trend in detergent effectiveness was observed
in that the HDL resulted in lower residue percentages of MeP at both
49°C and 60°C than did the other detergents evaluated.

     Since emulsifiable concentrate formulations are oil-based and
HDL detergents are noted for oil-removing ability, this formulation-
detergent combination may have provided for more complete removal.

     It had been theorized that higher detergent alkalinity would
produce more pesticide removal during laundering (10). In this
laboratory investigation, such was not the case. The pH readings of
the detergent solutions varied from 6.4 for HDL detergent to 10.1
for carbonate detergent. Examination of detergent's effectiveness
in lowering MeP residue raised a question about the alkalinity
theory.

Water Temperatures. There was significant evidence of heterogeneity
between amounts of MeP residues attributable to water temperature.
Mean amounts of MeP residues, across four detergents and two fabrics,
ranged from 24% to 60°C water laundering to 51% in 30°C water washing. Residue after washing in 49°C averaged 29% of contamination.
Statistical contrasts of the data by wash temperature revealed no
significant difference between 60°C and 49°C laundering, while 30°C
laundering resulted in significantly greater residues (p < 0.05).
Bioassays revealed that MeP residues on laundered contaminated denim
fabrics were toxic to 100% of the German cockroaches confined on
these fabrics. Regardless of water temperature or detergent used,
all cockroaches died within 24 hours.

Pesticide Concentration Levels. As anticipated, a linear relationship was found between the initial MeP concentrations and the amounts
of residue remaining following laundry (Table III). The doubling of
concentrations (i.e. 0.25% to 0.5%, 0.5% to 1%, and 1% to 2%)
generally caused decreasing rates of removal.

Table III. Impact of Laundering on Removing Varied
Concentrations of MeP EC from Contaminated Denim Fabric

MeP Concentration	ng/cm Residue		% Residue
0.25%	1.25 +	.48	4.4
0.50%	2.84 +	.46	4.2
1.0%	10.90 +	2.09	8.3
2.0%	65.64 +	6.48	25.3
54.0%	5025.00 +	1179.35	80.5

These findings emphasize the difficulty in removing MeP residues from fabric as the concentration level increases. While
lower-level concentrations were more readily removed, the full
strength or undiluted concentration was particularly difficult to
remove. The fact that less than 20% of the concentrated pesticide
was removed by one laundry cycle indicates that pesticide applicators
need to use extreme caution when working with full-strength chemicals.

Multiple Launderings. Distinct differences can be noted between the
two concentration levels used in this experiment (Table IV). Although the amount of MeP residues generally decreased over ten
launderings, the dissimilarity between 1.25% a.i. and 54% a.i. concentrations emphasized the difficulty in residue removal with
increased pesticide concentration.

The 1.25% concentrate was more completely removed during
laundering. Significant differences ($p \leq .05$) were found between
subsequent wash cycles up to, and including, the third laundry cycle.
After the third cycle, the amount of MeP residues was consistently
less than 1%. But the undiluted 54% concentrate was almost impossible to remove due to retention of MeP in the fabric. Even after ten
cycles, 33.3% of the full-strength (54% a.i.) MeP residue and the
detected residue on the fabric was 2,435 $\pm$ 406.8 g/cm^2. MeP residues
in this range on laundered fabric have been reported as contributing
to the death of an adult man (28).

Table IV. Effects of Multiple Launderings on Residues
in Contaminated Denim Fabric

Laundry Cycle	1.25%		54%	
	ng/cm	% Residue	ng/cm	% Residue
1	29.26 $\pm$ 7.31	18.31	6153 $\pm$ 1029.8	84.21
2	6.36 $\pm$ 3.48	3.98	4780 $\pm$ 336.8	65.42
3	0.83 $\pm$ 0.23	0.58	4355 $\pm$ 482.2	59.60
4	0.56 $\pm$ 0.11	0.35	3746 $\pm$ 244.0	51.27
5	0.47 $\pm$ 0.04	0.30	3634 $\pm$ 216.4	49.73
6	0.48 $\pm$ 0.04	0.30	3326 $\pm$ 434.5	45.52
7	0.43 $\pm$ 0.14	0.27	3617 $\pm$ 933.1	49.50
8	0.40 $\pm$ 0.12	0.25	2789 $\pm$ 344.7	39.17
9	0.44 $\pm$ 0.08	0.27	2608 $\pm$ 442.6	35.69
10	0.59 $\pm$ 0.28	0.37	2435 $\pm$ 406.8	33.32

Nontechnical Summary

Once contaminated usual textile items in pesticide applicators' wardrobes are difficult to decontaminate through laundering procedures
currently in use. The laundering procedures reduced residues to less
than one percent to as much as 20 percent of the original contamination, depending upon MeP formulation. Residues were lower after
laundering when the contamination had been from encapsulated and
wettable powder formulation and were greater for the emulsifiable
concentrate formulation. The nature of the soil, its particulate
make up, or its oil-based emulsion are felt to contribute to limited

effectiveness of laundering, dependent upon water temperature and detergent used.

The percentages of MeP transferred in laundry were miniscule; however, care should be exercised in laundering of pesticide-contaminated clothing in the home. WP formulations may be most easily removed from the original fabric and most readily transferred to the clean fabric due to the particulate nature of their composition. Rinsing the laundry apparatus is recommended. Although the percentage of pesticide transferred by contaminated laundry apparatus may be slight in relation to active ingredient made available in laundry of contaminated clothing, this amount may affect particularly susceptible individuals.

The level of MeP concentration is inversely related to the amount of residue removed through laundry. As a result, higher pesticide concentrations or undiluted chemicals require utmost care in handling. Even after ten multiple launderings, residues of an undiluted MeP contaminant can be readily detected in fabrics, as well as cause mortality to German cockroaches within 24 hours. It is recommended, therefore, that clothing contaminated with high pesticide concentrations be disposed of by burning or burial, as the fabric remains unsafe to the wearer. Fabrics contaminated with lesser MeP concentrations (i.e. field strength) require a minimum of three launderings.

Acknowledgments

This paper was published as Paper Number 7467, Journal Series, Nebraska Agricultural Experiment Station.

Literature Cited

1. Wolfe, H. R.; Durham, W. F.; Armstrong, J. F. Arch. Environ. Health 1967, 14, 622.
2. Occ. Saf. Heal. Stand. 1973, 1910.267a, FR 38.
3. Matthews, G. A. Pesticide Application Methods. New York: Longman Group, Inc., 1979.
4. "Apply Pesticides Correctly," Department of Agriculture and Environmental Protection Agency, 1975, 055-004-0007.
5. "Occupational Exposure During the Manufacture and Formulation of Pesticides. U. S. Department of Health, Education and Welfare (NIOSH), 1978.
6. Hayes, J. Toxicology of Pesticides. Baltimore, Maryland: Williams and Williams Co., 1975.
7. Finley, E. L.; Graves, J. B.; Hewitt, F. W. Bull. Environ. Contam. Toxicol, 1979, 22, 598.
8. Easley, C. B.; Laughlin, J. M.; Gold, R. E. and Schmidt, K. L. Bull. Environ. Contam. Toxicol. 1982, 28, 239.
9. Easter, E. Tex. Chem. Color. 1983, 47, 29.
10. Finley, E. L.; Metcalfe, G. I.; McDermott, F. G.; Graves, J. B.; Schilling, P. E.; Bonner. F. L. Bull. Environ. Contam. Toxicol. 1974, 12, 268.
11. Graves, J. B.; Schilling, P. E.; Baker, F. B. LA Agric. 1975, 19, 4.

12. Finley, E. L.; Graves, J. B.; Summers, T. A.; Schilling, P. E.; Morris, H. F. LA Agr. Expt. Sta. Circ. 1977, 104, 7.

13. Easley, C. B.; Laughlin, J. M.; Gold, R. E.; Tupy. D. R. Bull. Environ. Contam. Toxicol. 1981, 27, 101.

14. Laughlin, J. M.: Easley, C. B.; Gold, R. E.; Tupy, D. Bull. Environ. Contam. Toxicol. 1982, 27, 518.

15. Easley, C. B.; Laughlin, J. M.; Gold, R. E.; Hill, R. M. Bull. Environ. Contam. Toxicol. 1982, 29, 461.

16. Kim, C. J.; Stone, J. F.; Sizer, C. E. Bull. Environ. Contam. Toxicol. 1982, 29, 95.

17. Finley, E. L.; Graves, J. B.; Hewitt, F. W. Bull. Environ. Contam. Toxicol. 1979, 22, 599.

18. Applehans, F. Proc. 3rd Conf. Environ. Chem., Colo. St. Univ., 1974.

19. Hebeish, A.; Waly, A.; Abou-Zeid, N. Y.; El-Alfy, E. Amer. Dye Rept. 1982, 72, 15

20. Raheel, M. Tex. Chem. Color. 1983, 47, 216.

21. Obendorf, S. K.; Klemash, N. A. Tex. Resea. J. 1982, 52, 434.

22. Finley, E. L.; Rogillio, J. R. B. Bull. Environ. Contam. Toxicol. 1969, 4, 343.

23. Easley, C. B.; Laughlin, J. M.; Gold, R. E.; Hill, R. M. Bull. Environ. Contam. Toxicol. 1982, 29, 461.

24. Easley, C. B.; Laughlin, J. M.; Gold, R. E.; Tupy, D. Arch. Environ. Contamin. Toxicol. 1983, 12, 71.

25. Offic. Meth. Anal. of Assoc. Offic. Anal. Chem. 13 ed., Washington, D. C.: Assoc. Office Annal Chem.

26. AATCC Tech. Man., Amer. Assoc. Text. Chem. and Col., 1984, 59, 204.

27. Loveday, R. M. T. M. S. Thesis, University of Nebraska, Lincoln, 1979.

28. Southwick, J. W.; Mecham, H. D.; Cannon, P. M.; Gortatowski, M. J. Proceed. 3rd Conf. Environ. Chem. Human Animal Health, 1974.

RECEIVED August 25, 1984

Pesticide Drift and Quantification from Air and Ground Applications to a Single Orchard Site

G. B. MacCOLLOM, W. W. CURRIER, and G. L. BAUMANN

Vermont Agricultural Experiment Station, University of Vermont, Burlington, VT 05405

Eight applications of carbaryl and/or captan were made by air and ground equipment to an orchard site over a 2-year period. Two climatic parameters were used; calm conditions with temperature inversion, and wind velocities of 3 to 10 KPH with no inversion. Regardless of atmospheric stability, in the presence of an inversion, carbaryl deposits from air application were found at 500 m downwind, and at 300 m in absence of an inversion. Ground application gave deposits no further than 150 m downwind during inversion, and no detectable deposits at 50 m in absence of inversion. Captan applied by air gave detectable deposits 150 m downwind, with an inversion present, whereas ground application resulted in deposits at only 50 m downwind. Percent of total pesticide attributable to drift from both air and gound application is relatively small. In quantification studies deposition was measured from total foliage, bark, fruit, orchard floor, and off-target areas as well as from volatilization.

The drift and deposition of pesticide particulates outside of target areas is a concern of both the public and regulatory agencies. Studies by Currier et al (3) indicated drift residues from aerially applied carbaryl were greater during a temperature inversion. These findings were consistent with the results of Akesson and Yates (1) using air applied sprays on alfalfa and by MacCollom et al (4) using air applied dusts on orchards. That air application is a greater contributor to drift has been implied by numerous investigators. A report by the Council on Environmental Quality entitled "Environmental Trends" anonymous (2) states that two thirds of the insecticides used in agriculture are applied by aircraft, but only 25 to 50% reaches the crop, implying that a large amount is lost through drift.

In the Northeast, a substantial amount of orchard acreage is treated by air. This technique has distinct advantages over ground

0097-6156/85/0273-0189$06.00/0
© 1985 American Chemical Society

equipment during wet weather as reported by MacCollom (2). Ware
et al (6) indicated that ground air blast applications on
alfalfa resulted in greater drift deposits than similar air
application. The applicability of these studies, conducted on a low
growing crop on flat terrain, to sloping orchard terrain with trees
growing from 5 to 9 m in height is unknown.
    Studies were initiated in 1980 to determine drift differences
between air and ground applications, using one orchard location.
Two climatic parameters were used, the presence and absence of a
temperature inversion at the time of application. In 1980, as shown
in Table I, five applications of a carbaryl/captan mixture, were
made and in 1981, three applications of captan. The selection of
carbaryl and captan was based on the need for exposure studies due
to the uncertain registration status of the pesticides at the time
of the studies.

Table I. Air and Ground Application Summary with Prevailing
          Meteorological Conditions, Cornwall, VT

Date	Equipment Used	WV KPH	WD	%RH	Pesticide Used	Temperature Inversion
7/17/80	Air	4.8/9.7	S	80	carbaryl/captan	NO(+0.1°C)
7/24/80	Air	1.6/2.5	calm	68	carbaryl/captan	Yes(-3.6°C)
7/31/80	Ground	1.6/3.2	S	60	carbaryl/captan	Yes(-1.7°C)
8/7/80	Ground	3.2/6.4	S	50	carbaryl/captan	NO(+2.0°C)
8/12/80	Air	3.2/12.9	N	68	carbaryl/captan	NO DIFFERENCE
7/1/81	Air	1.6/3.1	Calm	90	captan	YES(-0.6°C)
7/15/81	Ground	1.6/4.8	NW	44	captan	NO(+1.0°C)
8/10/81	Ground	3.2/4.8	S	75	captan	YES(-2.1°C)

*Temp measured at 9.75 m and 2.45 m above ground level at time of
application difference (T9.75 -T 2/45) given in ( ).

Material and Methods

Site and Application Procedures. The orchard site and air
application equipment were the same as described by Currier (1982).
In 1980, ground applications were made with an Ag-Tech low volume
air blast sprayer, calibrated to deliver 187 1/ha, and in 1981, with
a Kinkelder low volume air blast sprayer calibrated to deliver 94.6
1/ha. From previous studies of MacCollom et al (5) and
Currier (3) it was known that the air application gave a median
droplet size diameter of 100 to 150 µm. Estimation of particle
size, as measured on water sensitive paper, for ground equipment was
75 to 110 µm. Application rates for captan 80W in both years was
3.12(AI) Kg/ha, and for carbaryl 80S, 2.24(AI) kg/ha.
    Drift deposition samplers consisted of 15 cm diameter petri
dishes holding a pre-cleaned film of teflon FEP. Three deposition
samplers were placed at each field sampling location in order to
receive impinging spray components and any subsequent fallout from
our spray operation. The deposition samplers were located at 50,
150, 300 and 500m radians (N, NE, E, SE, S, SW, W, NW) from the
orchard. Previous work by Currier et al (3) had shown that

sampling at 300 m was insufficient to completely define drift parameters. The samplers were placed on one meter stands, just above ground cover, and left uncovered for the duration of the experiment, about three hours. At the conclusion of the experiment dishes were covered and held at -4°C to await analysis. Storage of these samples with known standard deposits show little variation over a 12 week period.

Meteorological Measurements. Detailed meteorological data were taken during each study and during air sampling procedures 24H after application. This information consisted of: wind direction, wind velocity, temperature at 9.75 m and at 2.45 m, R.H., and barometric pressure. Ambient temperatures were measured in the orchard by shielded thermistors placed at 9.75 m and 2.45 m above the ground. Higher temperatures at the 9.75 m level indicated meso-scale temperature inversions. A sensitive hot wire anemometer was used at 6.1 m to measure wind velocity. A Thornthwaite Assoc. instrument indicated wind indicated wind directions. A summary of the prevailing meteorological conditions is shown in Table I.

Analytical Methods. In 1980 where carbaryl/captan were applied in combination, a simultaneous quantitative analysis for the mixture was developed using a Water's system (model M-45 pump, 6K injector and Model 450 variable wavelength detector) high pressure liquid chromatograph system and Hewlett-Packard 3380-A integrator. A 25 cm C_{18} μBondapak (Waters) column eluted with 1.3 ml/min of 70% acetonitrile: 30% H_2O and with the detector set at 205 nm gave good separation and detection of the carbaryl/captan mixture. The elution of the carbaryl in 3.15 min gave a .01 ng detection limit. The elution of captan in 3.96 min gave a 5-10 ng detection limit. Studies in 1981 where only captan was applied utilized the same procedure.

Recovery of deposits on the teflon discs were made by washing the disc in 70% acetonitrile for 30 min. During the course of these studies, a total of 395 carbaryl analyses, and 519 captan analyses were made.

Pesticide Quantification

Tree deposits. Recovery of deposits from the components for fruit, foliage, and bark were estimated by exposure of 5 x 10 cm strips of teflon film placed in tree canopy to mimic tree surfaces. Two sets of four teflon films attached to .95cm diameter wooden dowels were placed in the tops, and at shoulder height in the trees. The dowels were mounted 30.5cm into the canopy on the N, E, S, and W sides of the tree. This procedure was followed for two of the captan applications, one by air on 7/1/81, and the other by ground on 7/15/81. One tree was sampled in the center of the orchard for each application.

Volatilization sampling. One m^3 of air was drawn through Millipore filters (type glass depth A/E) for impingement of airborne particulates greater than 2 microns in diameter. Smaller particulates in the air were then drawn through a C_{18} Sep-pak

(Waters) for retention as well as any volatilized portion in the atmosphere. The air sampling Sep-Pak filter devices were placed 4.9 meters in the air, at 3 locations, one at the orchard and two at predetermined distances downwind. Due to equipment needed, this portion of the study was limited to 3 sampling sites. Total volume of atmosphere above the orchard was determined in m^3 using length, and width of area treated by 9.75 m, the height at which inversion, if present, was measured.

Tree Modeling. Work was initiated in 1983 based in part on a technique by Dr. L. A. Hull of the Pennsylvania State University, Biglerville Laboratory (1982 personal communication), to model the trees at the site of application studies conducted in 1980 and 1981. Using the cultivar McIntosh, 10 trees were measured for height and width within the site. Using a paraboloid of revolution, where volume = $\frac{1}{2}iib^2a$ (b= $\frac{1}{2}$ width, a= height) the total tree volume in m^3 was determined. A hollow cone in tree center, devoid of foliage, was measured, volume determined and substracted from total. Ten 2.83 x 10^4 cm^3 samples (1 ft^3) were collected throughout the tree, and leaves counted and measured for total area in cm^2, using a LI-COR model 3100 area meter. This permitted a determination of total foliar surface/tree. At the same time the 2.83 x 10^4 cm^3 leaf samples were collected, all fruit within the sample were also collected, and surface area ascertained.

Total bark surface of 3 McIntosh trees was determined from 1983 studies, by measuring length and circumference of trunk, branches, and twigs <1 cm in and >.5 cm diameter were measured with calipers and a tape measure. Total bark/tree surface area was determined by geometrical formula for a frustum. Both bark, foliage and leaf surface determinations were made within 10 days of application to minimize growth effects.

Orchard floor and off target drift deposits. The total deposit on the orchard floor was determined by deposition on teflon discs within 15 cm diameter petri dishes. Similarly, off- target deposition, as previously described, was determined by the same technique. Total deposition off-target was ascertained by assigning known values to off-target areas. The values assigned to each area were the average of the amounts in $\mu g/cm^2$ found at the near edge and at the most distant point of the area. The sampling distances of 50, 150, 300 and 500m were used to delineate the areas in either rectangular or triangular blocks.

Discussion

The ability to conduct field research dependent on similar climatic conditions prevailing over a prescribed time frame is extremely difficult. We desired applications be made under 2 climatic parameters, the presence and absence of a temperature inversion. Our premise was that the absence of a temperature inversion was generally associated with wind velocities of 5 to 10 KPH resulting in atmospheric turbulence. Hence, airborne particulates would be expected to mix into the atmosphere giving lesser amounts detectable off-target. Presence of an inversion was generally associated with slight winds (< 4 KPH) with reduced off-target carry and deposition of airborne particulates in proximity to the target area.

Despite careful attention to weather forecasts, never were we able to duplicate weather patterns exactly. On several occasions, after a day's preparation, a shift in wind direction or a sudden shower negated all our efforts.

In 1980, five applications of a carbaryl/captan mixture were used, two by ground and three by air, as indicated in Table I. Analyses of off-target depositions showed that carbaryl consistently drifted further than captan when applied by air (Figure 1). One would expect that the drifting particulates would have both pesticides present, and that levels of each would be detected wherever drift occurred. This unexpected result cannot be readily attributed to sensitivity of the analyses since all samples were well above the sensitivity limits (10 ng for captan and 0.01 ng for carbaryl). The vapor pressure of captan is appreciably lower than that of carbaryl and if volatilization from drifting minute particulates was a factor, captan should have been found in greater quantities than carbaryl.

The presence of a temperature inversion at the time of application resulted in off-target deposition at greater distances and/or in greater amounts than those found from applications made in absence of a temperature inversion. Comparison of two air applications of carbaryl/captan (Figure 1) show that regardless of wind or atmospheric stability carbaryl deposits were found at 500 m off-target downwind during an inversion with deposits 20 times (5.38 μg plate SE-radian) those of deposits (.25 μg/plate E-radian) at 300 m in the absence of an inversion.

A similar air application made in absence of an inversion resulted in carbaryl deposits (2.29 μg S-radian) at a maximum of 300 m and off-target downwind. In no instances was captan deposits detected with the carbaryl deposits found at the furthest off-target sites.

Comparison of two ground carbaryl/captan applications, (Figure 2) showed that in absence of an inversion no off-target deposits were seen, whereas the application during an inversion resulted in maximum off-target downwind deposits of both captan (.62 μg N-radian) and carbaryl (.58 μg N-radian) at 150 m downwind.

In 1981 3 applications of captan were used, 2 by ground, and 1 by air. Comparison of ground applications (Figure 3) showed off-target downwind deposits with detectable levels found at 300 m (4.28 μg SE-radian) in absence of an inversion, and (12.95 μg NE-radian) at 50 m in presence of an inversion. Air application (Figure 3) during an inversion showed no detectable levels beyond 150 m.

In 1981 air samples showed detectable levels of captan in all samples collected 4.9 m above the orchard edge, and that levels persisted for at least 30 minutes following application (Table II).

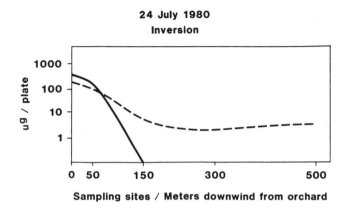

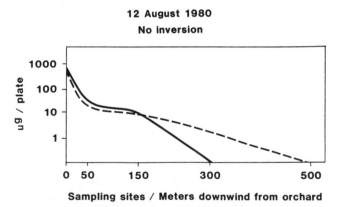

Figure 1. Carbaryl (broken line)/captan (solid line) applications by fixed wing aircraft in presence and absence of a temperature inversion.

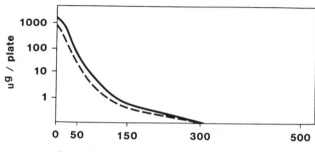

Ground application

31 July 1980
Inversion

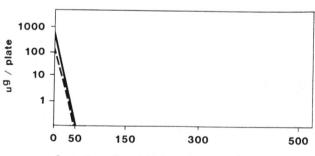

7 August 1980
No inversion

Figure 2. Carbaryl/captan applications by ground equipment in presence and absence of a temperature inversion.

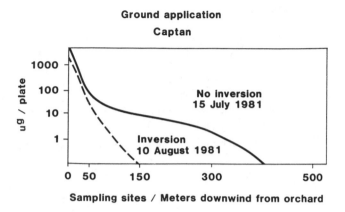

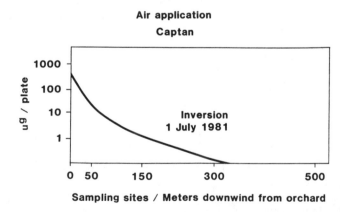

Figure 3.   Comparison of three captan applications, two by ground in presence and absence of a temperature inversion, and one by air with an inversion present.   Key: carbaryl, broken line; and captan, solid line.

Table II.   Atmospheric Levels of Captan (ug/m³) above Orchard
Downwind* Edge 1981

Type Application	Date	Before	During	30 Min After	60 Min After	24 Hrs. After
Air	7/1/81	ND**	50.62	52.36	ND*	ND
Ground	7/15/81	ND	11.21	16.65	T	ND
Ground	8/10/81	ND	3.03	3.66	7.80	ND

*Atmospheric samples also taken @ .5 and 1.0 Km downwind at same
time intervals with no detectable levels on 7/15 and 8/10 and only
trace amounts on 7/1/81.

**ND = Not detected, T = Trace

From these studies it is apparent that more drift occurs from
air application than ground equipment. The presence of a
temperature inversion at the time of application usually results in
greater off-target downwind deposition (regardless of slopes of <2%)
at the study site. The absence of an inversion with slight
turbulence results in reduced downwind drift and less variability in
deposits.

No suitable explanation can be offered to explain the detection
of carbaryl at consistently greater off-target distances than captan
when both were applied in combination by air.

Quantification of the two captan applications was based on means
of values derived for each component. Three McIntosh trees were
modeled for bark surface and 10 McIntosh trees were modeled for
foliage and fruit surfaces. The mean values per tree for each of
the components modeled are given in Table III. The mean deposit on
teflon film placed in one tree for each of the two applications was
1.56 μg/cm² for air, and 3.2 μg cm² for ground application.
These values were used in estimation of captan deposits assigned to
foliar, bark and fruit surfaces as shown in Table IV. The volatile
component was determined from atmospheric levels of captan detected
30 minutes after application as shown in Table II.

Table III.   Mean Values Used in Captan Quantification
Cornwall, VT 1983

AREA TREATED	2.1 HECTARES
NUMBER OF TREES	363
TREE SPACING	6.1 X 9.1 METERS
MEAN CANOPY VOLUME/TREE	51.14 m³
MEAN FOLIAR SURFACE/TREE	2,088,097.8 cm²
MEAN BARK SURFACE/TREE	78967.8 cm²
MEAN FRUIT SURFACE/TREE	21961 cm²
MEAN DEPOSIT OF CAPTAN(GRND)	3.2 μg/cm²
MEAN DEPOSIT OF CAPTAN(AIR)	1.56 μg/cm²

Table IV.   % Recovery from Two Captan Applications to Same
Orchard Site

	AIR 7/1/81	GROUND 7/15/81
FOLIAGE	30.30	31.30
BARK	1.14	1.20
FRUIT	0.32	0.33
FLOOR	18.10	62.40
DRIFT	1.90	2.12
VOLATILES	0.37	0.09
% RECOVERY	52.13	97.46

This preliminary study is based on a number of assumptions and mean values. However, it does show the methodology by which it is possible to quantify a pesticide application. Comparison of amounts (Table IV) attributable to all components except the orchard floor are similar, and account for 34.03% of the air application and 35.04% of the ground. The biggest difference is the amount recovered from the orchard floor. Both applications were made under differing climatic conditions, the air application with a strong temperature inversion, and the ground application made in absence of an inversion. These varying weather conditions might account for some of the differences noted.

Nontechnical Summary

During 1980-81, eight applications of captan and/or carbaryl were made by air and by ground to the same orchard site. Drift of the pesticides from the orchard site was measured by deposition at varying distances up to 500 m in the presence and absence of a temperature inversion. Generally drift was greater during a temperature inversion with air application. Surprisingly, when both pesticides were applied in combination by air, the pesticide with the higher vapor pressure (carbaryl) drifted further. The total amount of pesticide attributable to drift from either air or ground application was relatively small. Over 90% of captan applied by ground was accounted for, whereas slightly over 50% was recovered from air application. The greatest difference between air and ground was the amount recovered from the orchard floor.

Acknowledgments

We are indebted to Alphonse Quesnel of Dustaire, East Middlebury, Vermont and to Barney Hodges of Cornwall Orchards, Cornwall, Vermont, for their cooperation and assistance. This paper was published as Vermont Agricultural Experiment Station Journal Article No. 555.

Literature Cited

1. Akesson, N. B.; Yates, W. C. Annu. Rev. Entomol. 1964, 9, 285-318.
2. "Environmental Trends," Council on Environmental Quality, U.S. Govt. Printing Office, 1981, p. 92.
3. Currier, W. W.; MacCollom, G. B.; Baumann, G. L. J. Econ. Entomol. 1982, 75, 1062-8.
4. MacCollom, G. B.; Johnstone, D. B.; Parker, B. L. Bull. Environ. Contam. Toxicol. 1968, 3, 368-374.
5. MacCollom, G. B.; Gotlieb, A. R.; Calahan, C. L.; Baumann, G. L.; Eddy, D. Ag. Exp. Sta. Bull. 685, Univ. of Vt. 1980.
6. Ware, G. W.; Apple, E. J.; Cahill, W. P.; Gerhardt, P. D.; Frost, K. R. J. Econ. Entomol. 1969, 63, 844-6.

RECEIVED August 28, 1984

Exposure of Applicators and Mixer-Loaders During the Application of Mancozeb by Airplanes, Airblast Sprayers, and Compressed-Air Backpack Sprayers

RALPH O. MUMMA[1], GORDON A. BRANDES[2,3], and CHARLES F. GORDON[2]

[1] Pesticide Research Laboratory and Graduate Study Center, Department of Entomology, Pennsylvania State University, University Park, PA 16802
[2] Rohm and Haas Company, Independence Mall West, Philadelphia, PA 19105

The dermal and inhalation exposure of applicators and mixer-loaders to ethylenebisdithiocarbamate (EBDC) and ethylenethiourea (ETU) was determined during field applications of mancozeb by airplanes in Michigan, Minnesota and Oregon, by airblast sprayers in Ohio and by compressed air sprayers in a home yard setting. Absorbant pads were placed at prescribed locations outside and underneath protective clothing of workers and subsequently analyzed for mancozeb and ETU. Gloves and urine were also analyzed. Exposure was expressed in μg/body area, total μg/hour and total μg/Kg body weight/day. Mixer-loaders were exposed to mancozeb, especially the forearms (from 1125–9402 μg/body area). Pilots were minimumly exposed and their hands were the highest exposed (from 58–1409 μg/body area). Tractor driver-applicators were moderately exposed and again their forearms were highest (from nondetectable–1090 μg/body area). Home gardeners experienced little exposure except for their ankles and thighs (from nondetectable–4290 μg/body area). Protective clothing greatly reduced or eliminated exposure. ETU was usually not detectable. Mancozeb was not detected in the urine. Considerable variability existed between different persons performing the same task.

Persons involved in the application of pesticides have more opportunity to be exposed to the chemical than the average citizen. For consideration of the safety of the workers, it is important to determine just how much exposure is anticipated with each work assignment. It is also important to evaluate the effectiveness of protective clothing and to determine the expected variability of exposure of different persons performing the same task. The method of dispersal of the pesticide and the type of formulation also affects the overall exposure. These data are helpful to regulatory

[3] Current address: Advanced Genetic Sciences, Oakland, CA 94608

agencies to properly evaluate human exposure to a specific pesticide so reasonable guidelines for safe use can be established.

The purpose of this presentation is to describe the results of
field studies of dermal and inhalation exposure of applicators and
mixer-loaders to the fungicide mancozeb (DITHANE® M-45® fungicide,
80% active ingredient wettable powder, a product of Rohm and Haas
Company, Philadelphia, PA 19105, was used in these studies), a
coordination product of zinc ion and manganese ethylenebisdithiocarbamate, and ethylene thiourea (ETU). The latter compound is a
decomposition product of all EBDC's (mancozeb, maneb, metiram,
nabam and zineb) and also is produced from EBDC's as an artifact of
the analytical procedure for ETU.

Materials and Methods

General Conditions. All trials were performed under conditions of
actual commercial crop production or an urban homeyard environment.
Three trials were with fixed-wing aircraft (potato fields in Michigan, Minnesota and Oregon), one with a ground airblast sprayer (a
tomato field in Ohio), and two with a typical home garden compressed air tank sprayer (a homeyard in Ohio).

The subjects of study were three commercial aerial applicator-
pilots, one custom ground sprayer operator, four mixer-loaders, and
two home gardeners. Each trial was replicated twice with each
subject. Cotton gauze pads (10.16 x 10.16 cm) were stapled to subjects' clothing outside and underneath protective clothing at
specific locations (Table I). Cotton gloves were used as samplers
and worn underneath protective gloves for mixer-loaders, tractor
drivers and home gardeners. These gloves were worn by aircraft
pilots without protective gloves. Urine samples were collected
before and after spraying. Respirators with collecting pads (7.01
cm diameter) were used to measure inhalation exposure.

Table I. Positions of Samples Analyzed and Body Part Designation

Position Analyzed	Body Part Designation	Area of body part cm^2 (1,2)
Head	Face	650
Upper chest	Front of neck	150
Upper back	Back of neck	110
Forearms (R+L)	Forearms	1210
Hands (R+L)[a]	Hands	820
Ankles (R+L)	Ankles	560
Thighs (R+L)	Thighs	3482
Respirator (R+L)	Respirator	120

[a] cotton gloves

The exposure pads were removed from the garments and the pads, gloves and urine samples were immediately frozen and shipped with dry ice, by air, to the Pesticide Research Laboratory, Pennsylvania State University. Samples were stored at -20°C until analysis. Samples of the mancozeb formulation used in each test were also sent to the analytical laboratory.

Specific Spray Conditions. The field locations, equipment used and conditions for spraying potato fields with mancozeb by fixed-wing aircraft are presented in Tables II and III. Similar data for application of mancozeb by a ground airblast sprayer (tomatoes) and by a compressed air sprayer (home yard) are given in Tables IV and V respectively.

Table II. Field Locations and Equipment Used For Spraying Potato Fields with Mancozeb by Fixed-Wing Aircraft

Place	Investigators	Spray Equipment	Mixing Equipment
Michigan	Dr. Fred Tschirely Dr. H. Spender Potter	Piper Pawnee Brave, Ag Aircraft	1136 L tank
Minnesota	Dr. Howard L. Bissonette	Ag-Cat 450B Aircraft	1136 L tank
Oregon	Dr. James M. Witt Dr. Frank N. Dost	Cessna Ag-Wagon 300	208 L drum

Table III. Conditions for Spraying Potato Fields with Mancozeb by Fixed-Wing Aircraft

Place	Spray per 0.405 hectare	Rate A.I. per 0.405 hectare	Time of Work Mixer-Loader		Time of Work Pilot-Applicator	
			Rep I	Rep II	Rep I	Rep II
Michigan	15.1 L	725.7 g	9 min	17 min	12 min	15 min
Minnesota	18.9 L	725.7 g	15 min	15 min	30 min	30 min
Oregon	22.7 L	725.7 g	20 min	5 min	25 min	25 min

Table IV. Application of Mancozeb by a Ground Air-Blast Sprayer

---

Place: 4.05 hectare tomato field in Ohio
Investigator: Dr. James Farley
Spray Equipment: 1893 L air blast sprayer
Chemical: mancozeb, 80% wettable powder
Spray Volume: 189.3 L per 0.405 hectare
Rate: 1088 g A.I. per 0.405 hectare
Time of mixer-loader: Rep I = 6 min, Rep II = 6 min
Time of tractor-driver-applicator: Rep I = 20 min, Rep II = 19 min

---

Table V. Application of Mancozeb in a Home Yard With a Compressed
          Air Backpack Sprayer

Place: Urban home yard in Ohio
Investigator: Dr. Charles C. Powell
Spray Equipment: 7.57 L backpack compressed air sprayer
Object of Spray: shrubbery, small trees, flowers, lawn
Chemical: mancozeb, 80% wettable powder
Spray Volume: full coverage to point of run off
Rate: 22.5 mL per 3.785 L water
Time of first subject:
        Test No. 1. 5 min mixing, 20 min spraying
        Test No. 2. 5 min mixing, 11 min spraying
Time of second subject:
        Test No. 1. 5 min mixing, 20 min spraying
        Test No. 2. 5 min mixing, 20 min spraying

Preparation of Samples for Analysis. The cotton gauze pads, both garment and respirator, were prepared for analysis by halving the pads diagonally resulting in a 51.61 cm^2 and a 19.35 cm^2 sample, respectively. The urine samples were thawed and duplicate aliquots of 5 or 10 ml were removed for analysis.

Each glove pair (11 to 18 gm) was minced into pieces of less than 3.22 cm^2. The pieces were thoroughly mixed and a measured aliquot (approximately 2 gm) was analyzed in duplicate.

The freezer controls were prepared by suspending mancozeb formulation from each of the study areas in water by stirring. Aliquots of each solution were applied to control materials which were stored under the same conditions as the samples.

Analysis for Mancozeb. Residues of mancozeb on the cotton gauze pads (garment or respirator), cotton gloves and urine were determined by means of the Keppel procedure (3). Using this analytical procedure, a sample was suspended in 200 ml distilled water in a reaction flask (500 ml three-neck flask). Twenty ml of concentrated hydrochloric acid and 10 ml of freshly prepared stannous chloride reagent were added. By heating the solution at refluxing temperature for 30 minutes the mancozeb was decomposed liberating carbon disulfide (CS_2) which was swept through an absorption train. This closed system consisted of a drying tube filled with carbon dioxide absorbent, a U-shaped drying tube containing 15 ml of lead acetate reagent (0.8 M) to remove any hydrogen sulfide or carbon dioxide gases formed in the refluxing and a U-shaped drying tube with a stopcock opening at the bottom containing 10 ml of CS_2 trapping solution (0.0002 M cupric acetate and 1.0 M diethanolamine). Absorption of the CS_2 gas in the trapping solution resulted in the formation of a yellow complex, cupric N,N-bis(2-hydroxyethyl)dithiocarbamate. The intensity of the color was measured spectrophotometrically at 435 nm.

Analyses were performed using 8 decomposition-distillation apparatuses at a time. Controls were included in each run and consisted of a reagent blank, an untreated control of the same material and approximately the same size as the samples, and a "spiked" control in which a known amount of mancozeb was added to untreated pads or gloves or urine.

Analysis for ETU. Extraction and quantification of samples for ETU generally followed the procedures of Haines and Adler (4) but other references were used (5,6). Modifications in the procedure were performed since gauze pads and urine were analyzed. The cotton gauze pads or glove (sample) were placed in a 250 ml screw-top Erlenmeyer flask with 40 ml methanol. Samples containing double gauze pads required that 60 ml of methanol, rather than 40 ml, be added to the cut-up sample. The flask was sealed with a "polyseal" cap and shaken for 5 min on a wrist shaker. The sample was filtered through a medium grade sintered-glass filter funnel. The residue and flask were rinsed with portions of methanol. The filtrates were combined and made up to 100 ml total volume.

A 40 ml portion was taken and poured onto a column packed with 1 g 60/100 mesh Florisil, 4 g E. Merck Alumina II - III (middle layer), and 1 g Celite 545 (bottom layer). The sample was eluted with 20 ml of methanol and the effluent collected in a 250 ml round-bottom flask. Five ml of water and 3 ml of dimethylformamide were added to this flask and the solution was reduced to 3 ml using a rotary-evaporator with a 50°C water bath.

The contents of the round-bottom flask were transferred to a 25 ml concentration tube. The round-bottom flask was rinsed with several 1 ml portions of DMF to give a total volume of 6 ml in the concentration tube. Distilled 1-bromobutane (0.3 ml, important to redistill), approximately 0.1 g sodium borohydride and 1 ml 20% aqueous potassium hydroxide were added vortexing the sample after the addition of each reagent. The mixture was then let stand at room temperature for 5 min.

Exactly 4 ml of the upper layer was transferred to a pear-shaped 100 ml flask and a drop of concentrated hydrochloric acid was added. The solution was rotary-evaporated to dryness (90°C). The residue was dissolved in 0.5 ml of water, 0.5 ml of 20% aqueous potassium hydroxide, 1 ml of toluene, and then vortexed for 1 min. The toluene layer was removed with a pasteur pipet and placed in a vial for GLC analysis.

A Tracor MT-220 gas chromatograph was used with operating temperatures of: inlet – 230°C, detector – 180°C, and oven – 198°C. Injections (5 µl) were made onto a 10% carbowax 20 M 20% KOH column and swept through by nitrogen at a rate of 68 ml/min. The flame photometric detector was operated in the sulfur mode and flow rates of gasses used were 100 ml/min for hydrogen, 100 ml/min for air, and 10 ml/min for oxygen.

Urine samples were well-mixed and a 5 g aliquot was shaken for 2 min with 50 ml of methanol. The sample was applied to a Florisil column which had been pre-washed with 20 ml methanol. The sample was eluted with an additional 20 ml of methanol. The columns containing the urine samples took 5 hr to elute as opposed to 2 hr for the other samples.

A group of four people was used to complete 15 samples (which included a blank sample, a sample spiked with ethylenethiourea, and a sample spiked with mancozeb) in one day. All glassware used was washed in a "Micro-Clean" solution, rinsed with distilled water, and oven-dried immediately prior to use. To minimize conversion of mancozeb to ETU during analysis samples were worked up continuously from 8:30 a.m. until 10:00 p.m. On most days conversions were less than 1% and even undetectable on some days. Unfortunately on two extremely hot and humid days 3 and 5% conversions were experienced.

Results and Discussion

The amount of mancozeb present in each sample was calculated from the amount of CS_2 produced relative to a standard mancozeb sample. Spiked controls from freshly prepared standard solutions of mancozeb dissolved in EDTA were prepared daily and were run with each set of samples. Laboratory recoveries averaged 91.9% and samples were corrected for recoveries on a daily basis. The lower limit of detection for mancozeb was 10 µg per sample which resulted in an optical density change of 0.01 at 435 nm. Analysis of the cotton gauze freezer controls showed recoveries averaging 88% for low level spikes (20 µg) and 87% for high level spikes (100 µg). The recoveries for urine freezer controls averaged 61% for low level (20 µg) and 77% for high level (100 µg) spikes. The length of freezer storage was 8 months for gauze pads and 3 months for urine samples. Actual sample results were not corrected for freezer recoveries since their time in the freezer varied.

The ETU was quantified in the form of its butylated derivative and had a lower limit of detection of 7 ng. Recoveries averaged

88.6% and samples were corrected for recoveries on a daily basis. ETU is produced in part as an artifact of analysis through decomposition of mancozeb. This artificially produced ETU is reported to be found from 1–10% of the starting mancozeb depending on methods used and conditions. We found if the analyses were carried out in a cool room (airconditioned) and the sample continually worked up, we could average 1.1% conversion of mancozeb to ETU. Hot humid days seemed to increase the percentage conversion of ETU. Redistilling the bromobutane was found to be critical for good derivatization. Samples were corrected for ETU conversion on a daily basis. Freezer recoveries for ETU averaged 44% for a 3 µg spike to 72% for a 15 µg spike with gauze pads, 87–100% for gloves (15–75 µg) and 54 to 93% for urine (3–15 µg). Samples were not corrected for freezer controls.

The total µg per body areas was calculated from the µg/cm^2 determined per pad times the area of the body considered as expressed in Table I (2). The µg/hr was calculated by multiplying the total µg/body area by 60 (minutes) and dividing by the exposure time (minutes). The total µg/Kg body wt/day assumed a spraying day of 6 hours for commercial applicators and one hour for home gardeners and a 60 Kg average body weight.

The exposure of mixer–loaders and pilots during the airplane application of mancozeb to potato fields in Michigan, Minnesota and Oregon is given in Tables VI, VII and VIII. Mixer–loaders were exposed to mancozeb with forearms being most exposed (1125–9402 µg/body area). Pilots experienced very little exposure, but their hands did range from 58 to 1409 µg/body area.

Table IX presents the exposure of persons involved in the ground application of mancozeb by an airblast sprayer to a tomato field in Ohio. Mixer–loaders again experienced exposure to mancozeb with forearms predominating (2856–3485 µg/body area). Tractor driver–applicators did not experience much exposure, but forearms did range from nondetectable to 1090 µg/body area. Home gardeners using a compressed air sprayer in a homeyard setting experienced little exposure to mancozeb (Table X), except for their ankle and thigh pads (nondetectable–4290 µg/body area).

A number of overall generalizations can be made: 1) in all tests protective clothing greatly reduced or eliminated exposure, 2) of the persons examined in these studies mixer–loaders experienced the most exposure, 3) exposure to ETU was generally minimal or not detectable, 4) considerable individual variation in exposure was evident, and 5) no mancozeb was detected in urine.

Nontechnical Summary

The dermal and inhalation exposure of applicators and mixer–loaders to ethylenebisdithiocarbamate and ethylenethiourea (ETU) was determined during field applications of mancozeb by airplanes in Michigan, Minnesota and Oregon, by airblast sprayers in Ohio and by

Table VI. Exposure of Mixer-Loaders and Pilots to Mancozeb and ETU During the Application of Mancozeb by Airplanes in Michigan

	Mancozeb				ETU			
MIXER-LOADERS	Total µg/cm²	Total µg Body Area	Total µg/hr	Total µg/kg Body wt/day	Total µg/cm²	Total µg Body Area	Total µg/hr	Total µg/kg Body wt/day
Patches Outside Clothing								
1 - Face	0.28	182	1210	121	NDR[a]	NDR	NDR	NDR
1 - Neck front	NDR	NDR	NDR	NDR	NDR	NDR	NDR	NDR
1 - Neck back[b]	0.29	31.9	212	21.2	NDR	NDR	NDR	NDR
1 - Forearms[b]	1.19	1440	9590	959	NDR	NDR	NDR	NDR
1 - Respirator[b]	NDR	NDR	NDR	NDR	NDR	NDR	NDR	NDR
2 - Face	0.19	123	436	43.6	NDR	NDR	NDR	NDR
2 - Neck front	0.53	79.5	281	28.1	NDR	NDR	NDR	NDR
2 - Neck back[b]	0.17	18.7	66	6.6	NDR	NDR	NDR	NDR
2 - Forearms[b]	0.93	1125	3971	397	NDR	NDR	NDR	NDR
2 - Respirator[b]	NDR	NDR	NDR	NDR	NDR	NDR	NDR	NDR
Patches Under Clothing								
1 - Face	NDR	NDR	NDR	NDR	NDR	NDR	NDR	NDR
1 - Neck front	0.20	30	200	20.0	NDR	NDR	NDR	NDR
1 - Neck back[b]	0.29	32	212	21.2	NDR	NDR	NDR	NDR
1 - Forearms[b]	NDR	NDR	NDR	NDR	NDR	NDR	NDR	NDR
1 - Hands[bc]	0.085	69.7	464	46.4	NDR	NDR	NDR	NDR
2 - Face	0.20	130	459	45.9	NDR	NDR	NDR	NDR
2 - Neck front	NDR	NDR	NDR	NDR	NDR	NDR	NDR	NDR
2 - Neck back[b]	0.29	31.9	113	11.3	NDR	NDR	NDR	NDR
2 - Forearms[b]	0.82	992	3502	350	NDR	NDR	NDR	NDR
2 - Hands[bc]	0.037	30.3	107	10.7	NDR	NDR	NDR	NDR
Urine (1)(before)	NDR	NDR	NDR	NDR		NDR	NDR	NDR
Urine (1+2)(after)	NDR	NDR	NDR	NDR		NDR	NDR	NDR
Urine (1+2)(+12 hr)	NDR	NDR	NDR	NDR		NDR	NDR	NDR
Urine (1+2)(+24 hr)	NDR	NDR	NDR	NDR		NDR	NDR	NDR

PILOTS	Mancozeb				ETU			
	Total µg/cm²	Total µg Body Area	Total µg/hr	Total µg/kg Body wt/day	Total µg/cm²	Total µg Body Area	Total µg/hr	Total µg/kg Body wt/day
Patches Outside Clothing								
1 - Face	NDR[a]	NDR	NDR	NDR	NDR	NDR	NDR	NDR
1 - Neck front	0.16	24	120	12.0	NDR	NDR	NDR	NDR
1 - Neck back	NDR	NDR	NDR	NDR	NDR	NDR	NDR	NDR
1 - Forearms[b]	0.16	194	968	96.8	NDR	NDR	NDR	NDR
1 - Hands[bc]	0.19	155.6	778	77.8	NDR	NDR	NDR	NDR
2 - Respirator[b]	NDR	NDR	NDR	NDR	NDR	NDR	NDR	NDR
2 - Face	NDR	NDR	NDR	NDR	NDR	NDR	NDR	NDR
2 - Neck front	NDR	NDR	NDR	NDR	NDR	NDR	NDR	NDR
2 - Neck back	NDR	NDR	NDR	NDR	NDR	NDR	NDR	NDR
2 - Forearms[b]	NDR	NDR	NDR	NDR	NDR	NDR	NDR	NDR
2 - Hands[bc]	0.16	130.3	521	52.1	.0023	1.9	7.6	0.76
2 - Respirator[b]	NDR	NDR	NDR	NDR	NDR	NDR	NDR	NDR
Patches Under Clothing								
1 - Face	NDR	NDR	NDR	NDR	NDR	NDR	NDR	NDR
1 - Neck front	0.20	30.2	151	15.1	NDR	NDR	NDR	NDR
1 - Neck back	NDR	NDR	NDR	NDR	NDR	NDR	NDR	NDR
1 - Forearms[b]	NDR	NDR	NDR	NDR	NDR	NDR	NDR	NDR
2 - Face	NDR	NDR	NDR	NDR	NDR	NDR	NDR	NDR
2 - Neck front	NDR	NDR	NDR	NDR	NDR	NDR	NDR	NDR
2 - Neck back	NDR	NDR	NDR	NDR	NDR	NDR	NDR	NDR
2 - Forearms[b]	NDR	NDR	NDR	NDR	NDR	NDR	NDR	NDR
Urine (1)(before)		NDR	NDR	NDR		NDR	NDR	NDR
Urine (1+2)(+12 hr)		NDR	NDR	NDR		NDR	NDR	NDR
Urine (1+2)(+24 hr)		NDR	NDR	NDR		0.2	0.8	0.08

[a] No detectable residue. [b] Value for right and left. [c] Total µg per two gloves.

Table VII. Exposure of Mixer-Loaders and Pilots to Mancozeb and ETU During the Application of Mancozeb by Airplanes in Minnesota

MIXER-LOADERS	Mancozeb				ETU			
	Total μg/cm²	Total μg Body Area	Total μg/hr	Total μg/kg Body wt/day	Total μg/cm²	Total μg Body Area	Total μg/hr	Total μg/kg Body wt/day
Patches Outside Clothing								
1 – Face	0.71	462	1850	185	NDR[a]	NDR	NDR	NDR
1 – Neck front	1.75	263	1050	105	NDR	NDR	NDR	NDR
1 – Neck back[b]	0.20	22.0	88	8.8	NDR	NDR	NDR	NDR
1 – Forearms[b]	3.61	4368	17470	1747	NDR	NDR	NDR	NDR
1 – Respirator[b]	2.62	314.4	1258	125.8	NDR	NDR	NDR	NDR
2 – Face	0.25	163	65.0	6.5	NDR	NDR	NDR	NDR
2 – Neck front	0.39	58.5	234	23.4	NDR	NDR	NDR	NDR
2 – Neck back[b]	0.29	31.9	128	12.8	NDR	NDR	NDR	NDR
2 – Forearms[b]	2.14	2589	10360	1036	NDR	NDR	NDR	NDR
2 – Respirator[b]	2.87	344.4	1378	137.8	NDR	NDR	NDR	NDR
Patches Under Clothing								
1 – Face	0.62	93	372	37.2	NDR	NDR	NDR	NDR
1 – Neck front	0.22	24.2	96.8	9.7	NDR	NDR	NDR	NDR
1 – Neck back[b]	0.47	569	2270	277	NDR	NDR	NDR	NDR
1 – Forearms[b]	0.220	180.6	722.4	72.24	NDR	NDR	NDR	NDR
1 – Hands[bc]	NDR	NDR	NDR	NDR	0.0017	1.4	5.6	0.56
2 – Face	NDR	NDR	NDR	NDR	NDR	NDR	NDR	NDR
2 – Neck front	NDR	NDR	NDR	NDR	NDR	NDR	NDR	NDR
2 – Neck back[b]	NDR	NDR	NDR	NDR	NDR	NDR	NDR	NDR
2 – Forearms[b]	0.64	774	3078	309	NDR	NDR	NDR	NDR
2 – Hands[bc]	0.800	656.1	2624	262.4	NDR	NDR	NDR	NDR
Urine (1)(before)		NDR				NDR		
Urine (1+2)(+12 hr)		NDR				NDR		
Urine (1+2)(+24 hr)		NDR				NDR		

PILOTS	Mancozeb Total μg/cm²	Mancozeb Total μg Body Area	Mancozeb Total μg/hr	Mancozeb Total μg/kg Body wt/day	ETU Total μg/cm²	ETU Total μg Body Area	ETU Total μg/hr	ETU Total μg/kg Body wt/day
Patches Outside Clothing								
1 - Face	1.69	1099	2197	219.7	NDR[a]	NDR	NDR	NDR
1 - Neck front	0.20	30.2	60.4	6.04	NDR	NDR	NDR	NDR
1 - Neck back	NDR	NDR	NDR	NDR	NDR	NDR	NDR	NDR
1 - Forearms[bc]	NDR	NDR	NDR	NDR	NDR	NDR	NDR	NDR
1 - Hands[bc]	1.717	1408.6	2817.2	281.7	NDR	NDR	NDR	NDR
2 - Respirator[b]	NDR	NDR	NDR	NDR	NDR	NDR	NDR	NDR
2 - Face	NDR	NDR	NDR	NDR	NDR	NDR	NDR	NDR
2 - Neck front	0.40	60.0	120	12.0	NDR	NDR	NDR	NDR
2 - Neck back	NDR	NDR	NDR	NDR	NDR	NDR	NDR	NDR
2 - Forearms[b]	0.47	569	1140	114	NDR	NDR	NDR	NDR
2 - Hands[bc]	0.421	344.9	689.8	68.98	NDR	NDR	NDR	NDR
2 - Respirator[b]	0.23	27.6	55.2	5.52	NDR	NDR	NDR	NDR
Patches Under Clothing								
1 - Face	NDR	NDR	NDR	NDR	NDR	NDR	NDR	NDR
1 - Neck front	NDR	NDR	NDR	NDR	NDR	NDR	NDR	NDR
1 - Neck back	NDR	NDR	NDR	NDR	NDR	NDR	NDR	NDR
1 - Forearms[b]	NDR	NDR	NDR	NDR	NDR	NDR	NDR	NDR
2 - Face	NDR	NDR	NDR	NDR	NDR	NDR	NDR	NDR
2 - Neck front	NDR	NDR	NDR	NDR	NDR	NDR	NDR	NDR
2 - Neck back	NDR	NDR	NDR	NDR	NDR	NDR	NDR	NDR
2 - Forearms	NDR	NDR	NDR	NDR	NDR	NDR	NDR	NDR
Urine (1)(before)		NDR	NDR	NDR		NDR	NDR	NDR
Urine (1+2)(+12 hr)		NDR	NDR	NDR		NDR	NDR	NDR
Urine (1+2)(+24 hr)		NDR	NDR	NDR		0.22	0.44	0.044

[a] No detectable residue.   [b] Value for right and left.   [c] Total μg per two gloves.

Table VIII. Exposure of Mixer-Loaders and Pilots to Mancozeb and ETU During the Application of Mancozeb by Airplanes in Oregon

MIXER-LOADERS	Mancozeb				ETU			
	Total $\mu g/cm^2$	Total μg Body Area	Total $\mu g/hr$	Total $\mu g/kg$ Body wt/day	Total $\mu g/cm^2$	Total μg Body Area	Total $\mu g/hr$	Total $\mu g/kg$ Body wt/day
Patches Outside Clothing								
1 − Face	0.59	384	1150	115	NDR[a]	NDR	NDR	NDR
1 − Neck front	3.52	528.0	1584	158.4	NDR	NDR	NDR	NDR
1 − Neck back	0.36	39.6	119	11.9	NDR	NDR	NDR	NDR
1 − Forearms[b]	7.77	9402	28210	2821	NDR	NDR	NDR	NDR
1 − Respirator[b]	1.26	151.2	453.6	45.36	NDR	NDR	NDR	NDR
2 − Face	0.23	150	1794	179	NDR	NDR	NDR	NDR
2 − Neck front	0.54	81.0	972	97.2	NDR	NDR	NDR	NDR
2 − Neck back	0.26	28.6	343	34.3	NDR	NDR	NDR	NDR
2 − Forearms[b]	1.86	2251	27010	2701	0.014	16.9	203	20.3
2 − Respirator[b]	0.98	118	1411	141	NDR	NDR	NDR	NDR
Patches Under Clothing								
1 − Face	0.33	214	644	64.4	NDR	NDR	NDR	NDR
1 − Neck front	0.71	107	320	32.0	NDR	NDR	NDR	NDR
1 − Neck back	0.36	39.6	119	11.9	NDR	NDR	NDR	NDR
1 − Forearms[b]	0.45	545	1630	163	NDR	NDR	NDR	NDR
1 − Hands[bc]	0.108	88.8	266	26.6	NDR	NDR	NDR	NDR
2 − Face	NDR	NDR	NDR	NDR	NDR	NDR	NDR	NDR
2 − Neck front	0.19	28.5	342	34.2	NDR	NDR	NDR	NDR
2 − Neck back[b]	NDR	NDR	NDR	NDR	NDR	NDR	NDR	NDR
2 − Forearms[b]	0.93	1125	13500	1350	NDR	NDR	NDR	NDR
2 − Hands[bc]	0.0563	46.2	554.4	55.4	0.0029	2.4	28.8	2.88
Urine (1)(before)		NDR	NDR	NDR		NDR	NDR	NDR
Urine (1+2)(+12 hr)		NDR	NDR	NDR		NDR	NDR	NDR
Urine (1+2)(+24 hr)		NDR	NDR	NDR		NDR	NDR	2.88

PILOTS	Mancozeb Total µg/cm²	Total µg Body Area	Total µg/hr	Total µg/kg Body wt/day	ETU Total µg/cm²	Total µg Body Area	Total µg/hr	Total µg/kg Body wt/day
Patches Outside Clothing								
1 - Face	NDR[a]	NDR	NDR	NDR	NDR	NDR	NDR	NDR
1 - Neck front	NDR	NDR	NDR	NDR	NDR	NDR	NDR	NDR
1 - Neck back	NDR	NDR	NDR	NDR	NDR	NDR	NDR	NDR
1 - Forearms[b]	NDR	NDR	NDR	NDR	NDR	NDR	NDR	NDR
1 - Hands[b,c]	0.182	149.5	358.8	35.88	0.00127	1.044	2.50	0.25
1 - Respirator[b]	0.19	124	296	29.6	NDR	NDR	NDR	NDR
2 - Face	NDR	NDR	NDR	NDR	0.03	3.3	7.9	0.79
2 - Neck front	NDR	NDR	NDR	NDR	NDR	NDR	NDR	NDR
2 - Neck back	NDR	NDR	NDR	NDR	NDR	NDR	NDR	NDR
2 - Forearms[b]	NDR	NDR	NDR	NDR	NDR	NDR	NDR	NDR
2 - Hands[b,c]	0.0296	24.3	58.20	5.82	0.00449	3.68	8.83	0.88
2 - Respirator[b]	NDR	NDR	NDR	NDR	NDR	NDR	NDR	NDR
Patches Under Clothing								
1 - Face	NDR	NDR	NDR	NDR	NDR	NDR	NDR	NDR
1 - Neck front	NDR	NDR	NDR	NDR	NDR	NDR	NDR	NDR
1 - Neck back	NDR	NDR	NDR	NDR	NDR	NDR	NDR	NDR
1 - Forearms[b]	NDR	NDR	NDR	NDR	NDR	NDR	NDR	NDR
2 - Face	NDR	NDR	NDR	NDR	NDR	NDR	NDR	NDR
2 - Neck front	NDR	NDR	NDR	NDR	NDR	NDR	NDR	NDR
2 - Neck back	NDR	NDR	NDR	NDR	NDR	NDR	NDR	NDR
2 - Forearms[b]	NDR	NDR	NDR	NDR	NDR	NDR	NDR	NDR
Urine (1)(before)	NDR				NDR			
Urine (1+2)(+12 hr)	NDR				NDR			
Urine (1+2)(+24 hr)	NDR				NDR			

[a] No detectable residue. [b] Value for right and left. [c] Total µg per two gloves.

Table IX. Exposure of Mixer-Loaders and Tractor Driver-Applicator to Mancozeb and ETU During the Application of Mancozeb by Airblast Sprayer in Ohio

	Mancozeb				ETU			
MIXER-LOADERS	Total µg/cm²	Total µg Body Area	Total µg/hr	Total µg/kg Body wt/day	Total µg/cm²	Total µg Body Area	Total µg/hr	Total µg/kg Body wt/day
Patches Outside Clothing								
1 - Face	0.25	161	1610	161	NDR[a]	NDR	NDR	NDR
1 - Neck front	7.22	1083	10830	1083	NDR	NDR	NDR	NDR
1 - Neck back	0.26	28.6	286	28.6	NDR	NDR	NDR	NDR
1 - Forearms[b]	2.36	2856	28560	2856	NDR	NDR	NDR	NDR
1 - Respirator[b]	2.42	290.4	2904	290.4	NDR	NDR	NDR	NDR
2 - Face	0.98	637	6370	637	NDR	NDR	NDR	NDR
2 - Neck front	1.49	223.5	2235	223.5	NDR	NDR	NDR	NDR
2 - Neck back	20.70	2277	22770	2277	NDR	NDR	NDR	NDR
2 - Forearms[b]	2.88	3485	34850	3485	NDR	NDR	NDR	NDR
2 - Respirator[b]	1.92	230.4	2304	230.4	NDR	NDR	NDR	NDR
Patches Under Clothing								
1 - Face	NDR	NDR	NDR	NDR	NDR	NDR	NDR	NDR
1 - Neck front	0.16	24.0	240	24.0	NDR	NDR	NDR	NDR
1 - Neck back	NDR	NDR	NDR	NDR	NDR	NDR	NDR	NDR
1 - Forearms[b]	0.43	520	5200	520	NDR	NDR	NDR	NDR
1 - Hands[bc]	0.2025	166.1	1661	166.1	0.0008	0.66	6.6	0.66
2 - Face	0.81	1177	11770	1177	NDR	NDR	NDR	NDR
2 - Neck front	0.53	79.5	795	79.5	NDR	NDR	NDR	NDR
2 - Neck back[b]	0.25	27.5	275	27.5	NDR	NDR	NDR	NDR
2 - Forearms[b]	0.28	339	3390	339	NDR	NDR	NDR	NDR
2 - Hands[bc]	0.801	657	6570	657	NDR[d]	NDR	NDR	NDR
Urine (1)(before)					NDR	NDR	NDR	NDR
Urine (1+2)(after)					NDR	NDR	NDR	NDR
Urine (1+2)(+12 hr)					NDR	NDR	NDR	NDR
Urine (1+2)(+24 hr)					NDR	NDR	NDR	NDR

TRACTOR DRIVER–APPLICATORS	Mancozeb				ETU			
	Total μg/cm²	Total μg Body Area	Total μg/hr	Total μg/kg Body wt/day	Total μg/cm²	Total μg Body Area	Total μg/hr	Total μg/kg Body wt/day
Patches Outside Clothing								
1 – Face	0.88	572	1720	172	NDR	NDR	NDR	NDR
1 – Neck front	0.25	37.5	113	11.3	NDR	NDR	NDR	NDR
1 – Neck back	NDR	NDR	NDR	NDR	NDR	NDR	NDR	NDR
1 – Forearms[b]	0.90	1090	3270	327	NDR	NDR	NDR	NDR
2 – Respirator[b]	NDR	NDR	NDR	NDR	NDR	NDR	NDR	NDR
2 – Face	NDR	NDR	NDR	NDR	NDR	NDR	NDR	NDR
2 – Neck front	0.20	30.0	94.7	9.47	NDR	NDR	NDR	NDR
2 – Neck back[b]	NDR	NDR	NDR	NDR	NDR	NDR	NDR	NDR
2 – Forearms[b]	NDR	NDR	NDR	NDR	NDR	NDR	NDR	NDR
2 – Respirator[b]	NDR	NDR	NDR	NDR	NDR	NDR	NDR	NDR
Patches Under Clothing								
1 – Face	NDR	NDR	NDR	NDR	NDR	NDR	NDR	NDR
1 – Neck front	NDR	NDR	NDR	NDR	NDR	NDR	NDR	NDR
1 – Neck back[b]	NDR	NDR	NDR	NDR	NDR	NDR	NDR	NDR
1 – Forearms[b]	0.22	266	799	79.9	NDR	NDR	NDR	NDR
1 – Hands[bc]	0.111	91.2	273.6	27.36	0.00048	0.39	1.17	0.12
2 – Face	NDR	NDR	NDR	NDR	NDR	NDR	NDR	NDR
2 – Neck front	NDR	NDR	NDR	NDR	NDR	NDR	NDR	NDR
2 – Neck back[b]	0.16	17.6	55.6	5.56	NDR	NDR	NDR	NDR
2 – Forearms[b]	NDR	NDR	NDR	NDR	NDR	NDR	NDR	NDR
2 – Hands[bc]	0.0273	22.4	70.7	7.07	NDR	NDR	NDR	NDR
Urine (1)(before)	NDR	NDR	NDR	NDR			NDR	NDR
Urine (1)(after)	NDR	NDR	NDR	NDR			NDR	NDR
Urine (1)(+12 hr)	NDR	NDR	NDR	NDR			NDR	NDR
Urine (1+2)(+24 hr)	NDR	NDR	NDR	NDR			NDR	NDR

[a] No detectable residue. [b] Value for right and left. [c] Total μg per two gloves. [d] Sample spilled.

Table X. Exposure of Mixer-Applicators to Mancozeb and ETU During the Application of Mancozeb to a Homeyard in Ohio

MIXER-APPLICATORS	Mancozeb				ETU			
	Total μg/cm²	Total μg Body Area	Total μg/hr	Total μg/kg Body wt/day	Total μg/cm²	Total μg Body Area	Total μg/hr	Total μg/kg Body wt/day
Patches Outside Clothing								
1 - Face	NDR[a]	NDR	NDR	NDR	NDR	NDR	NDR	NDR
1 - Neck front	0.20	30	72	1.2[d]	NDR	NDR	NDR	NDR
1 - Neck back[b]	0.48	52.8	127	2.1	NDR	NDR	NDR	NDR
1 - Forearms[b]	NDR	NDR	NDR	NDR	NDR	NDR	NDR	NDR
1 - Respirator[b]	NDR	NDR	NDR	NDR	NDR	NDR	NDR	NDR
1 - Ankles[b]	3.04	1702	4085	68.1	0.00022	0.18	0.43	0.007
1 - Thighs[b]	0.47	1636	3928	65.5	NDR	NDR	NDR	NDR
2 - Face	NDR	NDR	NDR	NDR	0.0011	0.9	3.4	0.056
2 - Neck front	NDR	NDR	NDR	NDR	NDR	NDR	NDR	NDR
2 - Neck back[b]	NDR	NDR	NDR	NDR	NDR	NDR	NDR	NDR
2 - Forearms[b]	NDR	NDR	NDR	NDR	NDR	NDR	NDR	NDR
2 - Respirator[b]	NDR	NDR	NDR	NDR	NDR	NDR	NDR	NDR
2 - Ankles	NDR	NDR	NDR	NDR	NDR	NDR	NDR	NDR
2 - Thighs	NDR	NDR	NDR	NDR	NDR	NDR	NDR	NDR
Patches Under Clothing								
1 - Face	NDR	NDR	NDR	NDR	NDR	NDR	NDR	NDR
1 - Neck front	NDR	NDR	NDR	NDR	NDR	NDR	NDR	NDR
1 - Neck back[b]	NDR	NDR	NDR	NDR	NDR	NDR	NDR	NDR
1 - Forearms[b]	NDR	NDR	NDR	NDR	NDR	NDR	NDR	NDR
1 - Hands[bc]	0.0687	56.3	135.1	225	0.0054	4.4	10.6	0.176
1 - Ankles[b]	NDR	NDR	NDR	NDR	NDR	NDR	NDR	NDR
1 - Thighs[b]	NDR	NDR	NDR	NDR	NDR	NDR	NDR	NDR

MIXER APPLICATORS	Mancozeb				ETU			
	Total µg/cm²	Total µg Body Area	Total µg/hr	Total µg/kg Body wt/day	Total µg/cm²	Total µg Body Area	Total µg/hr	Total µg/kg Body wt/day
2 – Face	NDR	NDR	NDR	NDR	NDR	NDR	NDR	NDR
2 – Neck front	NDR	NDR	NDR	NDR	NDR	NDR	NDR	NDR
2 – Neck back	NDR	NDR	NDR	NDR	NDR	NDR	NDR	NDR
2 – Forearms[b]	NDR	NDR	NDR	NDR	NDR	NDR	NDR	NDR
2 – Hands[bc]	NDR	NDR	NDR	NDR	0.0041	3.4	12.8	0.21
2 – Ankles[b]	NDR	NDR	NDR	NDR	NDR	NDR	NDR	NDR
2 – Thighs[b]	NDR	NDR	NDR	NDR	NDR	NDR	NDR	NDR
Urine (before)					NDR	NDR	NDR	NDR
Urine (+12 hr)					NDR	NDR	NDR	NDR
Urine (+24 hr)					NDR	NDR	NDR	NDR
Patches Outside Clothing								
3 – Face	0.26	169	406	6.8	NDR	NDR	NDR	NDR
3 – Neck front	0.36	54	130	2.2	NDR	NDR	NDR	NDR
3 – Neck back[b]	0.25	27.5	66	1.1	NDR	NDR	NDR	NDR
3 – Forearms[b]	0.54	653	1570	26.1	NDR	NDR	NDR	NDR
3 – Respirator[b]	0.29	34.8	83.5	1.4	NDR	NDR	NDR	NDR
3 – Ankles	0.74	414	995	16.6	NDR	NDR	NDR	NDR
3 – Thighs	0.95	3308	7939	132.3	NDR	NDR	NDR	NDR
4 – Face	NDR	NDR	NDR	NDR	NDR	NDR	NDR	NDR
4 – Neck front	NDR	NDR	NDR	NDR	NDR	NDR	NDR	NDR
4 – Neck back[b]	1.41	155.1	372.2	6.20	NDR	NDR	NDR	NDR
4 – Forearms[b]	0.59	714	1710	28.6	NDR[e]	NDR	NDR	NDR
4 – Respirator[b]	0.25	30	7.2	1.2	NDR	NDR	NDR	NDR
4 – Ankles	7.66	4290	10300	171.6	NDR	NDR	NDR	NDR
4 – Thighs	0.59	2054	4931	82.2	NDR	NDR	NDR	NDR

Continued on next page.

Table X. Continued

| | Mancozeb | | | | ETU | | | |
MIXER APPLICATORS	Total μg/cm²	Total μg Body Area	Total μg/hr	Total μg/kg Body wt/day	Total μg/cm²	Total μg Body Area	Total μg/hr	Total μg/kg Body wt/day
Patches Under Clothing								
3 – Face	NDR	NDR	NDR	NDR	NDR	NDR	NDR	NDR
3 – Neck front	NDR	NDR	NDR	NDR	NDR	NDR	NDR	NDR
3 – Neck back	NDR	NDR	NDR	NDR	NDR	NDR	NDR	NDR
3 – Forearms [b]	0.25	302	726	12.1	NDR	NDR	NDR	NDR
3 – Hands [b,c]	NDR	NDR	NDR	NDR	NDR	NDR	NDR	NDR
3 – Ankles	NDR	NDR	NDR	NDR	NDR	NDR	NDR	NDR
3 – Thighs	NDR	NDR	NDR	NDR	NDR	NDR	NDR	NDR
4 – Face	NDR	NDR	NDR	NDR	NDR	NDR	NDR	NDR
4 – Neck front	NDR	NDR	NDR	NDR	NDR	NDR	NDR	NDR
4 – Neck back	NDR	NDR	NDR	NDR	NDR	NDR	NDR	NDR
4 – Forearms [b]	NDR	NDR	NDR	NDR	NDR	NDR	NDR	NDR
4 – Hands [b,c]	0.060	49.3	118	2.0	NDR	NDR	NDR	NDR
4 – Ankles	NDR	NDR	NDR	NDR	NDR	NDR	NDR	NDR
4 – Thighs	NDR	NDR	NDR	NDR		NDR	NDR	NDR
Urine (before)		NDR	NDR	NDR		NDR	NDR	NDR
Urine (+12 hr)		NDR	NDR	NDR		NDR	NDR	NDR
Urine (+24 hr)		NDR	NDR	NDR		NDR	NDR	NDR

[a] No detectable residue.   [b] Value for right and left.   [c] Total μg per two gloves.
[d] Assumes one hour of work per day.   [e] Sample spilled.

compressed air sprayers in a home yard setting. Mixer-loaders were more exposed than applicators. Home gardeners experienced little exposure except for their ankles and thighs. Protective clothing greatly reduced or eliminated exposure. ETU was usually not detectable on the sample pads or in urine. Mancozeb was not detected in the urine.

Acknowledgments

Appreciation is expressed to Fredrick Tschirely and Spencer Potter of the Department of Botany and Plant Pathology, Michigan State University, East Lansing, Michigan 48823; Howard L. Bissonette of the Department of Plant Pathology, University of Minnesota, Minneapolis, Minnesota 55455; and James M. Witt and Frank N. Dost of the Department of Agricultural Chemistry, Oregon State University, Corvallis, Oregon 97331, for their direction of the experiments involving air application of mancozeb. Also thanks are given to James Farley and Charles C. Powell of the Department of Plant Pathology, Ohio State University, Columbus, Ohio 43210, for their direction of the air-blast sprayer and home yard application experiments. Edward Bogus, James Brady, David Kurtz, Kathleen Simmons and Remo Vallejo performed analytical analyses. Also, thanks is expressed to Linwood D. Haines of ROHM and HAAS Co. for his valuable advice. We appreciate the support of NAPIAP which financed all the field tests and the analyses. ROHM and HAAS Co. provided the mancozeb, contributed analytical apparatus and coordinated the field tests. Paper No. 7014 in the Journal Series of the Pennsylvania Agricultural Experiment Station.

Literature Cited

1. Davis, J. E. In "Residue Reviews"; Gunther, F., Ed.; Springer-Verlag New York Inc.: New York, 1980; Vol. 75, p. 33-50.

2. Wolfe, H. R.; Durham, W. F. Arch. Evn. Health 1961, V-3, Oct.

3. Keppel, G. E. J. Assoc. Off. Anal. Chem. 1977, 25, 561-7.

4. Haines, L.; Adler, I. L. J. Assoc. Off. Anal. Chem. 1973, 56, 333-7.

5. Onley, J. H.; Giuffrida, L.; Ires, N. F.; Watts, R.; Storherr, R. W. J. Assoc. Off. Anal. Chem. 1977, 60, 1105-10.

6. Pease, H.; Holt, R.F. J. Agric. Food Chem. 1977, 25, 561-7.

RECEIVED November 16, 1984

Inhalation Exposure of Grain Samplers and Grain Inspectors to Carbon Tetrachloride

HOWARD M. DEER[1,3], CHARLES E. MCJILTON[2], PHILLIP K. HAREIN[1], and WILFRED SUMNER[1]

[1] Department of Entomology, University of Minnesota, St. Paul, MN 55108
[2] Department of Environmental Health, University of Minnesota, Minneapolis, MN 55455

CCl_4 is a common ingredient of liquid grain fumigant mixtures. Exposure data for this registered use are needed in making regulatory decisions on continuing this registration. USDA's NAPIAP funded research on the CCl_4 inhalation exposure of grain samplers and grain inspectors in Minnesota. Ambient concentrations of CCl_4 in 7700 grain samples submitted for inspection were determined by colorimetric tube and are an estimator of peak grain inspector exposure to CCl_4. Concentrations ranged from nondetected to >60 ppm. Significant differences were determined for dates, locations, grain types, and grain transportation vehicles. Approximately 350 8-hour TWA CCl_4 exposures for grain samplers and grain inspectors were determined by using passive dosimeters. All TWA 8-hour exposures were <2 ppm.

Fumigants are applied to stored grain to control insect infestations. Many different formulations are available (Table I) (1) and selection for use is based on several considerations such as grain temperature, grain storage facility, time available for fumigation, fumigant cost, and others.

For many years the Environmental Protection Agency (EPA) has expressed interest in these grain fumigants, especially those that have met or exceeded the risk criteria of EPA's Rebuttable Presumption Against Registration (RPAR) Program (2).

[3] Current address: Interdepartmental Program in Toxicology, UMC 46, Utah State University, Logan, UT 84322

Ethylene dibromide (EDB) met or exceeded the risk criteria for oncogenicity, mutagenicity, and reproductive disorders, and an RPAR notice for EDB was issued in December 1977 (3). Approximately 6 years later EDB's pesticidal life as a grain fumigant ended by way of emergency suspension and intended cancellation (4, 5) when its presence in raw grain, flour and ready-to-eat grain products became common knowledge. The term "common knowledge" is used because literature reports of EDB in these food products were published several years earlier (6-8).

Carbon tetrachloride received an RPAR notice on October 15, 1980 with risk criteria of oncogenicity, hepatoxicity, and nephrotoxicity specified (9). CCl_4 has been shown to induce oncogenic effects in rats, mice, and hamsters after oral administration. CCl_4 has also been shown to have toxic effects on the liver of monkeys, rats, guinea pigs and rabbits after oral, inhalation or subcutaneous exposure. CCl_4 has caused liver damage in humans who were intermittently exposed. CCl_4 has been shown to cause toxic kidney effects in chronically exposed rats and to cause kidney dysfunction in occupationally exposed humans (Table II).

Carbon tetrachloride, or tetrachloromethane, is a nonflammable, noncorrosive, colorless liquid with a molecular weight or 153.84, a specific gravity of 1.58 ($25°C$), a boiling point of $76.76°C$, a freezing point of $-22.8°C$, a vapor pressure of 89.5 mm $20°C$, a vapor density of 5.6, water solubility of 0.28 g/kg at $25°C$, a miscibility with alcohol, benzene, chloroform, ether, carbon disulfide, petroleum ether, and oils and is generally inert but can be decomposed in water at high temperatures (10-12). The odor threshold for CCl_4 has been reported at 60-70 ppm (13), at 21-100 ppm (14), at approximately 50 ppm (15) and at a threshold of detection of 79 ppm with a strong odor at 176 ppm (10).

The anesthetic properties of carbon tetrachloride were reported by Smith (16) as early as 1867, but its potential for agricultural use was not reported until the start of the 20th century. Carbon tetrachloride's fumigant usage dates from approximately 1908 (17) when it may have been used to fumigate nursery stock (18), its primary use since that time has been as an industrial solvent and degreaser. CCl_4 was inexpensive and readily available (19), and it was popular for home use as a spot remover and general solvent (20). The dry cleaning industry used CCl_4 extensively, but this use has now been replaced by less toxic chemicals (21). Carbon tetrachloride's primary use today is for fluorocarbon manufacture and it is estimated that approximately 1 billion pounds are produced annually with 95% going into fluorocarbon production and the other 5% into pesticide products, degreasers, propellants, refrigerants, solvents, fire extinguishers, and semiconductors (9). CCl_4 is manufactured by the chlorination of methane or carbon disulfide (12), and principal manufacturers and formulators include Allied Chemical Corporation, Dow Chemical, Dupont and Company, FMC Corporation, Inland Chemical Corporation, Stauffer Chemical Company and Vulcan Materials Corporation (9). The National Institute for Occupational Safety and Health estimates that approximately, 160,000 people are potentially exposed to CCl_4 and that 25,000 of these are in the grain industry (12).

Table I.   Representative Grain Fumigants*

TRADE NAME	MANUFACTURER	% ACTIVE INGREDIENTS	
Weevil-Cide	Weevil-Cide	Carbon Tetrachloride	81.5
		Carbon Disulfide	16.2
		Sulfur Dioxide	1.5
Tetrakil Weevil Killer and Grain Conditioner	Douglas Chemical	Carbon Tetrachloride	77.7
		Carbon Disulfide	15.4
		Ethylene Dibromide	5.0
		Sulfur Dioxide	1.5
		Pentane	0.4
Max Kill 10 Liquid Grain Fumigant	Research Products	Carbon Tetrachloride	70.5
		Carbon Disulfide	16.5
		Ethylene Dibromide	6.6
		Methylene Chloride	6.4
Dawson 73	Ferguson Fumigants	Ethylene Dibromide	70.0
		Methyl Bromide	30.0
Fume-O-Death Gas No. 3	Knox Chemical	Carbon Tetrachloride	30.0
		Ethylene Dichloride	70.0
Selig's Selcofume	Selig Chemical	Carbon Tetrachloride	75.0
		Ethylene Dichloride	25.0
Lethogas Fumigant	Prentis Drug and Chemical	Carbon Tetrachloride	24.5
		Ethylene Dichloride	73.5
		Ethylene Dibromide	2.0
Topkote 77	Douglas Chemical	Carbon Tetrachloride	75.0
		Malathion	2.9
		Pyrethrins	0.04
		Piperonyl Butoxide	0.4
		Petroleum Distillates	19.7
Sircofume Liquid Fumigating Gas	Sirotta-Bernard	Ethylene Dichloride	96.0
		Tetrachloroethylene	1.0
		Trichloroethane	1.0
		Trichloroethylene	1.0
Staffel's High Life	The Staffel Co.	Carbon Disulfide	99.9
Frontier Chloro Fume Grain Fumigant	Vulcan Materials	Chloroform	72.2
		Carbon Disulfide	20.4
		Ethylene Dibromide	7.4
Fumitoxin	Pestcon Systems	Aluminum Phosphide	55.0
Fumi-cel	DeGesch America	Magnesium Phosphide	32.3

Continued on next page

Table I. Continued

TRADE NAME	MANUFACTURER	% ACTIVE INGREDIENTS	
Larvacide 100	Soweco	Chloropicrin	100.0
Methyl Bromide	Dow Chemical	Methyl Bromide	100.0
Calcium Cyanide Grain Fumigant	DeGesch America	Calcium Cyanide	42.0

Source: Adapted from Ref. 1.

Table II. Carbon Tetrachloride Toxic Effects

TEST ANIMAL	ROUTE	DOSE	RESPONSE	INVESTIGATOR
Mice (B6C3F1)	Gavage in corn oil	1,250 and 2,500 mg/ kg/day	98-100% liver carcinoma; 22 -57% adrenal pheochromocytoma.	NCI (1977)
Rats (Osborn-Mendel)	Gavage in corn oil	NR*	Liver tumors and cirrhosis	NCI (1977)
Hamsters (Syrian Golden)	Gavage in corn oil	125 ul/ kg for 7 weeks, then 62.5 ul/kg for 23 weeks	Carcinoma of liver.	Della Porta et al. (1961)
Rabbits	Oral	0.1-6.0 ml/kg	Centrilobular necrosis of liver.	Gardner et al. (1924)
Monkeys	Oral	1-2 ml/kg, 3 days/week for 176 days	Liver cell vacu- olation and swelling, fat accumulation in liver lobules.	Gardner et al. (1924)
Rats	Subcuta- neous	0.4 ml/kg, autopsies 2,4,8,16, 20,24,30, 36,42,48, 72,96,120, & 168 hrs after dose	Liver and kidney damage at 4 hrs. Kidneys normal at 48 hrs, livers normal at 120 hrs.	Lundh (1964)

Table II. Continued

		4 ml/kg, autopsies same as above	Kidney damage at 2 hrs. Liver damage at 4 hrs. Kidneys near normal at 120 hrs, liver still damaged.	
		0.4 ml/kg/ 3 days for 3 days - 12 weeks, autopsies 3 days, 2,3, 4,5,6,7,8,10, and 12 weeks	At 2 weeks kidney damage persisted and fibrotic and cirrhotic damage began.	
Rats	Inhalation	400 ppm, 3 min./day 94 days	No effect	Adams et al. (1952)
		400 ppm, 1 hr/day, 46 days	Decreased growth rate, signs of liver cirrhosis.	
		400 ppm, 1 hr/day, 173 days	Increased liver and kidney weights; increased clotting time; liver degeneration; slight tubular degeneration of the kidney.	
Monkeys, Rats, Guinea Pigs, Rabbits	Inhalation	1 ppm continuous for 90 days	No effects.	Prendergast et al. (1967)
		10 ppm continuous for 90 days	Enlarged livers, fatty infiltration.	
Humans	Inhalation	10-100 ppm intermittently	CNS and gastrointestinal effects; fatty degeneration of the liver.	Dellian and Wittgens (1962)
Humans	Inhalation	NR	Kidney dysfunction	Barnes and Jones (1967)

*NR = not reported
(9)

Carbon tetrachloride's pesticide usage includes fumigation of stored grain, seed stocks, and wool furnishings (9). It is a common constituent of liquid grain fumigants usually ranging from about 22% to 94% of contents (9). It is usually mixed with carbon disulfide, ethylene dibromide, or ethylene dichloride. CCl_4 has insecticidal properties but also acts as an explosion and flammability inhibitor and increases the penetration and diffusion of the fumigant mixture (22-26). There are approximately 110 federal registrations for pesticide products containing CCl_4 (1). One of the most popular formulations is a combination by volume of approximately 83% carbon tetrachloride and 17% carbon disulfide, or 80:20 as it is commonly known (1, 26).

Carbon tetrachloride has been exempted from food tolerance level requirements because no residues were detected in fumigated grains in 1956 when levels of detection were approximately 1 to 2 ppm (9) and because it was reasoned that no CCl_4 would remain in processed foods because of its volatility and such processing procedures as milling and baking. In 1980, however, it was detected in flour so, if the RPAR decision is to reregister CCl_4 for fumigation of stored grain, then food tolerance levels will have to be established (9).

During 1977-78 national off-farm usage of CCl_4 fumigants totaled 19,593,000 pounds and on-farm usage was estimated at 8,607,000 pounds (9). The estimated annual use of CCl_4-based grain fumigants on bulk stored grain is 30% of the wheat and 70% of the oats (27). Additionally, this report estimates a total annual use of CCl_4 in liquid grain fumigants of 13,521,178 pounds. A 1978 postharvest grain insecticide usage survey in Minnesota estimated that farmers treated about 5% of their stored corn, 10% of their wheat, 2% of their oats, and 20% of their barley with insecticides, including grain fumigants (28). This survey also reported that structural pest control operators applied more than 22,000 pounds of CCl_4 in fumigating stored grain, and various pesticide manufacturers reported CCl_4 fumigants usage in Minnesota at about 1,000,000 pounds. Another 1978 Minnesota farm use of pesticides survey reported that 12% of farmers used insecticides or fumigants to protect on-farm stored grain (29), and a 1980 Minnesota survey reported that 14% of farmers using grain fumigants to protect on-farm stored grain (30).

A 1980 Ohio survey on pesticides used on-farm stored grain (corn, oats, and wheat) reported 287,415 pounds of carbon tetrachloride used and also reported the time of year when the grain and(or) storage facilities were treated (31). During the months of June to September the greatest percentages of grain treatment occurred both by farmers and elevator operators. Elevator operators also reported treatments occurring during April and May.

Carbon tetrachloride, along with ethylene dichloride and ethylene dibromide, are also reported as the most commonly used grain fumigants in Great Britain (32).

These liquid grain fumigants are poured or pumped onto the grain while it is in storage or while it is flowing into a storage facility. Fumigating occurs in both on-farm and off-farm storage. Labels recommend dosages and fumigation time requirements, and dosages are based on the type of grain and type of storage facility and are usually calculated on a gallonage per 1,000 bushel basis (33–42). A general rate of application for carbon tetrachloride is from about 350 to 375 ml per metric ton of grain (43).

Pesticide labels must include directions for use, precautionary statements, EPA product registration and establishment numbers, a signal word such as "Caution, Warning, or Danger," and an active ingredient statement, a net contents statement, the name and address of the manufacturer and if it has been classified as a restricted use pesticide it must state "Restricted Use Pesticide" (44). There are approximately 45 pesticides presently classified as "Restricted Use Pesticides" (2). The 80:20 formulations are not classified as restricted use at this time but are proposed for such classification (45). Since 80:20 formulations are not "Restricted Use Pesticides" they may be purchased and used by anyone. Both federal and state laws require pesticide use to be consistent with labeling and violations are punishable by fines and(or) imprisonment (44).

Pesticide labels on 80:20 formulations require applicators to use respiratory protective equipment, such as a self-contained breathing apparatus or approved full face gas mask (33–42). Warning statements caution that high concentrations may exceed 2% by volume and thus necessitate air supplied equipment. Black for organic vapor canisters are required and they must be approved by the U.S. Bureau of Mines. Labels are less specific in requirements that the grain be aerated or that the fumigant be removed from the grain after fumigation. One label (36) stated "Do not use fumigated material or feed it to livestock until aeration has eliminated the odor of fumigant." Another (41) states "Avoid Toxic Gases, Do Not Enter Bin During or After Treatment." Another (38) states "Do not enter any treated structure until it has been aired for at least 24 hours. Do not feed treated feed or grain to livestock until it has been aired enough to remove all fumigant odor."

When the fumigation time requirement has passed, usually 72 hours, the fumigated grain may be moved through transportation and processing channels and frequently is in need of grading so that a basis for price can be established. The grading process involves sampling the grain and assigning it a grade according to established standards (45). Factors, such as grain temperature, ambient temperature, grain type, length of time from fumigant application, type of storage facility, grain moisture and others, affect the dosage rate of fumigant and the rates of sorption and desorption (6, 7, 46–54).

The Occupational Safety and Health Administration (OSHA), the National Institute for Occupational Safety and Health (NIOSH), and the American Conference of Governmental Industrial Hygienists (ACGIH) have each published standards or guidelines for exposure to carbon tetrachloride concentrations. The OSHA standards are the legal standards that must be observed whereas those of NIOSH and ACGIH are only recommended, but are considered to be based on more current information and may better reflect the level of exposure that should be strived for.

OSHA (15) standards for carbon tetrachloride are a 10 ppm level for the time-weighted average (TWA) exposure over an 8-hour period, a 25 ppm acceptable ceiling, and a 200 ppm maximum ceiling exposure that should not be exceeded for more than 5 minutes in any 4 hour period. NIOSH (55) recommends a 2 ppm ceiling for 60 minutes. Liver cancer is the primary health effect listed as considered in setting NIOSH's recommended limits. ACGIH (56) recommends a 5 ppm threshold limit value (TLV) TWA for 8-hour workdays and a 20 ppm Short Term Exposure Level (STEL), which is a 15-minute TWA and should not be exceeded at any time during a work day. Exposures at the STEL should not exceed 15 minutes in length and should occur only four times per day with at least 60 minutes between exposures. Furthermore, ACGIH identifies carbon tetrachloride as having a "skin" exposure hazard and lists carbon tetrachloride in its A-2 table, which states "Industrial Substances Suspect of Carcinogenic Potential for Man."

The Immediately Dangerous to Life and Health (IDLH) level for carbon tetrachloride is set at 300 ppm (57).

In 1981 the North Central Region of the National Agricultural Pesticide Impact Assessment Program (NAPIAP) funded a project entitled "Inhalation Exposures of Grain Samplers and Grain Inspectors to the RPAR Pesticide Carbon Tetrachloride."

Objectives

The objectives for this project were to:

1. Develop a method to assess the workday exposure of Minnesota Department of Agriculture grain samplers and grain inspectors to CCl_4;

2. Detect by instrumentation atmospheric concentrations of CCl_4 above standards in order to reduce human exposure;

3. Reduce the reliance of "fumigant-like" odors as a method for determining CCl_4 presence; and

4. Develop a program that could be adopted by the Minnesota Department of Agriculture for continued CCl_4 exposure assessment.

Materials, Methods, and Procedures

Objective #1 was accomplished by the use of NIOSH approved for carbon tetrachloride 3M Brand #3500 Organic Vapor Monitors. These were chosen because of their simplicity of design, lack of interference for the worker being monitored, cost, and ease of analysis. These

passive monitors were attached to the shirt collars of various grain
samplers and grain inspectors working in grain sampling and
inspection locations at Duluth, Mankato, and Minneapolis, Minnesota.
The organic vapor monitors were unpacked by the researcher; the badge
number, initial time, and employee identification number were
recorded; and the badges were attached to the worker or to an object
in close proximity to the worker. The worker was asked to perform
his job functions as usual and the badge was collected at the end of
the sampling period. When the sampling period was over, the
researcher removed the badge from the worker, recorded the end time,
and followed the manufacturer's directions for securing the badge for
subsequent analysis. All badges for a given sampling period were
collected by the researcher and delivered as quickly as possible to
the GC-MS analysis facilities on the St. Paul Campus of the
University of Minnesota. Analysis was performed by personnel
assigned to operate this facility and to assist research projects
conducted at this institution.

Carbon tetrachloride vapors enter the monitor by diffusion and
are adsorbed onto an active adsorbent medium inside the badge.
Badges are to be worn near the breathing zone of personnel exposed to
organic vapors that are to be quantified. They are designed to
measure time-weighted average (TWA) concentrations over a measured
time interval. No sampling pump is required. The prinicples of the
method of using the passive monitor are:

1.   The organic vapor to be quantified enters the badge by
diffusion and is adsorbed by an active adsorbent medium inside of the
badge. The amount of organic vapor adsorbed is dependent on length
of exposure time and organic vapor concentration that is present in
the sampling area.

2.   After the sampling period has been completed and the
monitors collected and secured, analysis is performed by adding 1.5
ml of carbon disulfide through a center port of the badge to remove
the CCl_4 from the adsorbent medium. The badge is allowed to elute
for 30 minutes with occasional slight agitation.

3.   Then, an aliquot (4 ul) of the eluent is removed by syringe
and injected into the GC-MS analyzer. The mass of organic vapor
adsorbed by the badge is determined by comparison to injection of
known standards taking into consideration the background values for
CCl_4.

4.   The mass in micrograms of organic vapor adsorbed is used to
calculate the TWA for the individual workers who were monitored by
multiplying it by a calculation constant (manufactured supplied) and
then dividing by the recovery coefficient (manufacturer supplied)
times the number of minutes in the sampling period. The result is
the concentration in parts per million for the exposed worker for the
sampling period, and this value is then time adjusted for an 8 hour
TWA.

Objective #2 was accomplished by the use of Bendix/Gastec
Colorimetric Pumps & Tubes for detecting carbon tetrachloride. These

NIOSH approved tubes are direct reading and are graduated in parts per million from 0-60. The pump draws a measured volume of air through the tube, and contaminant reaction causes a color change within the direct reading tube.

When a grain sample is submitted for inspection it is handled by several persons. Samples are first received by an employee, who distributes them to inspectors for "breakdown", a process in which the grain is removed from the sample bag and run through a divider to collect an amount of grain that is sufficient for inspection and the assignment of a grain grade. This amount is then delivered by the inspector to a dockage mill operator, who mills the grain to separate the dust, chaff, and some of the other foreign materials from the grain itself. After milling, the grain sample is returned to the inspector for grading. In the grading process the inspector conducts the "cofo" test, or commercially objectionable foreign odor test, in which the inspector inserts his nose into the pan of grain to be graded and inhales to test for off odors, such as sourness, rancidity, and others. He then continues the grading procedure which includes visual inspection, weighing, and other procedures and assigns a specific grade to that sample of grain.

To determine the peak exposure potential for the grain inspector, it was necessary to determine at which point in the grain grading process this peak exposure occurred. The grain inspector's job function was broken down into components of 1) opening the grain sample bag, 2) passing the grain through the grain divider, 3) passing the grain through the dockage mill, 4) performing the "cofo" test, and 5) completing the grain grading process. Both a Miran 1A Infrared Analyzer and Bendix/Gastec CCl_4 Colorimetric Tube System were used to determine that the peak exposure potential occurred during peformance of the "cofo" test.

As grain pans were removed from the dockage mill and placed on a counter for the assigned inspector to retrieve and grade, a colorimetric tube for CCl_4 was placed in the grain in the pan. The concentration of CCl_4 was then determined by direct reading and recorded on a data entry card. These cards contained data on employee identification number, date, location of work, grain vehicle, grain type, and CCl_4 concentration. A data card was filled out for each grain sample checked.

The upper limit of concentration for the colorimetric tubes is 60 ppm. Samples that gave a reading >60 ppm were assigned the value of 100 ppm. This value was chosen as the concentration at which inspectors would no longer perform the "cofo" test. As reported in the literature, the odor threshold for CCl_4 is between 21 and 100 ppm, with most reports in the 50-80 ppm range. Inspectors interviewed stated they would perform the "cofo" test if the smell of CCl_4 was not evident to slight in odor strength. The literature reports the odor of CCl_4 to be strong at 176 ppm, so it was assumed that inspectors would perform the "cofo" test if the odor of CCl_4 was up to "slight" but not "strong." If the mean for the odor threshold is 64 ppm and the odor is strong at 176 ppm then it is assumed to be moderate at the midpoint, approximately 120 ppm, and slight at approximately one-third of the concentration between the threshold of detection and strong.

Tubes evidencing no CCl_4 in a particular sample were used in subsequent samples until a reading was determined or a lengthy time interval was to occur, such as lunch time. No tubes were carried over to another day. Tubes that showed streaking were recorded as an average between the high and low readings of the streak. Tubes showing questionable results, such as channeling, were discarded and no reading was recorded.

Since grain sample flow was extremely rapid, at times as many as six pumps and tubes were being used at one time. Maximum efficiency was mandatory in data recording, and tube preparation during these intervals. Lag times were used to check data entry cards, prepare additional tubes, check pumps for air leaks, and other activities.

Data entry cards for each day's testing were delivered to the computer services offices on the St. Paul Campus of the University of Minnesota for entry into a data storage bank, which was statistically analyzed at completion of the study period.

Objective #3 was accomplished by utilizing the colorimetric tube system to detect the presence of CCl_4 in grain samples to be inspected rather than relying on the olfactory senses of the various inspectors. Previous to this study, CCl_4 concentrations in grain samples were determined by inspectors who detected an odor that they had come to recognize as that of CCl_4. When grain samples to be inspected were checked with a colorimetric tube, samples that contained CCl_4 concentrations could be identified before the "cofo" test was performed.

Objective #4 was accomplished by selecting and designing a CCl_4 exposure assessment methodology that met the requirements of simplicity and cost effectiveness.

Results and Discussion

Monitoring of grain samples for ambient concentrations of carbon tetrachloride and monitoring workplace atmospheres for TWA concentrations of carbon tetrachloride were carried out in three Minnesota locations: Minneapolis, Duluth and Mankato. Monitoring was conducted on 73 days during the study period of July 14, 1981 through Ocotber 28, 1982.

Testing for CCl_4 peak concentrations in this research project was conducted just in front of the performance of the "cofo" test, because this was the point at which peak exposure occurred as evidenced by conducting laboratory testing of job function components with a Miran 1A Infrared Analyzer and the Bendix/Gastec Colorimetric Detection System. This peak determination was made for corn, wheat, rye, oats, and barley, and in each instance the "cofo" test had the highest potential for CCl_4 exposure. The second highest potential for exposure occurred during the opening of the grain sample bag for

corn, wheat, and barley and during passing the grain through the
dockage mill for rye and oats. The concentration range for the
"cofo" test was from approximately 15.5-71.0 ppm on the Miran 1A
Infrared Analyzer and from approximately 12->60 ppm on the
Bendix/Gastec Colorimetric Tubes. The range for opening the grain
sample bag for corn, wheat and barley on the Miran 1A was from 2.8-
3.0 ppm and on the Bendix/Gastec system the readings were
approximately 1.5-3.0 ppm. The results for passing the grain through
the dockage mill was 2 ppm for rye and 5 ppm for oats. Ambient air of
grain samples was checked as close to, but in front of, the grain
inspector performing the "cofo" test; and this value is used as an
estimator of peak grain inspector exposure.

Samples that contained high concentrations (>100 ppm) of CCl_4
were frequently detected at the time of "breakdown." Inspectors
could smell CCl_4 as soon as they opened the canvas and inner
polyethylene bags that held the grain sample. These relatively
infrequent samples contained such high levels of CCl_4 that inspectors
removed them from the inspection process at that time and held them
out until the odor dissipated to levels below detection by the
olfactory senses. Since the level of detection for CCl_4 is about 70
ppm there was the possibility that samples that had been held out
because of excessive CCl_4 concentrations were allowed back into the
inspection process as soon as their CCl_4 concentration had dropped
below the 70 ppm threshold of detection. Reliance on the olfactory
sense results in detection of samples containing high levels of CCl_4
but probably not of samples containing concentrations at or above the
OSHA acceptable ceiling of 25 ppm and the ACGIH STEL of 20 ppm but
below the odor threshold.

When the information on the odor threshold and colorimetric tube
methods were demonstrated to the various inspectors and their
supervisors, the colorimetric tube method was preferable for
detecting the presence of CCl_4 concentrations in grain samples to be
inspected. Inspectors who had been relying on CCl_4 odors as a method
of detection were shown that such a method was inadequate to keep
exposures below the OSHA and ACGHI ceilings. As a result of the
explanation as to why odor threshold detection was inadequate, the
inspectors could understand how a more sensitive detection system
could reduce their exposures to CCl_4.

The frequency of occurrence of concentrations of CCl_4 in the
ambient air of grain samples was determined (Table III).
Approximately 87% of the 7,749 samples checked showed no colorimetric
tube evidence of CCl_4, whereas 8.2% evidenced 5 ppm and 1.9% 10 ppm
CCl_4 concentration. All other concentrations in 5 ppm increment were
less than 1% frequency. Approximately 0.5% of the grain samples
checked evidenced a concentration of CCl_4 >60 ppm, which was the
upper limit of detection for the Bendix/Gastec Colorimetric Tube
System. This system is NIOSH approved for CCl_4 and has a $\pm$ 25%
accuracy rating.

Table III. CCl_4 Concentrations in Ambient
Air of Grain Samples*

PPM	N	%
0	6764	87.3
5	632	8.2
10	151	1.9
15	43	0.6
20	31	0.4
25	18	0.2
30	22	0.3
35	7	0.1
40	9	0.1
45	9	0.1
50	10	0.1
55	5	0.1
60	13	0.1
> 60	35	0.5
	7749	100.0

*Bendix/Gastec Colorimetric Tubes

The mean CCl_4 concentration for the 7,749 grain samples checked was 1.69 ppm with a standard deviation of 8.35.

The data collected on ambient air concentrations of CCl_4 in grain samples to be inspected were analyzed statistically for significant differences between means as related to location of work, type of grain, type of grain transportation vehicle, and date.

Results indicated that Duluth (8.78) had a significantly higher ppm mean than Minneapolis (1.24) or Mankato (0.66) at p=.05 (Table IV).

Table IV. CCl_4 CONCENTRATION IN GRAIN SAMPLE AMBIENT AIR BY SAMPLING LOCATION

	MEAN (ppm)	S.D.	N	%
Minneapolis	1.24	6.16	6443	83.1
Mankato	0.66	2.63	781	10.1
Duluth	8.78*	22.32	525	6.8
			7749	100.0

*Significantly different from other means at p=.05.

The data also indicated (Table V) that corn (0.64) had a significantly lower mean than the other tested grains and that oats, rye, and other grains had signficantly higher means than barley, corn and wheat at p=.05.

Table V. CCl_4 CONCENTRATION IN GRAIN SAMPLE AMBIENT AIR BY TYPE OF GRAIN

	MEAN (ppm)	S.D.	N	%
Barley	1.69	8.74	1491	19.2
Corn	0.64*	2.96	1853	23.9
Oats	4.24**	17.80	257	3.3
Rye	4.62**	17.24	326	4.2
Wheat	1.84	7.82	3676	47.4
Other***	4.24**	17.80	146	1.9
			7749	100.0

*Significantly different from all other means at p=.05.
**Significantly different from barley, corn, and wheat means at p=.05.
***Other-Buckwheat, Flax, Sorghum, Soybeans, and Sunflowers.

When analyzed by grain transportation vehicle (Table VI), boats
had a mean that was significantly (p=.05) higher than other transportation vehicle means. Analysis by date (Table VII) revealed a
significant increase in the fall months of 1981. September (4.71),
October (4.20), and December (5.17) 1981 were significantly different
from the other means, and August (2.96) 1981 was different from other
means except for November (2.44) 1981 and April (2.03) 1982.
November (2.44) 1981 was different from the other means except for
August (2.96) 1981 and April (2.03) and October (1.06) 1982. April
(2.03) 1982 was different from the means except for July (.96),
August (2.96), and November (2.44) 1981 and October (1.06) 1982.

Table VI. CCl_4 CONCENTRATION IN GRAIN SAMPLE AMBIENT
AIR BY GRAIN TRANSPORT VEHICLE

	MEAN (ppm)	S.D.	N	%
Barge	1.43	5.47	237	3.1
Boat	32.10*	35.68	112	1.4
Boxcar	1.26	8.74	167	2.2
Hoppercar	1.21	6.53	5144	66.4
Truck	1.45	5.40	1826	23.6
Other	.40	2.17	263	3.4
			7749	100.0

*Significantly different from other means at p=.05.

Table VII. CCl$_4$ CONCENTRATION IN GRAIN SAMPLE AMBIENT
AIR BY DATE

DATE	MEAN (ppm)	S.D.	N	%
7/81	0.96	3.24	250	3.2
8/81**	2.96	7.86	312	4.0
9/81*	4.71	13.23	450	2.8
10/81*	4.20	13.90	541	7.0
11/81***	2.44	11.25	398	5.1
12/81*	5.17	19.40	464	6.0
1/82	0.78	3.20	465	6.0
2/82	0.45	1.69	566	7.3
3/82	0.76	4.59	810	10.5
4/82****	2.03	9.35	481	6.2
5/82	0.52	1.98	474	6.1
6/82	0.20	1.09	490	6.3
7/82	0.42	2.04	608	7.8
8/82	1.08	4.08	1023	13.2
9/82	0.50	1.93	308	4.0
10/82	1.06	4.96	109	1.4

*Significantly different from other means at p=.05.
**Significantly different from other means except
  11/81 & 4/82 at p=.05.
***Significantly different from other means except 8/81,
  4/82 and 10/82 at p=.05.
****Significantly different from other means except 7/81, 8/81
  11/81 and 10/82 at p=.05.

According to information supplied by the Division of Grain
Inspection, Minnesota Department of Agriculture, the frequency of
sample collection and sample inspection per employee can be
determined. During fiscal 1980 the Division of Grain Inspection had
144 samplers that collected 484,107 samples, or 3,361 samples per
grain sampler. With approximately 240 work days per year, this is
equal to 14 samples collected per day for each grain sampler. The
Division of Grain Inspection also employed 103 inspectors who
inspected 648,656 samples, or 6,297 samples per grain inspector.
This is equal to approximately 26 samples inspected per day for each
grain inspector. Therefore, the average grain inspector performs the
"cofo" test 26 times per day. During each "cofo" test the inspector
inserts his nose into the pan of grain that he is grading and inhales
for 1-2 seconds to check the grain for rancidity, sourness and other
off odors. The inhaled air is held by the inspector for another 1-2
seconds and then released. This peak exposure period lasts
approximately 3-4 seconds per "cofo" test or on the average from 1-2
minutes in each work day.

Determination for 8-hour time weighted averages (TWAs) evidenced
a range from nondetected to 1.88 ppm based on 379 vapor monitor
badges. Sensitivity ranged from .01 to .09 ppm. The highest reading

of 1.88 ppm occurred for the principal investigator on this research project. The date was December 22, 1981 at Mankato when corn samples collected from hopper cars were being inspected. The second highest value of 1.61 ppm occurred on October 5, 1981 at Mankato when corn samples collected from hopper cars were being inspected. This badge was attached to the pants cuff of the dockage mill operator. Another badge that was attached to his shirt collar had a concentration of 0.15 ppm.

The third highest value of 1.18 ppm, and also the only other value above 1 ppm, occurred on October 22, 1981 at Duluth when wheat samples collected from a boat being filled were being inspected. This badge was attached to the grain divider that samples were passed through just after collection. The badge on the grain sampler who performed this function had a concentration of 0.075 ppm. On this same day and in this same location a badge attached to the pants cuff of the grain inspector had a concentration of 0.25 ppm, a badge attached to the shirt collar of the inspector was 0.055 and an employee designated as the "rover" had a concentration of 0.18 ppm. The "rover" moves about within the grain handling facility checking on automatic sampling systems and performing other duties. The researcher's badge on this day had a value of 0.70 ppm.

Other TWA concentration that were greater than 0.5 ppm included an inspector (0.71) in Minneapolis on April 22, 1982 who was inspecting oats samples collected from hopper cars and a grain sampler (0.82) in Duluth on December 13, 1981 who was sampling trucks of wheat. The sampling of the wheat was done automatically and the sampler remained in a small cinder block room to which the sample was pneumatically delivered. Periodically, he would bag up some of the wheat and send it on to an inspector for the grading process.

All of the other badges had 8-hour TWA concentrations of less than 0.5 ppm. This amount is at least 20 times below the OSHA 8-hour TWA value of 10 ppm. ACGIH recommends a Threshold Limit Value of 5 ppm and NIOSH recommends a 2 ppm ceiling for 1 hour.

The 3M #3500 Organic Vapor Monitor is very simple in design and function. It is NIOSH approved for CCl₄. Badge preparation is easy and its use does not interfer with job performance. The Minnesota Department of Agriculture has laboratory facilities capable of analyzing these badges. Badges cost about $6 each. Results of this research indicate which employees should wear badges based on date, location, type of grain, and type of grain vehicle.

The Bendix/Gastec Colorimetric Pump and Tube method is easily understandable and functionally simple. It is NIOSH approved for CCl₄. Preparing the apparatus to test for CCl₄ is also easy. Pumps cost approximately $100 each and the double tube system costs $4 for both tubes, or approximately $20 for a box of 5 testing systems. Results of this research indicate which samples have the greatest potential for CCl₄ presence based on date, location, type of grain, and type of grain vehicle. These samples would be the ones that should be checked most often, although continued random checking would still be advised.

Conclusion

There was evidence of grain sampler and grain inspector exposure to carbon tetrachloride from its use as a grain fumigant based on the results of colorimetric tube and passive dosimeter monitoring. Peak exposure for the grain inspector occurred during the commercially objectionable foreign odor "cofo" test. The average ambient CCl_4 concentration per sample was 1.69 ppm. There were significant differences in peak exposure potentials between locations, by type of grain, by type of grain vehicle, and by date.

Time Weighted Average (TWA) breathing zone exposures for both grain samplers and grain inspectors were below 1 ppm.

These exposure results were within the limits of the OSHA standards for TWA, ceiling, and peak exposure and the ACGIH TLV standard of 5 ppm. The peak exposures determined sometimes exceeded the ACGIH Short Term Exposure Limit maximum of 20 ppm and the NIOSH 2 ppm for 1-hour ceiling exposure limit.

Continued monitoring of grain samples, especially Duluth boat samples and rye and oats samples and late summer and fall (August-December) samples, is recommended.

Nontechnical Summary

The inhalation exposure of Minnesota Department of Agriculture Grain Samplers and Grain Inspectors to carbon tetrachloride from its use as a grain fumigant was studied over a 16 month period from July 1981 to October 1982 in three locations; Minneapolis, Mankato, and Duluth. Peak exposures were determined by the use of colorimetric tubes and work day exposures were determined by use of passive dosimeters attached to worker's shirt collars. Peak exposures occurred during performance of the commercially objectionable foreign odor or "cofo", test. The ambient air of approximately 7,700 grain samples submitted for inspection were checked by colorimetric tube and these values are indicators of peak exposure for grain inspectors. Approximately 87% of the samples checked showed no evidence for CCl_4 while approximately 8% indicated 5 ppm and 2% indicated 10 ppm. One half of 1% showed a CCl_4 concentration of greater than 60 ppm which was the upper limit of detection for colorimetric tube system. The average CCl_4 concentration per sample was 1.69 ppm.

Data collected was analyzed statistically for significant mean differences according to location, type of grain, type of grain transportation vehicle, and date. Duluth was significantly higher than Minneapolis or Mankato in its ppm mean per sample. Oats, rye, and other grains (buckwheat, flax, sorghum, soybeans, and sunflowers) were significantly higher than barley, corn, and wheat. Boats had a significantly higher CCl_4 concentration than barges, boxcars, hoppercars, and trucks. The fall months of September, October, and December were significantly higher than other months.

All work day exposures were less than 2 ppm on a time weighted average. Most were less than 1 ppm. The Occupational Safety and Health Administration's (OSHA) time weighted average (TWA) standards is set at 10 ppm, while the American Conference of Governmental Industrial Hygienists' standard is 5 ppm and the National Institute for Occupational Safety and Health's standard is set a 2 ppm for 1 hour.

The methodology used in this research showed the advantages of using a system such as the colorimetric tube rather than olfactory senses for determining the presence and concentration of CCl_4 in grain samples. The simplicity and cost effectiveness of the methodology makes it adaptable by the Minnesota Department of Agriculture for continued monitoring of CCl_4 exposure to grain samplers and grain inspectors.

Acknowledgments

This project was supported through the North Central Region Pesticide Impact Assessment Program. Acknowledgment is given to Tom Krick and Dave Baloga, University of Minnesota, who conducted the GC-MS vapor monitor analysis.

Literature Cited

1. National Pesticide Information Retrieval System (NPIRS), 1983.
2. "Protection of Environment." Code of Federal Regulations, Chapter 10, 1983.
3. "Ethylene Dibromide; Rebuttable Presumption Against Registration and Continued Registration of Certain Pesticide Products." Federal Register Vol 42, No. 240, December 14, 1977.
4. "Ethylene Dibromide; Decision and Emergency Order Suspending Registrations of Pesticide Products Containing EDB." Federal Register, Vol. 49, No. 25, February 6, 1984.
5. "Ethylene Dibromide; Intent to Cancel Registrations of Pesticide Products Containing Ethylene Dibromide;..." Federal Register, Vol. 48, No. 197, October 11, 1983.
6. Berck, B. J. Agric. Food Chem., 1974, 22, 977-984.
7. Jagielski, J.; Scudamore, K.A.; Heuser, S.G. Pestic. Sci.1978, 9, 117-126.
8. Olomucki, E.; Bondi, A. J. Sci. Food Agric. 1955, 6, 592.
9. "Carbon Tetrachloride; Rebuttable Presumption Against Registration and Continued Registration of Certain Pesticide Products." Federal Register. Vol. 45, No. 201, October 15, 1980.
10. Clayton, G.D.; Clayton, F.E. "Patty's Industrial Hygiene and Toxicology,", John Wiley and Sons, New York, 1981; 3472-3478.
11. Hayes, W.J. "Toxicology of Pesticides", The Williams and Wilkins Company, Baltimore, MD 1975.
12. "Criteria For a Recommended Standard - Occupational Exposure to Carbon Tetrachloride." National Institute for Occupational Safety and Health, 1975.
13. Torkelson, T.R.; Hoyle, H.R.; Rowe, V.K. Pest Control, 1966, 6.

14.   Leonardos, G.; Kendall, D.; Barnard, N. J. of Air Pollution,
      1969, 19, 91-95.
15. "NIOSH/OSHA Occupational Health Guidelines for Chemical Hazards."
      National Institute for Occupational Safety and Health, 1981.
16.   Smith, P. Lancet 1867, 6, 660-62, 693, 762-63, 791-92.
17.   Thomson, W.T. "Agricultural Chemicals - Book III, Miscellaneous
      Chemicals (Fumigants, Growth Regulators, Repellents, and Roden-
      ticides)," Thomson Publications, Fresno, CA, 1978; p. 8.
18.   Britton, W.E. Connecticut Agricultural Experiment Station
      Report No. 31.
19.   Patty, F.A. "Industrial Hygiene and Toxicology," 2nd Edition,
      Interscience Publishers, New York, 1963; Vol II; p. 1264-1269.
20.   Casarett, L.J.; Doull, J. "Toxicology, The Basic Science
      of Poisons"; Macmillan Publishing Company, New York, 1975; p.472.
21.   "Documentation of the Threshold Limit Values for Substances in
      Workroom Air." American Conference of Governmental Industrial
      Hygienists, 3rd ed, 1971.
22.   Berck, B. X Int. Congr. Entomol. Proc., 1956, p. 94-104.
23.   Berck, B. Canadian Dept. of Agriculture, Publication Number
      1004, 1961.
24.   Harein, P.K. Unpublished data. "A Review of Fumigant Residues on
      Grain and Cereal Products as Hazards to Domestic Livestock."
      Agricultural Experiment Station, University of Minnesota, St.
      Paul, MN, 1981.
25.   Metcalf, C.L.; Flint, W.P. "Destructive and Useful Insects,"
      McGraw-Hill Book Company, New York, 1962; p. 382,383.
26.   Storey, C.L.; Martin, C.R.; Sukkestad, D.R. J. Econ. Entomol
      1981, 74:188-190.
27.   "The Biologic and Economic Assessment of the Pesticide Carbon
      Tetrachloride." United States Department of Agriculture, (in
      preparation).
28.   Harein, P.K.; Deer, H.M.; Barak, A., Minnesota Cooperative Ex-
      tension Service, University of Minnesota, St. Paul, MN, 1979.
29.   "Farm Use of Minnesota Pesticides 1978." Minnesota Crop & Live-
      stock Reporting Service, St. Paul, MN, 1980.
30.   "Pesticides Used on Minnesota Farms in 1980." Minnesota Agri-
      cultural Statistics Service, St. Paul, MN, 1981.
31.   "The Use of Pesticides For Stored Grain In Ohio 1980." Ohio
      Cooperative Extension Service, Ohio State University, Columbus,
      Columbus, OH, 1982.
32.   Heseltine, H.K. Chem. Ind., 1969, 41:1405-1408.
33.   Douglas Chemical Co. "Douglas Tetrafume Weevil Killer and Grain
      Conditioner", EPA Reg. NO. 1015-10. Liberty, Missouri, 1983.
34.   Douglas Chemical Co. "Douglas Tetrakill Weevil Killer and Grain
      Conditioner, EPA Reg. No. 1015-20. Liberty, Missouri, 1983.
35.   Dow Chemical Co. "Vertifume," EPA Reg. NO. 464-188-AA, Midland
      MI., 1981.
36. Research Products Co."Max Kill High Life Liquid Grain Fumigant,"
      EPA Reg. No. 2548-22. Salina, KS., 1983.
37.   Stauffer Chemical Co. "F.I.A. 80-20 Grain Fumigant With SO_2,"
      EPA Reg. No. 476-1113. NY, 1983.
38.   TH Agriculture and Nutrition Co. "De Pester Fumigant 82 FR,"
      EPA Reg. No. 46946-105. Kansas City, MO., 1983.

39. TH Agriculture and Nutrition Co. "De Pester Fumigant No. 2," EPA Reg. No. 46946-149. Kansas City, MO., 1983.
40. TH Agriculture and Nutrition Co. "De Pester Super Fumigas," EPA Reg. No. 46946-21. Kansas City, MO., 1983.
41. Vulcan Materials Co. "Vulcan Formula 82-H Grain Fumigant," EPA Reg. No. 5382-6. Birmingham, AL., 1983.
42. Vulcan Materials Co., "Vulcan Terminal Grain Fumigant," EPA Reg. No. 5382-31. Birmingham, AL., 1983.
43. Hayes, Jr., W.J. "Pesticides Studied In Man"; Williams and Wilkins, Baltimore, MD., 1982.
44. "The Federal Insecticide, Fungicide, and Rodenticide Act As Amended." United States Environmental Protection Agency, 1978.
45. "Regulations for the Enforcement of the Federal, Insecticide, Fungicide and Rodenticide Act; Notification to the Secretary of Agriculture of a Proposed Regulation Classifying Certain Uses of Four Pesticide Active Ingredients for Restricted Use." Federal Register, Vol. 48, No. 145, July 27, 1983.
46. "The Official United States Standards for Grain." United States Department of Agriculture, 1978.
47. Bielorai, R.; Alumot, E. J. Agric. Food Chem. 1973, 23, 426-429.
48. Dhaliwal, G.S. J. Food Sci. Technolo. 1974, 12, 1-5.
49. Harein, P.K. Minnesota Cooperative Extension Service, University of Minnesota, St. Paul, MN, 1979.
50. Heuser, S.G. Proc. 1st International Working Conference, 1974.
51. Lindgren, D.L.; Vincent, L.E. J. Econ. Entomol., 1960, 53, 1071-1077.
52. Scudamore, K.A.; Goodship, G. Pestic. Sci., 1982, 13, 149-155.
53. Scudamore, K.A.; Heuser, S.G. Pestic. Sci., 1973, 4, 1-12.
54. Storey, C.L. J. Econ. Entomol., 1971, 64, 227-230
55. "Summary of NIOSH Recommendations for Occupational Health Standards." National Institute for Occupational Safety and Health, 1980.
56. "Threshold Limit Values for Chemical Substances and Physical Agents in the Work Environment With Intended Changes for 1983-84." American Conference of Governmental Industrial Hygienists 1983.
57. "NIOSH/OSHA Pocket Guide to Chemical Hazards." National Institute for Occupational Safety and Health, 1978.

RECEIVED September 16, 1984

Inhalation Exposure of Museum Personnel
to Ethylene Dichloride–Carbon Tetrachloride Fumigant

TERRY D. SPITTLER, JOHN B. BOURKE, PAUL B. BAKER[1], and GEORGE W. HELFMAN

Pesticide Residue Laboratory, New York State Agricultural Experiment Station, Cornell University, Geneva, NY 14456

Prior to the semiannual fumigation of the private study collections in the Division of Birds and Mammals, National Museum of Natural History, Smithsonian Institution, five staff members were monitored for inhalation exposure to Dowfume 75 (70% ethylene dichloride plus 30% carbontetrachloride) using activated carbon traps. The one-week study was repeated seven days following fumigation and again 30 days thereafter. Personnel in both the Mammals and Birds divisions, and also in the adjacent, non-fumigated, Division of Anthropology, wore battery operated air monitors throughout their daily routines. Eight-hour time weighted average exposure was found by GLC analysis to be within the 50 ppm and 10 ppm OSHA standards allowed for EDC and CCl_4, respectively.

Museum and archive specimens demand and warrant a level of protection from pests (primarily insects, occasionally fungi) that approaches absolute. Historical artifacts and preserved members of extinct species are not, unlike commercial products, renewable commodities. Consequently, a damage threshold or allowable loss level is not possible if valuable collections are to be maintained. Most collections are, however, dynamic, with the addition of new items, and the removal of others for loan or study, constantly taking place. Both the storage and the flux of a viable collection have the potential for infestation and irreparable damage. Therefore, pest protection is an important and constant responsibility of a museum's staff.

[1] Current address: Department of Entomology, New York State Agricultural Experiment Station, Cornell University, Geneva, NY 14456

0097–6156/85/0273–0243$06.00/0

A recent survey of museum personnel regarding problems and pesticide usage elucidated the full range of troubles that beset institutions of all sizes, and the remedies (both legal and illegal) that they use (1). Because the loss of some chemicals due to the RPAR (Rebuttable Presumption Against Registration) process could remove certain protection methods from the preservation scene, we were investigating the potential impact of this at selected Northeastern museums and libraries. The dominant question (or concern) that emerged was the one of personnel exposure to those approved chemicals already in use. And of particular interest was Dowfume 75, a widely used fumigant composed of two volatile materials, ethylene dichloride (70%) and carbontetrachloride (30%). These materials have OSHA standards of 50 ppm and 10 ppm, respectively, for eight-hour time weighted average exposure (2).

Dowfume 75 is used on a semiannual basis to protect the study specimens in the Bird and Mammal Divisions of the National Museum of Natural History, Smithsonian Institution, Washington, DC. Although the study collections are not open to the public and are frequented only by the museum staff and authorized visiting scholars, there was concern on the part of the administration and staff that exposure to these chemicals might be in excess of the recognized safe levels cited. So, with the cooperation of the Museum of Natural History, a personnel exposure study was initiated using volunteers who gave their informed written consent; additionally, the study was reviewed and approved by the Cornell University Human Subjects Committee. Verification that label-specified uses of this fumigant were yielding exposures below permissible amounts would both reassure current personnel and provide valuable data in the event these compounds and their uses fell under the spectre of re-evaluation by OSHA and/or EPA.

Housed on the floors of the Museum of Natural History above those open to the general public, the study collections consist of several million bird and mammal specimens contained in over 4900 sealed, wooden or metal quarter case equivalents. These vary in size from 1 M x 1 M x .75 M quarter cases for small specimens to 2 M x 2 M x .75 M full cases for whole body mounts. Each case contains drawers and/or shelves according to the item(s) it accommodates. Cases have one or more reservoirs holding approximately 200 mL of liquid fumigant and a cotton wick attached to the door or mounted on the inner walls. Reservoirs are refilled, as needed, when repeated opening of individual cases allows the fumigant to dissipate. In addition, new and loan-return specimens are fumigated in a separate area before being brought into the range (case area) or returned to a case. Every six months all cases are opened and the reservoirs are replenished--an empty reservoir is indicative of excessive loss through the seal and is cause for a complete inspection of the case and its contents.

This fumigation is always done on Saturdays by qualified staff members, thus allowing for proper ventilation of the premises prior to the return of the full staff Monday AM. Two-man teams wearing charcoal-filter respirators, gloves, and rubber aprons open each case and refill the reservoirs from a three-gallon canister which is in turn refilled from a 50 gallon drum stored in the receiving area. Cases which have not been opened since the last fumigation/inspection generally require the addition of less than 50 mL/reservoir. Cases receiving intermittent use would require more. The amount of Dowfume 75 used in each semiannual proceeding averages 35 gallons for Mammals and 25 gallons for Birds.

However, the workers performing this operation were experienced and well protected and not really the primary objects of concern. Rather, the staff who work unprotected throughout the collection range forty hours a week were. The Division of Mammals and the Division of Birds are the only sections employing Dowfume 75; Anthropology, located between these two divisions, does not fumigate, but its staff has indicated its awareness of the chemicals used by the others, and the Divisions of the Entomology, Crustacea, etc., employ alternative control methods.

Exposure Monitoring

Two subjects each from Birds and Mammals were fitted with Accuhaler Model 808 Personal Sampling Pumps (MDA Scientific Inc., Glenview, IL 60025). A fifth Accuhaler was hung in the Anthropology section, contiguous to Birds and Mammals. Each unit was worn on a belt clip and measured 17 cM x 8 cM x 3.5 cM. The battery operated air pump (rechargeable) drew air at a rate of approximately 100 cc/min. through a 2 mM x 1 M Tygon tube, to the end of which was attached an activated charcoal-containing glass tube. This tube was secured in a protective plastic holder which was clipped to the shirt collar so as to sample the breathing air available to the subject. Tubes were of two sizes, containing either 100 mg or 400 mg of charcoal adsorbent, the size selected being dependent upon the levels of material expected to be encountered.

At the start of each work day subjects were given a recharged unit with a fresh charcoal tube to wear during the performance of their usual routine. The time and machine cycle counts were recorded at the start and finish of the day. Each PSP had a calibration factor unique to its cycle counts (e.g. 5.4 cc/cycle) such that the exact volume of air sampled was determined. If the subject had to leave the building for any period of time the unit was turned off and the time and counts recorded. Likewise, they were recorded when the unit was restarted upon reentry. At day's end, final readings were made by the technician in charge who also took each charcoal tube, sealed it with plastic endcaps, and tagged it for analysis. Tubes were kept frozen until extracted.

After a five-day survey (April 6, 7, 8, 9, & 12, 1982) using four mobile subjects and one stationary location, fumigation of the Bird Division took place on April 24, 1982 and of the Mammal Division on May 1, 1982. Following the fumigation of the Mammals section, a five-day monitoring was performed May 4, 5, 6, 7, & 10, 1982, and a third assessment was made thirty

days later on June 2, 3, 4, 7 & 8, 1982. Four subjects were
employed in these trials due to the malfunctioning of one of the
PSP units.

Sample Analysis

Sample ampullas were sent to the Pesticide Residue Laboratory,
Cornell University, Geneva, NY for analysis using modifications
of standard methods(3). Each 100 mg tube was eluted with 6 mL
of anhydrous diethyl ether (400 mg tubes, 10 mL) and this
solution was chromatographed as 5 μL injections on a Tracor MT-
220 Gas Chromatograph; Column 15% OV-17 on CW-HP, 80-100 mesh, 6
ft. x 1/4 in. glass; Oven temperature program $55_6^{\circ}C$ to $170^{\circ}C$ @
$5^{\circ}C/min.$; inlet $210^{\circ}C.$, detector $300^{\circ}C.$ using a ^{63}Ni electron
capture detector. Sensitivity: 0.41 ng CCl_4 gave 5% full scale
deflection (90% recovery), whereas 1.6 ng EDC gave 5% full scale
deflection (95% recovery).

Results and Discussion

Monitoring parameters, subject location, and analytical data are
contained in Table 1. EDC and CCl_4 are expressed in ppm as the
average concentration encountered over the duration (min) of a
particular days tasks. These are equivalent to the eight-hour
time weighted average OSHA standards. Normally calculated using
Equation 1, where E is the sum of a finite number of products of
a concentration(C) times a time interval(T), divided by eight,
our determinations were made over the entire (ca 480 min) shift.

$$E = (C_a T_a + C_b T_b \dots C_n T_n)/8 \qquad (1)$$

Figures 1, 2 and 3 summarize the results obtained for the
three monitoring periods, i.e. pretreatment, post-treatment, and
30 days post-treatment. What is immediately obvious is that no
eight-hour exposure exceeds or even approaches the 50 and 10 ppm
allowable levels for EDC and CCl_4, respectively. Subject 02
received an average exposure of 18 ppm EDC on May 4, 1982, and
CCl_4 exposures of 1.3 and 1.2 ppm were noted for subjects 02 and
07 on May 5, and May 7, 1982, but even these are well within
tolerances. Other measurable exposures are evident for certain
personnel but these are even less significant than those shown
for subjects 02 and 07. Points clustered in the non-detectable
to 0.10 ppm range are plotted for illustrative purposes only.
Inspection of Figures 1, 2 & 3 suggests that background levels
were raised the week following fumigation, but that they had
dropped to background levels by 30 days post-treatment.
        A brief, task-oriented study in which subjects performed
typical operations in and near treated cases for one-hour
intervals while wearing PSP's showed no detectable levels.
Insufficient data are available to speculate as to what events
and of what duration are necessary to produce periodic
exposures exceeding even 1 ppm.
        The conclusion to be draw from this study was that exposure
to EDC and CCl_4, the components of Dowfume 75, in the Birds,
Mammals and Anthropology Divisions of the Museum of Natural

Table I. Monitoring of Museum Personnel and Sites for Exposure
to EDC and CCl$_4$

DATE	SUBJ-DIV*	TIME(min)	AIR(Liters)	EDC(ppm)	CCl4(ppm)
4-6-82	01-M	441	38.70	0.27	0.10
4-7-82	01-M	425	36.95	--	0.15
4-8-82	01-M	430	38.91	0.95	0.01
4-9-82	01-M	513	46.07	0.81	0.006
4-12-82	01-M	373	33.44	0.017	0.005
4-6-82	02-M	472	41.41	0.012	0.002
4-7-82	02-M	415	37.14	--	0.077
4-8-82	02-M	571	47.05	0.16	0.027
4-9-82	02-M	472	37.55	0.15	0.016
4-12-82	02-M	416	34.90	**	0.009
4-6-82	03-B	455	38.93	--	0.007
4-7-82	03-B	438	38.28	--	0.038
4-8-82	03-B	502	41.54	--	0.021
4-9-82	03-B	402	35.60	--	0.030
4-12-82	03-B	493	41.20	--	0.007
4-6-82	04-B	380	24.71	0.029	--
4-7-82	04-B	442	27.78	--	0.005
4-8-82	04-B	438	27.33	--	--
4-9-82	06-B	457	28.36	0.051	--
4-12-82	06-B	480	25.77	0.048	--
4-6-82	05-A	363	37.81	--	--
4-7-82	05-A	469	47.84	**	**
4-8-82	05-A	500	49.22	--	--
4-9-82	05-A	**	36.51	--	--
4-12-82	05-A	**	38.92	--	0.005
5-4-82	07-M	506	44.27	--	0.68
5-5-82	07-M	500	43.53	0.57	0.41
5-6-82	07-M	525	44.84	--	0.10
5-7-82	01-M	375	33.34	0.65	0.19
5-10-82	01-M	388	33.28	--	0.59
5-4-82	02-M	527	44.35	18	0.085
5-5-82	02-M	446	37.18	--	1.3
5-6-82	02-M	403	33.49	--	0.099
5-7-82	07-M	518	42.04	--	1.2
5-10-82	07-M	515	42.04	--	0.031
5-4-82	03-B	490	41.07	--	0.88
5-5-82	03-B	488	40.94	--	0.074
5-6-82	03-B	427	35.88	--	0.028
5-7-82	03-B	402	33.45	--	0.076
5-10-82	03-B	512	42.87	--	0.027
5-4-82	05-A	521	32.13	--	0.039
5-5-82	05-A	508	31.41	--	0.027
5-6-82	05-A	518	31.92	--	0.023
5-7-82	05-A	515	30.07	--	0.065
5-10-82	05-A	524	31.78	--	0.008

Continued on next page.

Table I. Continued

DATE	SUBJ-DIV*	TIME(min)	AIR(liters)	EDC(ppm)	CCl4(ppm)
6-2-82	07-M	430	38.21	--	--
6-3-82	07-M	493	43.18	--	0.020
6-4-82	07-M	545	47.03	--	0.032
6-7-82	07-M	499	43.93	--	0.020
6-8-82	07-M	464	40.55	--	0.029
6-2-82	02-M	439	35.30	--	0.14
6-3-82	02-M	467	37.25	0.63	0.060
6-4-82	02-M	428	35.08	--	0.081
6-7-82	02-M	493	39.52	--	0.003
6-8-82	02-M	373	29.54	--	0.28
6-2-82	03-B	444	37.69	--	0.014
6-3-82	03-B	493	41.61	--	0.010
6-4-82	03-B	509	42.20	--	0.035
6-7-82	03-B	456	37.47	--	0.012
6-8-82	03-B	380	31.45	--	0.012
6-2-82	05-A	430	26.31	--	--
6-3-82	05-A	487	29.16	--	0.006
6-4-82	05-A	604	35.37	--	--
6-7-82	05-A	493	29.66	--	--
6-8-82	05-A	460	27.66	**	**

*M=Mammals, B=Birds, A=Anthropology
**Datum lost
--Nondetectable; <0.01 EDC, <0.001 CCl$_4$

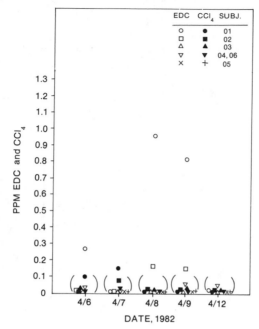

Figure 1. Exposure monitoring of museum personnel, pre-fumigation.

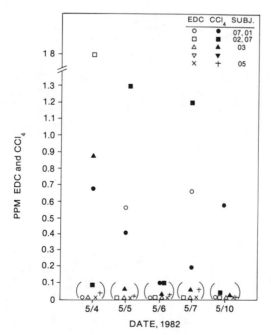

Figure 2. Exposure monitoring of museum personnel, post-fumigation.

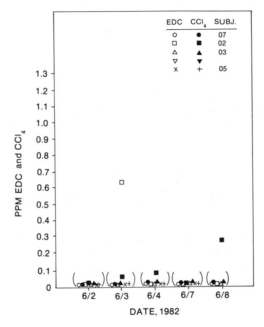

Figure 3.   Exposure monitoring of museum personnel, 30 days post-fumigation.

History was well within the limits allowed by OSHA. No judgement as to the inherent safety and effectiveness of these chemicals is inferred, and it is recognized that exposure standards are subject to revision.

Nontechnical Summary

When Dowfume 75 was used as a fumigant insecticide in closed specimen cases to protect the study collections of the National Museum of Natural History, Smithsonian Institution, the exposure of museum personnel to its components, ethylene dichloride and carbontetrachloride, was found to be well within OSHA's Standards of 50 and 10 parts per million, respectively. The highest exposures measured for persons working in the case range and occasionally opening and closing the cases were 18 ppm for ethylene dichloride and 1.3 ppm for carbontetrachloride. Monitoring was conducted by having volunteer staff members wear battery operated air inhalation devices for their entire working day(s). The activated carbon collection devices were analyzed by gas chromatography. Five-day studies were conducted the week before, the week after, and 30 days after a semiannual fumigation.

Acknowledgments

The assistance Dr. C. W. Hart, F. M. Greenwell, D. Schmitt and the staff of the National Museum of Natural History was greatly appreciated. Funding for this project was through the Northeast Pesticide Impact Assessment Program.

Literature Cited

1.   Edwards, S.R.; Bell, B.M.; King, M.E. "Pest Control in Museums"; Association of Systematic Collections: Lawrence, Kansas, 1981.

2.   Title 29, Code of Federal Regulations; Part 1910, Section 254 (29 CFR 1910.1000); Washington, D.C.

3.   "Pesticide Analytical Manual" II; Food and Drug Administration: Washington, D.C., 1982.

RECEIVED August 28, 1984

Dermal and Respiratory Exposure of Applicators and Residents to Dichlorvos-Treated Residences

ROGER E. GOLD[1] and TERRY HOLCSLAW[2]

[1] University of Nebraska, Lincoln, NE 68583–0802
[2] University of Nebraska Medical Center, Omaha, NE 68105

Applicators and residents of dichlorvos (DDVP) treated structures were monitored for evidence of insecticide exposure using exposure pads, air samplers, serum and red blood cell acetylcholinesterase (AChE) tests, and urine analysis. There was no evidence of DDVP or dichloroacetic acid (DCAA) in the urine of applicators or cooperators. There were slight but significant differences ($P \leq 0.05$) in serum AChE activity of residents of treated units, but erythrocyte AChE was unchanged. Applicator AChE test results were inconclusive. It was concluded that there was not a significant risk, in terms of acute toxicity, to either the pesticide applicators or the residents of treated structures.

Pesticides are toxicants that are deliberately added to the environment in an effort to insure our food and fiber supply, protect our homes and structures, and guard our health. Pesticide use is considered essential by many groups, but it is impossible to overlook the hidden costs (externalities) associated with their use. In 1962, Durham and Wolfe (1) expressed the opinion that there was not a single pesticide for which there is definitive information concerning the interrelationships between occupational exposure by different routes, the fate of the compound in the human body, and its chemical effects. Although that statement can no longer be made unconditionally, this premise remains valid for dichlorvos [2,2-dichlorovinyl dimethyl phosphate (DDVP)], a pesticide used both in agricultural and urban settings.

DDVP is an insecticide that has been subjected to the "special review" process by the U.S. Environmental Protection Agency (USEPA) based on reported mutagenicity, reproductive and fetotoxic effects, oncogenicity and neurotoxicity (2-5). Studies have been conducted on the respiratory and dermal exposure of humans to DDVP formulated in resin strips (6-9); however, limited research data are available on the exposure of humans to other formulations of DDVP used by commercial pest control applicators and homeowners (10) within structures.

Materials and Methods

The dermal exposure of applicators who applied DDVP in these replicated trials was monitored by using the techniques described by Durham and Wolfe (1), Gold et al. (10-12), and Leavitt et al. (13). Applicators wore a one-piece polyester jumpsuit with an open collar and long sleeves, a hard hat, respirator, and rubber gloves. They were fitted with both inside and outside dermal exposure pads placed on the outer clothing and on the skin beneath the clothing. Internally located pads (those beneath the clothing) were positioned carefully to avoid overlap with the external pads (those attached to the outer clothing). Pad locations were: head (both under and on top of the hard hat), forearm (just above the wrist), leg (just above the ankle), chest, and back.

Exposure pads were constructed in three layers. The bottom layer was a 10.2 by 10.2 cm glassine paper. An equal sized sheet of filter paper (Whatman Chromatography Paper, 0.16 mm thickness) was used as a second layer. Top layer was an eight-ply gauze pad (Steri-Pad). Layers were fastened together with strips of masking tape with a 6.4 by 6.4 cm area left exposed. Preliminary analysis indicated exposure pads contained no materials that would interfere with DDVP detection. Following pesticide applications, the exposure pads were removed from the applicators and were placed in Ziplock Sandwich Bags and stored on ice in an insulated cooler until frozen in the laboratory. Total amount of DDVP found on the exposure pads was divided by the exposed area of the pads and elapsed application time to give an estimated rate of exposure ($\mu g/cm2/hr$).

Dermal exposure was further monitored by washing both of the hands of each applicator in 200 ml of a 50:50 mixture of ethanol: water. Each hand was placed in the solution and shaken vigorously for approximately 30 seconds. Wash solutions were sealed in a glass jar and immediately placed on ice in an insulated cooler until they could be stored at 5°C in the laboratory. Preliminary experimental results indicated that DDVP was soluble in the washing solution. The amount of DDVP found on the hands following each application was divided by the area of both hands to give an estimate of hand exposure ($\mu g/cm^2/hr$).

Applicator respiratory exposure was monitored with a battery-powered personnel air pump (Telmatic Model 150A) fitted with a 30 ml glass midget impinger (Houston Glass Fabricating). The impinger was of the straight shank type with the shank end embedded in a plastic bubbler (Bendix). The impinger was filled with 5 ml of water plus 15 ml of ethylene glycol. Preliminary test results showed this mixture was effective in scrubbing DDVP from the air. The air sampler was bolted to a fiber belt and worn on the lower back. One end of a Tygon tube (15 mm internal diameter) was attached over the shoulder to rest on the upper chest. Air samplers pumped a mean of 44.6 liters/hr when worn by the applicators. At the end of the exposure period, the impinger was removed and immediately stored in ice. In the laboratory, the solution was transferred to a capped glass vial and held at 5°C until analysis. Data resulting from respiratory monitoring was expressed as µg DDVP/liter of air, calculated by dividing the amount of DDVP in the impinger by the length of application time and the pumping rate. The respiratory rate of the applicators was assumed to be 1,740 liters/hr (1).

Both blood and urine samples were collected from the applicators prior to (time 0) and then at regular intervals throughout the study period. Each subject had two 5 ml blood samples taken from the antecubital vein via Vacutainer. One blood sample was used to derive serum and the other was used as whole blood. Both the serum fraction and erythrocytes derived from the whole blood were assayed for acetylcholinesterase (AChE) activity by the spectrophotometric method of Ellman et al. (14) using acetylthiocholine as substrate. Urine samples were collected from each applicator at the time blood samples were drawn. Each urine sample was frozen for later analysis of DDVP and dichloracetic acid (DCAA) by a modification of the gas chromatographic method of Schultz et al. (15).

One resident from each of the 20 DDVP treated units was involved in pesticide exposure monitoring. Each cooperator provided both urine and blood samples before (time 0) and 24 hrs after their residence had been treated. At the time the initial and posttreatment samples were collected, each resident was interviewed to collect data on age, sex, health history, medications taken (including use of alcohol and tobacco), pesticides used, amounts of time spent in the treated units for the 24 hrs following DDVP application, and any adverse health effects noted as a result of the treatment.

Environmental exposure was monitored by placement of the same type of exposure pads as used in dermal monitoring on top of the refrigerator, stove, kitchen table, and kitchen floor (center). Pads were in place prior to insecticide application and were collected 2 hrs posttreatment. Pads from all locations (within each unit) were combined and analyzed using the procedures for dermal pads. Room air samplers were used to monitor DDVP concentrations prior to, during, and following DDVP application. The air samplers were designed and constructed specifically for this work and utilized a vacuum pump (Neptune Dyna-Pump Model 4K) connected in series with a Dwyer Model RMA-14-TMV flow meter, and a double impinger assembly with 5 ml ethanol and 15 ml ethylene glycol (total volume of each impinger was 20 ml). The air pumps were calibrated to operate at 66 liters/hr, and a Cramer Conrac Type 635 G minute meter was used to record the actual time the pump was in operation. Air samplers were operated in residences scheduled for treatment for 24 hrs to measure background levels of DDVP. On the day of treatment, air samplers were operated for 24 hrs; however, the impingers were replaced at 2 hrs, with the last sample at 24 hrs posttreatment (samples taken at 2 and 24 hrs). It was therefore possible to determine the amount of DDVP in ambient air both during treatment and the 24 hr posttreatment interval. Extraction and analysis of the room air samples were as described for personnel air samples.

A total of 20 single-family residences were treated with a
0.5% water emulsion spray of DDVP prepared from Vaponite 2EC (24.7%
Vapona). Application was made with a 3.8 liter B & G hand sprayer
operated at 137.9 kPa pressure fitted with a multi-tip nozzle set
for fan spray. Insecticide was applied in a continuous band along
the baseboards; around the doorways, windows and all entrances;
beneath the sink, stove and refrigerator; in and on all shelves and
cabinets; and around plumbing and other utility installations.
Cooperators were required to remove materials from all shelves,
closets and storage areas prior to treatment, and were asked to
stay out of the treated residences during treatment and for 2 hrs
posttreatment. Records were maintained as to the amount of DDVP
applied per residence and the time required to make the treatment.

Exposed dermal and environmental monitoring pads were kept at
-10°C until analysis to reduce volatilization and degradation of
DDVP. Prior to extraction, the tape edge of each pad was cut away
leaving the exposed gauze surface. The glassine backing was
discarded and pads (internal and external pads were extracted
separately) were folded and pushed into a 33 by 94 mm Whatman
single thickness cellulose thimble. Extraction proceeded for 3
hrs in 150 ml of glass-distilled acetone in a soxhlet extractor
fitted with a boiling flask. Following extraction, acetone was
concentrated to 5 ml with a vacuum rotary evaporator (Model R Buchi
Rotovapor) in a 40°C water bath. The extract was transferred to a
12 ml graduated centrifuge tube to which 2.5 ml of toluene was
added. A nitrogen stream and 40°C water bath was used to evaporate
the extract to a volume of 2.0 ml. After all acetone had
evaporated and the sample was in toluene, analysis was accomplished
by gas chromatography (GC).

Personnel air pump samples (20 ml) were poured into a 60 ml
separatory funnel. Distilled water (20 ml), part of which had been
used to rinse the sample container, was added. Two grams of reagent grade sodium chloride plus 9 ml of glass-distilled dichloromethane were added. Contents of the funnel were shaken vigorously
for two minutes. After phase separation, the lower dichloromethane
phase was decanted into a 12 ml graduated centrifuge tube. A second
extraction was made with 5 ml of dichloromethane and the extracts
combined. A nitrogen stream in conjunction with a 40°C water bath
was used to reduce the volume of the extracts to 5 ml, whereupon
2.5 ml of reagent toluene was added. Evaporation was continued to
a final volume of 2.0 ml. Following evaporation, 0.5 grams of
anhydrous sodium sulfate was added to the toluene to absorb moisture. Analysis proceeded using a GC.

Hand wash samples were poured into a 500 ml separatory funnel
to which was added 200 ml of water. Fifteen grams of reagent grade
sodium chloride plus 20 ml of glass-distilled dichloromethane were
added to the funnel. After shaking vigorously for two minutes,
phase separation was achieved. The dichloromethane phase was drawn
off into a 250 ml flask. Original handwash solution was once again
extracted with 10 ml of dichloromethane, the extracts combined, and
volume reduced to 5 ml with a vacuum rotary evaporator. Toluene
(2.5 ml) was added and extraction, evaporation and analytical
procedures were as for pads and air samples.

Analysis of all residue samples was performed with a Hewlett-
Packard 5840A gas chromatograph equipped with a nitrogen-

phosphorous specific thermionic detector. The separation column was a 180 cm by 2 mm I.D. glass column packed with 3% OV-25 on 100-120 mesh Chromosorb W HP. Temperatures were as follows: detector, 300°C; inlet, 165°C; and column oven, 155°C. Gas flows were 1.02 liters/hr for the nitrogen carrier, 0.18 liter/hr for hydrogen, and 0.30 liter/hr for air. Quantitation was accomplished with external standardization methodology by frequent recalibration and peak area measurement.

Serum pseudo-cholinesterase (referred to hereafter as serum cholinesterase) activities were determined from a five minute reaction period at room temperature with a modification of the method of Ellman et al. (14). Briefly, a 10 μl aliquot of serum was added to both a reference and sample cuvette containing 3.0 ml of 5,5-dithiobis-(2-nitrobenzoate) (DTNB) buffer (0.25 mM in ph 8.0, 0.1 M sodium phosphate buffer) and mixed with a micro-stirring rod. The reaction was started in the sample cuvette by the addition of 20 μl of acetylthiocholine iodide (78 mM) and stirred. The reference cuvette received 20 μl of distilled water in place of substrate. Absorbance was measured at 412 nm over a five minute period and the rate calculated from the slope of the derived curve.

Erythrocytes were prepared from whole blood samples to measure acetylcholinesterase activity. A 7.0 ml aliquot of 0.9% saline was added to 1.0 ml of whole blood from each subject in a screw cap culture tube. Tubes were shaken for two minutes at high speed in a reciprocal shaker after which they were centrifuged for 10 minutes at 2000 RPM. The clear supernatant was discarded and an additional 7.0 ml of saline (0.9%) was added to the tubes and the above procedure repeated. The wash step was repeated a third time prior to analysis of enzyme activity. To the erythrocyte pellet was added 1.0 ml of 0.9% saline which was gently vortex mixed. A 10 μl aliquot of the erythrocyte suspension was then added to 6.0 ml of sodium phosphate buffer (0.1 M, pH 8.0). A 3.0 ml aliquot of the erythrocyte suspension was placed in the sample and reference cuvettes to which 25 μl DTNB buffer (10 mM) were added and mixed with a micro-stirring rod. Finally, 20 μl of substrate acetylthiocholine (78 mM) or water was added to the appropriate cuvettes. Absorbance was measured as for serum assays over a five minute period. Enzyme activity was expressed as change in absorbance per gram of hemoglobin.

Urine samples were thawed at room temperature and centrifuged for 30 minutes at 2,000 rpm to separate salts and proteins. The clear urine was collected and divided into fractions for DDVP and DCAA extraction. In order to extract DDVP, 10.0 ml of sample urine was added to a centrifuge tube containing 2.0 ml of ethanol (95%) and mixed. This was followed by the addition of 18.0 ml of hexane. Tubes were shaken for 15 minutes at high speed on an Eberbach reciprocal shaker and then centrifuged for 10 minutes at 2,000 RPM. A 17.0 ml aliquot of the n-hexane phase was removed and added to another tube containing 2.0 grams of anhydrous sodium sulfate and stored overnight at 4°C. A 16.0 ml aliquot was placed in a tube and evaporated under a nitrogen stream to a final volume of 1.0 ml. A 1.5 ml aliquot of toluene was added to the 1.0 ml hexane. The remaining hexane was evaporated until the sample was in toluene which was injected directly into the GC. A standard curve for DDVP was prepared using diluted stock solutions ranging from 0.1-100 μg/ml in ethyl acetate. Recovery samples were obtained by spiking urine samples with varying amounts (1.35, 2.69, 3.40, 10.80 μg) of DDVP in ethyl acetate. Recoveries were 85-90% with minimum detectability for DDVP at 1.0 ppb.

Dichloracetic acid (DCAA) was quantitated in urine samples following derivitization. A 5.0 ml aliquot of urine was added to a 50 ml screw cap centrifuge tube containing 2.0 g of sodium chloride and mixed. To each tube was added 5.0 ml of sulfuric acid (16N) while the tubes were held in an ice bath. After removal from the ice bath, 25.0 ml of ethyl ether were added to each tube after which they were shaken at high speed for 15 minutes. Following extraction of DCAA into ether phase, the ether was removed and dried over 10 grams of anhydrous sodium sulfate in a 50 ml centrifuge tube. Samples were allowed to stand for at least 30 minutes. Following extraction, a 9.5 ml aliquot of the ether phase was placed in a test tube and evaporated under a stream of nitrogen at 40°C in a water bath to a final volume of 1.0 ml. To each tube was added 3.0 ml of boron trifluoride (BF^3) in methanol (14% V:V) and vortexed for 10 seconds. All tubes were heated in a 70°C water bath for 15 minutes and then allowed to cool to room temperature. After cooling, 5.0 ml of aqueous saturated sodium chloride solution were added to each tube followed by 10.0 ml of reagent grade benzene. Samples were vortexed for one minute. After phase separation, the organic phase containing the derivatized DCAA was held for injection directly into the GC column. This column was a 1.83 m by 3.18 mm I.D. glass column packed with 10% carbowax TPA on 80-100 mesh Gas Chrom Q. Carrier gas was 5% methane in argon at a flow rate of 1.02 liter/hr. Detector temperature was 250°C while inlet and column temperatures were 130°C and 124°C, respectively.

Controls were urine samples without DCAA carried through the entire extraction and derivatization procedures. Recovery determinations were made with 1.0 ml of methanol containing various amounts of DCAA (0.1-10 μg) added to urine blanks and carried through the procedures. Recovery values routinely averaged 89.4% with a minimum detectability for DCAA of 1.5 ppb.

Total dermal exposure was calculated by multiplying the sum of the unclothed body areas by the appropriate exterior exposure rate and adding to the product the total clothed areas multiplied by the appropriate interior exposure rate and then adding to this total the hand exposure value. Total body surface areas were calculated from the applicator height and weight using the formula of Dubois and Dubois (16) with specific body surfaces apportioned by the Berkow method (17). Total respiratory exposure was calculated by multiplying the air concentration of DDVP by the mean ventilation rate of a man doing light work (1). Total percent of a toxic dose per hr was calculated according to the formula of Durham and Wolfe (1) assuming that the dermal LD$_{50}$ of DDVP to humans is 107 mg/kg body weight (18).

Results and Discussion

Applicators took a mean of 25.5 minutes to apply 0.19 gm (A.I.)/m^2 of DDVP (38.7 ml/m^2 of finished spray) to each of the 20 residences included in this study. Residences size averaged 103.0±33.2 m^2 and received a mean of 19.6 gm (A.I.) DDVP based on the floor area of each structure. Applications were made at a mean temperature of 26.1°C and 82% relative humidity.

Applicators who applied DDVP in this study were exposed to the insecticide. Dermal exposure as determined by measurement of DDVP on gauze pads attached to the applicators during treatment was 0.499 ± 0.274 $\mu g/cm^2/hr$ on exterior pads, 0.102 ± 0.062 $\mu g/cm^2/hr$ on interior pads (those located beneath the clothing), and 0.024 ± 0.021 $\mu g/cm^2/hr$ on the hands. Recovery of DDVP on interior pads was interpreted to indicate movement of insecticide through the clothing with approximately 20% of the chemical contacting the outer garments penetrating to the skin beneath ([10]). This penetration is approximately 2-3 times more than noted in similar experiments with carbaryl (Sevin WP) insecticide ([11], [13]).

Rubber gloves worn by applicators apparently minimized hand exposure; DDVP application and handling resulted in 0.024 $\mu g/cm^2/hr$. Hand contamination accounted for 0.9% of total dermal exposure (Table 1) as compared with 87% in carbaryl exposure studies ([11], [13]) where hand protection was not worn. The fact that DDVP was recovered from the hands of the applicators in all 20 treatments demonstrated the need to stress hand protection and decontamination even when rubber gloves are worn.

Potential applicator respiratory exposure as measured by the personnel air samplers was 0.021 ± 0.019 $\mu g/liter$, 2.1% of the threshold limit value (TLV) set by the American Conference of Governmental Industrial Hygienists ([18]) at 1 mg/m^3. There was clear evidence of potential applicator exposure to DDVP through respiration based on the sampler data, but the values ranged from 0.4-6.4% of the TLV indicating that minimal negative impact would be expected ([10]).

Total applicator exposure (Table 1) was estimated based on measurements of both total dermal and respiratory exposure. Total dermal exposure was 2.354 mg/hr or 0.028 mg/kg/hr for an applicator weighing 84 kg and wearing an open-neck, long-sleeve shirt, full length pants, shoes and socks, head gear, and rubber gloves ([10]). Potential respiratory exposure for the applicators was 0.037 mg/hr or 0.0004 mg/kg/hr assuming a ventilation rate of 1740 liters/hr ([1]). The percent toxic dose of DDVP to applicators was $0.028 \pm 0.021\%/hr$ as calculated by the formula of Durham and Wolfe ([1]) where respiratory exposure is considered 10 times more toxic than dermal exposure. A "worst case" estimate of percent toxic dose for a completely unprotected applicator would have been 0.11%/hr.

DDVP and its hydrolysis products (dimethylphosphate, des-methyldichlorvos, dichloroethanol, dichloroacetic acid) are known to appear in the urine of animals including man following signifi-cant exposure ([19-22]). However, our results on urine samples of applicators of DDVP failed to demonstrate detectable quantities of insecticide at any of the experimental time periods. This occurred in spite of known applicator exposure as indicated by dermal and respiratory results. Assay sensitivity (1 ppb) was well within the range for detecting DDVP in trace amounts. As a result of not detecting DDVP in urine and considering its known rapid metabolism in mammals, urine samples were examined for the metabolite DCAA. No significant amounts of DCAA were identified in urine samples of any of the subjects (applicators or residents). It was believed

Table I. Total Exposure of Applicators of DDVP in Residences [1]

Exposure Route	Body Part	Surface Area[2] (S.A. in cm^2)	Exposure Calculation (mg/hr)	Total Exposure[3] mg/kg/hr	% Toxic Dose/hr
Dermal	Face, front "V" chest	910	0.454		
	Head (minus face)	460	0.047		
	Back neck	120	0.060		
	Back trunk (minus back neck)	3420	0.349		
	Front trunk (minus front neck, "V" chest)	3790	0.387		
	Upper arms	1340	0.137		
	Forearms	1390	0.142		
	Thighs	3660	0.373		
	Legs and feet	3760	0.383		
	Hands	930	0.022		
Total Dermal Exposure		19,708	2.354	0.028	
Respiratory	Lungs (Ventilation rate "V.R." liters/hr)[4]	1740	0.037	0.0004	
TOTAL EXPOSURE			2.391	0.0284	0.028

[1] Applicator wore head gear, an open neck, long sleeve shirt, pants and gloves (10).

[2] Total body surface was calculated from the height and weight of the applicators using the formula of Dubois and Dubois (16), and then apportioned by the Berkow method (17) for specific body areas.

[3] Total exposure calculations based on a 84 kg applicator applying DDVP with a dermal LD_{50} of 107 mg/kg (18). The percent toxic dose per hour was calculated by the formula of Durham and Wolfe (1).

[4] Ventilation rate of a man doing light work (1).

that the assay for DCAA was appropriately sensitive and selective
for the analysis. It is recognized that two other major metabolites are formed and excreted in urine, but they were not examined.
    The effects of DDVP on both serum and erythrocyte acetyl-
cholinesterase (AChE) have been well documented in the literature.
In the present study when DDVP applicators were evaluated for serum
cholinesterase activity at various time periods following initiation
of applications (Applicator 1 at 7 and 30 hrs; Applicator 2 at 8,
24, 30, 48, and 56 hrs), significant reductions in AChE activity
were noted (10). Applicator 1 was forced, due to illness, to
discontinue DDVP applications during the 7th hour of the experiments. The exact cause of the illness was not confirmed by the
medical staff overseeing the experiments, but pesticide poisoning
could not be ruled out. His serum AChE activity was reduced by 59%
by the 7th hours of exposure, but had rebounded significantly by 30
hrs post-initiation. Applicator 2 experienced a 21% reduction in
serum AChE activity in the first exposure period, but enzyme
activity returned to baseline within 48 hrs. Erythrocyte AChE
activity results were difficult to interpret due to inconsistent
response to DDVP. Applicator 1 had an increase in AChE activity
during a period of decreased serum AChE activity. With the rebound
in his serum AChE activity was noted a similar but disproportionate
increase in erythrocyte AChE activity. Applicator 2 was noted to
have a general decline in erythrocyte AChE activity which was
correlated with increased exposure to DDVP. Decreases in erythrocyte AChE activity were considered slight but consistent with what
would have been expected for low dermal and respiratory exposure
(10).
    A total of 20 residents of DDVP-treated structures were
included in the study population. From questionnaires completed by
cooperators when blood and urine samples were taken, it was determined that: mean age of the participants was 40.7 ± 16.2 years
(range 19-64 yrs); 70% were female; none had taken cholinesterase
inhibiting medications during the 24 hrs of the study, but 5% and
10% had used tobacco and alcohol, respectively; 70% had used pesticides in their residence within the preceeding 3 months; the mean
time spent in the DDVP-treated structure was 15.8 ± 3.3 hrs prior to
final blood and urine samples; and 15% indicated that the treatment
to their residence had caused a feeling of illness (headache was
only symptom indicated).
    Results of the environmental monitoring indicated that DDVP
was present in the treated residences up to 24 hrs following initial treatments. Air samplers operated in the structures for 24
hrs, including the time of application, collected measurable DDVP
residues. Greatest concentrations of DDVP were collected during
the first 2 hrs post-initiation with 0.548 ± 0.297 µg/liter recovered.
This is 54.8% of the TLV and represents a 26-fold increase over the
concentrations recovered by the personnel air sampler worn by the
applicator who spent a mean of 25.5 minutes in the structure. The
fact that the room air sampler collected significantly more DDVP
than personnel air samplers is explained in part by the fact that
the room air samplers were positioned in the kitchen/utility areas
which received approximately 50-60% of the total volume of finished
spray applied to the residence (23), and that the applicator was
constantly moving to areas of the structure that were at that point

untreated.   Of the 337.5 μg DDVP collected by the room air samplers, 21.4% was attributed to the time of application and the two
hrs following initiation of treatments.   Concentration of DDVP in
the treated residences was 0.21 μg/liter or 21.3% of the TLV through
the 24 hrs of the study.   Residents who spent a mean of 15.8 hrs in
the treated structures would have been exposed to 0.08 mg/kg,
assuming the same ventilation rate as the applicators and a mean
body weight of 75 kg. Potential respiratory exposure to residents
was 10 times that of the applicators who mixed and applied DDVP to
the structures.   Even though the potential respiratory exposure was
significantly greater to the residents than applicators, the level
of exposure was considered to be slight based on either the oral
(80 mg/kg) or dermal (107 mg/kg) LD_{50} of DDVP (18).

Dermal exposure to residents to DDVP could not be assessed;
however, it was noted that the environmental exposure pads received
0.319 ± 0.183 μg/cm^2/hr during the application and the two hrs post-
initiation.   This represents 63.9% of the total dermal exposure of
the applicators.

The serum and erythrocyte acetylcholinesterase activity
measurement in this work basically confirm the findings of Cavagna
et al. (8) who investigated the effects of DDVP plastic resin
strips on human subjects.   Data analysis revealed a slight but
statistically significant ($P\leq0.05$) reduction in serum
cholinesterase activity in the overall resident population at 24
hrs posttreatment.   Mean enzyme activity prior to spraying was
1.400 ± 0.348 International Units (I.U.), whereas the mean activity
dropped to 1.296 ± 0.316 I.U. by the end of the 24 hr period (10).
Mean difference between enzyme activities was slight (0.104 I.U.)
representing a 7.9% decrease suggesting only minor exposure of the
population to the insecticide.   Fluctuations in activity of this
magnitude are not unusual even in the absence of pesticide exposure
(13).   Analysis of erythrocyte acetylcholinesterase activity
before (0.36 ± 0.10 absorbance change/minute/gram hemoglobin X 10^{-2})
and following treatment (0.36 ± 0.10) revealed no significant
differences for the test population; however, there were decreases
in activity ranging from 5.3 to 37.5%.   These decreases could
represent normal fluctuations for the study population.

Conclusions

There was evidence of pesticide exposure to applicators based on
results of dermal and respiratory monitoring, but the percent toxic
dose (0.028%/hr) and results of serum and erythrocyte acetylcholinesterase testing were interpreted to indicate low probability of
significant acute exposure to DDVP when label directions were
followed.   It was demonstrated that normal work apparel does provide an effective barrier to the penetration of DDVP to the skin of
applicators and that hand protection is strongly recommended.

Residents of DDVP-treated structures were noted to have exposure to DDVP based on results of room air sampler data analysis and
serum and erythrocyte acetylcholinesterase determinations. Resident
exposure was estimated at 0.03% toxic dose/hr had they been present
during application of DDVP and remained in the treated structure
for the full 24 hrs posttreatment.   Based on these results it is
recommended that unprotected residents not be allowed in structures

during application (<u>10</u>) and that exposure be further reduced by
thoroughly ventilating treated areas.

Nontechnical Summary

Twenty residential structures were treated with dichlorvos
insecticide (DDVP) for German cockroach control. Dermal exposure
pads, air samplers, blood tests for serum and erythrocyte acetylcholinesterase (enzyme) activity and urine analyses were used to
monitor both applicators and residents for evidence of exposure to
DDVP.

There was evidence of pesticide exposure to applicators based
on results of dermal and respiratory monitoring. However, the
percent toxic dose (0.03%/hr) and results of serum and erythrocyte
acetylcholinesterase testing were interpreted to indicate low
probability of significant acute exposure to DDVP when label
directions were followed. It was demonstrated that normal work
apparel does provide an effective barrier against DDVP penetrating
to an applicator's skin; however, hand protection is strongly
recommended.

Based on analysis of room air samples, and serum and erythrocyte acetylcholinesterase tests, it was concluded that residents of
DDVP-treated structures were exposed to the pesticide. Resident
exposure was estimated at 0.03% toxic dose/hr had the person been
present during the DDVP application and remained continuously in
the treated structure for 24 hours after the pesticide was applied.
Based on these results, it is recommended that unprotected
residents not be allowed in structures during application and that
exposure be further reduced by thoroughly ventilating treated
areas.

Acknowledgments

This project was supported through the North Central Region
Pesticide Impact Assessment Program. The authors wish to express
their appreciation to Dr. James Ballard and Duane Tupy of the
University of Nebraska for their assistance in the collection and
analysis of samples.

Literature Cited

1. Durham, W. F.; Wolf, H. R.   <u>Bull. W.H.O.</u> 1962, 26, 75–91.
2. Kimbrough, R. D.; Gaines, T. B.   <u>Arch. Environ. Health</u> 1968,
   16, 805–8.
3. Krause, W; Homola, S.   <u>Bull. Environ. Contam. Toxicol.</u> 1974,
   11, 177–81.
4. Voogd, C. E.; Jacobs, J. J. J. A. A.; Van Der Stel, J. J.
   <u>Mutation Res.</u> 1972, 16, 417–9.
5. Ashwood-Smith, M. J.; Trevino, J; Ring, R.   <u>Nature</u> 1972, 20,
   418–20.
6. Leary, J. S.; Keane, W. T.; Fontenot, C.; Feichtmeir, E. S.;
   Shultz, D; Koos, D. A.; Hirsch, L.; Lavor, E. M.; Roan, C. C.;
   Hine, C. H.   <u>Arch. Environ. Health</u> 1974, 29, 308–14.
7. Cavagna, G.; Locati, G.; Vigliani, E. C.   <u>Arch. Environ.
   Health</u> 1969, 19, 112–23.

8. Gillet, J. W.; Harr, J. R.; Linstrom, F. T.; Mount, D. A.; St. Clair, A. D.; Weber, L. J. Residue Rev. 1972a, 44, 115-59.
9. Gillet, J. W.; Harr, J. R.; St. Clair, A. D.; Weber, L. J. Residue Rev. 1972b, 44, 161-84.
10. Gold, R. E.; Holcslaw, T.; Tupy, D.; Ballard, J. B. J. Econ. Entomol. 1984, 77, 430-436.
11. Gold, R. E.; Leavitt, J. R. C.; Ballard, J. J. Econ. Entomol. 1981, 74, 552-4.
12. Gold, R. E.; Leavitt, J. R. C.; Holcslaw, T.; Tupy, D. Arch. Environ. Contam. Toxicol. 1982, 11, 63-7.
13. Leavitt, J. R. C.; Gold, R. E.; Holcslaw, T.; Tupy, D. Arch. Environ. Contam. Toxicol. 1982, 11, 57-62.
14. Ellman, G. L.; Courtney, K. D.; Valentino, A.; Featherstone, R. M. Biochem. Pharmacol. 1961, 7, 88-95.
15. Schultz, D. R.; Marxmiller, R. L.; Koos, B. A. J. Agr. Food Chem. 1971, 19, 1238-43.
16. Dubois, D.; Dubois, E. F. Arch. Intern. Med. 1916, 17, 863-6.
17. Berkow, S. G. Am. J. Surg. 1931, 11, 315.
18. "Documentation of the Threshold Limit Values for Substances in Workroom Air," American conference of Governmental Industrial Hygienists, 1971, 3rd ed.
19. Arthur, B. W.; Casida, J. E. J. Agric. Food Chem. 1957, 5, 186-92.
20. Casida, J. E.; McBride, L.; Niedermeier, R. P. J. Agric. Food Chem. 1962, 10, 370-7.
21. Tracy, R. L.; Woodcock, J. G.; Chodroff, S. J. Econ. Entomol. 1960, 53, 593-601.
22. Teicher-Kuliszewska, K.; Szymezyk, T. Bromatol. Chem. Toksykol. 1980, 13, 37-40.

RECEIVED September 6, 1984

Subterranean Termite Control: Chlordane Residues in Soil Surrounding and Air Within Houses

R. B. LEIDY, C. G. WRIGHT, H. E. DUPREE, JR., and T. J. SHEETS

Pesticide Residue Research Laboratory and Department of Entomology, North Carolina State University, Raleigh, NC 27695

A study was undertaken to determine concentrations of chlordane in soils and the air of houses treated for subterranean termite control by commercial applicators over a 5-year period. Sixty houses, each with known histories of chlordane application were divided into two groups; one from predominately sandy regions and the other from predominately clay-soil regions of North Carolina. The houses were divided further into those with a crawl space (15/region), those with a combination crawl space and slab (15 on clay soils), and those on a full slab (15 on sandy soils). Chlordane residues averaged 1052 and 1475 ppm in sandy and clay soils, respectively; air samples from crawl spaces averaged 14 and 12 $\mu g/m^3$ from sand and clay regions, respectively. In the sandy region air samples from kitchens averaged 2.5 (range: 0.05 to 5.7) and those from bedrooms averaged 3.1 (range of 0.05 to 7.2) $\mu g/m^3$. In the clay region average levels in air were 3.0 (range of 0.05 to 9.9) and 3.2 (range of 0.05 to 9.8) $\mu g/m^3$, for kitchens and bedrooms, respectively.

Field experiments to determine the efficiency of chlordane (1,2,4,5, 6,7,8,8-octachloro-3a,4,7,7a-hexahydro-4,7-methano-1H-indene) to control subterranean termites have been conducted since the 1940's (1),(2). This insecticide continues to be used widely today by commercial pest-control firms in houses and in industrial buildings. In many instances, chlordane is applied with heptachlor (1,4,5,6,7, 8,8-heptachloro-3a,4,7,7a-tetrahydro-4,7-methano-1H-indene) as a preventative and remedial treatment in buildings. This combination, called Termide (EPA Reg. No. 876-233AA contains 39.22% chlordane and 19.60% heptachlor) contains 0.5% technical chlordane and 0.25% heptachlor when diluted for application. Chlordane is applied at a 1.0% emulsion with water as the diluent. Relatively large quantities (ca. 378-756 liters) are applied in trenches dug into soil around crawl-space walls and chimney bases and into pilasters and wall voids. In addition many structures built on concrete slabs are treated before the foundation is poured. Because of the persistent

0097-6156/85/0273-0265$06.00/0

nature of these two insecticides, and the large quantities applied, one would expect to find residues in soil and the ambient air of the treated structures.

In an early study, the chlordane level in the air of five treated houses was below the detectable levels (3). An inadvertent application at a US air-force (USAF) base caused chlordane to be dispersed throughout a house when the furnace was activated (4). Similar incidents were reported in other base houses, which led to a large scale sampling at several USAF bases. Some 500 ground-level apartments were sampled at a midwest base in 1980 and chlordane was found in the air at concentrations up to 379 $\mu g/m^3$ (5).

Seven USAF bases were examined during the winter of 1980-81, and in 408 units (86%) of 474 which had been treated with chlordane using subslab injection or exterior ditching after construction, the airborne chlordane concentrations were less than 3.5 $\mu g/m^3$. The levels in 2% of the units were greater than 6.5 $\mu g/m^3$. The chlordane in the other 12% of the houses fell between these two levels (6). Wright and Leidy (7) determined chlordane and heptachlor levels in air for one year following a prescribed application to six single-flamily houses by commercial pest control firms. Residues of chlordane varied widely between 0.3 and 5.8 $\mu g/m^3$, and heptachlor residues varied between 0.01 and 1.8 $\mu g/m^3$. Because residue levels varied, it was concluded that a number of factors including construction type, temperature, humidity, and air movement due to cooling and heating probably influenced the concentrations. There are no established tolerances for chlordane or heptachlor in the ambient air in home environments. An interim guideline level of 5.0 $\mu g/m^3$ (chlordane) and 2.0 $\mu g/m^3$ (heptachlor) has been recommended by the Committee on toxicology of the National Academy of Sciences (8). The maximum allowable limit in work-space air during a 40 h workweek (Threshold Limit Value, Time Weighted Average) (TLV-TWA) is 500 $\mu g/m^3$ for chlordane and heptachlor (9).

Few data are available on soil and airborne residues of chlordane and heptachlor from homes treated by commercial pest control firms. Thus, a study was undertaken to determine chlordane and heptachlor residues in clay and sand soils and in the air of selected houses.

Materials and Methods

House Selection and Sampling Procedure.

Sixty single-family houses were selected by commercial pest control firms located in North Carolina. The following criteria were required for selection: a willingness of the homeowner to allow both soil sampling and air monitoring; and either a remedial or preventative treatment for termites within the last 5 years (1978-1983) and either chlordane or Termide as the termiticde used. Houses were divided into two groups: 30 in the Coastal Plain of North Carolina with predominately sandy soils, and 30 in the Piedmont region with predominately clay soils. In the sandy-soil region, 15 houses having a full concrete slab and 15 having crawl-space construction were selected; in clay-soil regions, 15 houses with a combination crawl space/slab (i.e. split level) and 15 with crawl-space construction were chosen.

No observations were made of the application, because all had been completed at the time of selection; thus it was assumed that the proper amount of either chlordane or Termide was applied following prescribed label directions. The amounts of termiticides applied were obtained from records of the pest control firm that treated the house. Temperatures and relative humidities were measured in each house during sampling, and a soil temperature was taken from houses with crawl spaces. In addition, observations were made as to whether air conditioning fans were operating or if windows were open.

Composite soil samples were taken from all houses with crawl spaces. Sampling sites around each house were selected based upon the type of structure which determines the method of application. Using a coring device (30 by 2.5 cm), samples were taken from two locations along each of the four longest foundation walls and from soils around the base of two pillars in the crawl space area. An attempt was made to obtain samples from 0 to 10 cm and 10 to 20 cm depths, but in some instances the locations of the foundation footing interfered with sampling at the 10 to 20 cm depth. Soils were placed in 950 mL glass jars. The jars were sealed, and stored at -20C until analyzed.

Air samples were taken in a central location of the crawl space, the kitchen, and a bedroom with personal-type air samplers (10). Polyurethane foam plugs (2 cm od. by 3 cm) contained in a glass holder were attached to the sampler. A 2-h sample was taken at a flow rate of 2.8 L of air/min. The holder and foam were removed, placed in plastic bags, and stored at -20C until analyzed.

Soil Particle-Size Analysis. The hydrometer method was used to perform a mechanical analysis of the soils (11).

Analytical Procedures. Soil samples were extracted using a modified procedure described by Bennett et al (12). Soils were screened through a No. 10 mesh sieve to remove rocks and debris. Two grams of soil were tared into a 500-mL glass jar, 5 mL of deionized water and 50 mL of 2-propanol were added, and the sample was shaken mechanically for 15 min. One hundred mL of hexane were added, and the sample was shaken for an additional 2 h and allowed to sit overnight. Samples were filtered under reduced pressure through a 300-mL membrane filter apparatus containing a GF/B fiberglass filter (4.7 cm o.d.) topped with 10 g Na_2SO_4 (ANHYD) and 5 g Celite. The filtrate was placed in a 500-mL separatory funnel, 200 mL of deionized water added, and the contents were shaken gently for 1 min. After the layers separated, the aqueous layer was discarded and the procedure was repeated twice more. The hexane layer was filtered through Na_2SO_4 (ANHYD) and concentrated to 2 to 3 mL under reduced pressure at 40C. Samples were brought to final volume with hexane for analysis.

Air samples were extracted as described by Leidy et al., (13). Foam plugs were placed in a 250-mL beaker containing 150 mL of ethyl acetate, and an additional 50 mL of ethyl acetate were poured through the glass sample holder. The plug was squeezed against the side of the beaker using a 20-cm glass rod at 10 min intervals for 30 min. The solvent was poured into a 500-mL boiling flask and the beaker and foam plug were rinsed with an additional 50 mL of ethyl acetate. The combined extract was concentrated under reduced pressure to 2 to 3 mL and diluted to volume with ethyl acetate.

The pesticide concentrations were determined by gas-liquid chromatography (GLC) using a Tracor Model 222 chromatograph equipped with a ^{63}Ni electron capture detector. The column was U-shaped glass (183 by 0.2 cm id) packed with a 1:1 mixture of 1.5% OV-17 + 3% QF1 and 3% OF-1 on Supelcoport (80/100). The carrier gas was N_2 at a flow rate of 70 mL/min through the column and 20 mL/min to the detector. Temperatures were as follows: oven, 190 C; detector, 285 C; inlet, 225 C. Data were quantitated by the peak-height method using the peaks of compound O (RT 7.4 min) compound E (RT 10.8 min) trans-cnlordane (RT 16.2 min); cis-chlordane (RT 18.4 min), and trans-nonachlor (RT 19.2 min). The peaks were added together and divided by the injection volume. Heptachlor was not measured in chlordane samples but was in the Termide samples. The normal concentration of heptachlor in technical chlordane averaged 10% and this amount was substracted from the heptachlor peak in samples containing Termide. The low detectable limits were: chlordane, 0.01 µg; heptachlor, 0.005 µg.

Samples were injected by a Dynatech Model GC 211V Precision Sampler (Dynatech Precision Sampling Corp; P. O. Box 15119; Baton Rouge, LA 70895) controlled by a Lindberg Enterprises Control Model "CD" Timer. (Lindberg Enterprises, Inc.; 9707 Candida St., San Diego, CA 92126). Injection volumes were 3 µL and time between injections was 35 min. Two analytical standards, one containing chlordane and the other heptachlor, were placed after every 5 samples for quantitation purposes.

Efficiency of the extraction processes was monitored by fortifying untreated soils and foam plugs with known amounts of chlordane or heptachlor and carrying these through the analytical process. Two fortified samples were extracted with each set of soil or foam-plug samples.

All data were subjected to an analysis of variance, and the resulting statistical parameters were used in pointing out differences between means.

Results and Discussion

Houses were numbered consecutively from 1 to 60, and all sample numbers in all Tables refer to the same house. Samples were collected over a 3-month period between June and September, 1983. Average temperatures in clay soils and the surrounding crawl space were 20.6 and 22.9 C, respectively; for sandy soils and the associated crawl space temperatures averaged 19.8 and 23.6 C, respectively. House temperatures varied widely between 21 and 31 C, because of the use of air conditioning in a number of dwellings and the 3-month sampling interval. For these same reasons the relative humidities in homes ranged from 49 to 79% while in the crawl spaces, the range was from 52 to 96%. Humidities normally were 20 to 30% higher in the crawl spaces than in the dwellings. Eight of the houses, four on each soil type, had a polyethylene barrier laid over the soil.

Recoveries of chlordane from fortified clay and sand soils averaged 102% (range of 83 to 143%) and 90% (range of 80 to 100%), respectively at fortification levels varying from 1 to 3000 ppm. Heptachlor recoveries from clay and sand soils averaged 95% (range of 88 to 113%) and 91% (range of 79 to 114%). It is possible that the high recoveries in clay soils resulted from the presence of some chlordane prior to fortifying the soil or improper soil mixing.

Known amounts of chlordane and heptachlor were added to untreated foam plugs and two fortified samples were extracted with each set of experimental samples. The average chlordane recovery was 89% (range of 73 to 111%) and heptachlor recoveries averaged 91% (range of 81 to 102%) at fortification levels varying from 0.04 to 16.0 µg. None of the data were corrected to reflect recovery values.

Chlordane and heptachlor residues from clay soils from houses constructed with crawl spaces are shown in Table I. Concentrations varied widely. The average level of chlordane in the first 10 cm of soil was 1405 ppm (15 samples) and the average concentration in soil from the 10 to 20 cm depth was 806 ppm (7 samples). In many instances, it was impossible to obtain a 10 to 20 cm depth sample, because of the hardness of the soil, interfering foundation footings, or construction debris which had been buried under many of the dwellings. The amount of heptachlor found in the soil samples averaged 386 ppm from the 0 to 10 cm (11 samples) and 261 ppm from the 10 to 20 cm depth (3 samples).

Residues of chlordane and heptachlor in air from houses with crawl spaces constructed on clay soils are shown in Table II. The highest chlordane residues found were in the crawl space (8.7 µg/m^3) compared to the kitchen (2.3 µg/m^3) and bedroom (2.5 µg/m^3). Heptachlor residues in air averaged 1.7 µg/m^3 in crawl spaces compared to 0.6 µg/m^3 in kitchens and bedrooms.

Tables III and IV show residue levels of chlordane and heptachlor in soils and air, respectively, from crawl-slab constructed houses built on clay soils. Soil residues of chlordane averaged 1545 ppm (15 samples) from the 0 to 10-cm depth and 861 ppm (five samples) from the 10 to 20 cm depth. Heptachlor levels for the upper and lower soil layers were, respectively 441 ppm (11 samples) and 314 ppm (two samples). As was seen in crawl-space dwelling on clay soils, residues of chlordane were highest in air of the crawl space 14.4 µg/m^3) than in air of kitchens (3.4 µg/m^3) and bedrooms 3.4 µg/m^3). Heptachlor residues in air in crawl spaces averaged 2.2 µg/m^3 compared to 0.6 µg/m^3 in kitchens and 0.8 µg/m^3 in bedrooms.

When residues in crawl-space constructed houses were compared with those in houses built on a crawl-slab foundation, residues were equivalent in soils but higher in air samples of rooms. The average house size of the crawl-space constructed house was 135 m^2 and an average of 533 L of diluted termiticide were applied. The average size of the crawl-slab constructed house was 172 m^2 and an average 734 L of the emulsion were applied. It is possible that more termiticide was applied in a smaller area in the crawl-slab constructed houses than in crawl-space constructed ones which could produce the higher residue levels.

Table V shows residue levels of chlordane and heptachlor in soils and air, respectively, from crawl-space constructed dwellings built on sandy soils. Soil residues of chlordane and heptachlor in the 0 to 10-cm depth averaged 1052 (15 samples) and 414 ppm (seven samples) respectively, and in the 10 to 20-cm depth 204 (eight samples) and 82 ppm (one sample), respectively. The airborne concentrations of chlordane and heptachlor averaged 13.7 and 2.5 in crawl spaces; 2.7 and 1.0 in kitchens, and 3.6 and

Table I.   Chlordane and Heptachlor Residues in Clay Soils from Houses
with Crawl Spaces[a]

No	Termiticide treatment	Year treated	Amount applied (L)	Soil depth (cm)	Chlordane (ppm)	Heptachlor[d] (ppm)
1	Chlordane[b]	1983	927	0–10	283	
				10–20	161	
2	Chlordane	1980	757	0–10	1022	
				10–20	303	
3	Termide[c]	1979	757	0–10	2310	385
4	Termide	1979	492	0–10	1564	276
5	Termide	1979	378	0–10	1890	485
6	Termide	1979	378	0–10	852	333
7	Termide	1978	378	0–10	504	14
				10–20	42	2
8	Chlordane	1979	586	0–10	1124	
9	Chlordane	1979	378	0–10	1239	
				10–20	924	
10	Termide	1982	416	0–10	3324	565
				10–20	1138	236
11	Termide	1982	681	0–10	1643	441
				10–20	1787	299
12	Termide	1982	757	0–10	1805	635
				10–20	1289	248
13	Termide	1981	378	0–10	1948	532
14	Termide	1981	322	0–10	1053	373
15	Termide	1983	416	0–10	516	202

[a] Soils sampled between June and October, 1983.

[b] Chlordane applied as a 1.0% emulsion.

[c] Termide emulsion contains 0.5% chlordane and 0.25% heptachlor
after dilution for application.

[d] Heptachlor fraction not calculated.

1.0 $\mu g/m^3$ in bedrooms. The average dwelling size was 147 m^2 and 574
L of termiticide were applied.
      Slab-constructed dwellings were treated prior to the foundation
being poured, and soil samples could not be taken. The data for
airborne concentrations of termiticides are shown in Table VI. No
residues were detected in five of the houses sampled; and although
the average amount of termiticide applied was greater than that
applied to the crawl-space houses (613 L vs 574 L), average residues
in air in the kitchen and bedroom were lower. Residues of chlordane
and heptachlor in the kitchens averaged 2.3 and 0.7 $\mu g/m^3$ and those
for bedrooms were 2.6 and 0.5 $\mu g/m^3$, respectively.
      Air of eight of the rooms sampled during the study contained
chlordane residues above the recommended 5.0 $\mu g/m^3$ limit. Five of
these rooms were from houses treated in 1983, two were from houses
treated in 1980, and one was from a 1979-treated house. Both the
kitchen and bedroom in a 1983-treated home (crawl-space construction
on sandy soil) were higher than the recommended level, while the
other six rooms were in six different dwellings. The air concentrations in these rooms ranged from 5.3 to 9.9 $\mu g/m^3$.

Table II. Chlordane and Heptachlor Residues in Air from Houses with Crawl Spaces[a]

Sample no	Termiticide treatment	Year treated	Amount applied (L)	Crawl space chlordane ($\mu g/m^3$)	Crawl space heptachlor ($\mu g/m^3$)	Kitchen chlordane ($\mu g/m^3$)	Kitchen heptachlor ($\mu g/m^3$)	Bedroom chlordane ($\mu g/m^3$)	Bedroom heptachlor ($\mu g/m^3$)
1	Chlordane[b]	1983	927	10.8		2.2		<0.05	
2	Chlordane	1980	757	11.7		<0.05		<0.05	
3	Termide[c]	1979	757	1.2	0.1	0.5	0.1	0.7	0.1
4	Termide	1979	492	6.2	0.5	1.4	0.2	2.2	0.3
5	Termide	1979	378	8.4	0.5	1.6	0.2	1.4	0.1
6	Termide	1979	378	11.9	2.6	1.9	0.2	1.2	0.3
7	Termide	1978	378	9.7	1.5	4.7	0.7	3.2	0.3
8	Chlordane	1979	586	8.3	0.7	2.1	0.4	4.3	0.4
9	Chlordane	1979	378	6.0		1.6		1.4	
10	Termide	1982	416	23.4	5.5	1.5	0.5	1.0	0.3
11	Termide	1982	681	7.3	3.2	3.2	1.7	3.3	2.0
12	Termide	1982	757	7.5	2.5	3.9	1.3	3.5	1.2
13	Termide	1981	378	4.5	0.9	2.4	0.8	2.9	0.7
14	Termide	1981	322	8.6	0.7	1.1	0.1	1.4	0.1
15	Termide	1983	416	5.3	1.7	4.0	1.1	5.7	1.4

[a] Samples taken from houses located on clay soils between June and October, 1983.

[b] Chlordane applied as 1.0% emulsion.

[c] Termide emulsion contains 0.5% chlordane and 0.25% heptachlor

[d] Heptachlor fraction not calculated.

Table III.   Chlordane and Heptachlor Residues in Clay Soils from
Crawl-Slab Constructed Houses[a]

No	Termiticide treatment	Year treated	Amount applied (L)	Soil depth (cm)	Chlordane (ppm)	Heptachlor[d,e] (ppm)
16	Chlordane[b]	1983	700	0-10	303	
				10-20	100	
17	Termide[c]	1980	378	0-10	151	21
				10-20	ND	ND
18	Termide	1979	681	0-10	1495	276
19	Termide	1979	378	0-10	2504	206
20	Chlordane	1979	719	0-10	856	
				10-20	1458	
21	Termide	1982	492	0-10	1031	152
22	Termide	1983	1230	0-10	1219	254
				10-20	1903	569
23	Termide	1982	908	0-10	4020	491
24	Termide	1982	852	0-10	434	142
				10-20	415	58
25	Termide	1981	851	0-10	438	222
				10-20	ND	
26	Chlordane	1983	946	0-10	769	
				10-20	ND	
27	Termide	1979	1325	0-10	2483	557
28	Chlordane	1982	757	0-10	2092	
				10-20	431	
29	Termide	1983	851	0-10	3531	1452
				10-20	ND	ND
30	Termide	1982	568	0-10	1843	1073

[a] Houses sampled between June and October, 1983.

[b] Chlordane applied as a 1.0% emulsion.

[c] Termide emulsion contains 0.5% chlordane and 0.25% heptachlor

[d] None detected.

[e] Heptachlor fraction not calculated.

Some general conclusions can be drawn from this study. Although
the average residue of chlordane found in clay soils was higher than
sandy soils [2318 vs 1254 ppm (0 to 20 cm)], average concentrations
of the pesticides in air were equivalent in both crawl spaces (11.9
vs 13.7 $\mu g/m^3$) and in houses (3.0 vs 2.8 $\mu g/m^3$). These data indicate
that chlordane is more volatile from sandy soils, than clays, that
chlordane moves downward in sandy soils more readily than in clay, or
that both factors are involved. It is possible that equivalent
amounts of chlordane are present, generally in the two soil types but
in sandy soils the chemical is distributed in a larger volume of
soil. Concentrations of chlordane in air in houses built on clay
soils with crawl space construction were lower than those with crawl-
slab construction (2.4 vs 3.4 $\mu g/m^3$). Since an average of 180 L more
of the diluted termiticide were applied to a smaller area, it would
seem logical to find higher levels in the air of crawl-slab constructed dwellings. When airborne residues of chlordane from crawl-
space constructed houses on sandy soils were compared to those in air

Table IV. Chlordane and Heptachlor Residues in Air from Crawl-Slab Constructed Houses[a]

Sample no	Termiticide treatment	Year treated	Amount applied (L)	Crawl space chlordane (μg/m³)	Crawl space heptachlor (μg/m³)	Kitchen chlordane (μg/m³)	Kitchen heptachlor (μg/m³)	Bedroom chlordane (μg/m³)	Bedroom heptachlor (μg/m³)
16	Chlordane[b]	1983	700	3.6		<0.05		<0.05	
17	Termide[c]	1980	378	1.1	0.5	<0.05	0.2	<0.05	0.2
18	Termide	1979	681	5.7	0.5	0.8	0.1	0.7	0.1
19	Termide	1979	378	5.6	0.4	2.2	0.3	1.6	0.2
20	Chlordane	1979	719	47.2		9.9		4.9	
21	Termide	1982	492	7.5	4.7	3.6	0.7	3.4	0.3
22	Termide	1981	1230	7.0	2.6	2.7	1.5	3.4	1.5
23	Termide	1982	908	7.7	3.0	2.8	1.2	3.7	1.5
24	Termide	1982	832	11.1	5.2	2.8	0.5	4.6	1.7
25	Termide	1981	851	10.6	2.7	4.8	1.0	3.7	0.9
26	Chlordane	1983	946	46.6		3.4		9.8	
27	Termide	1979	1325	13.2	2.2	2.9	0.6	0.7	0.1
28	Chlordane	1982	757	31.1		2.6		4.0	
29	Termide	1983	851	6.9	0.7	1.7	0.1	0.7	0.02
30	Termide	1983	568	10.5	2.0	3.6	1.0	3.0	1.3

a Samples taken from houses located on clay soils between June and October, 1983.

b Chlordane applied as a 1.0% emulsion.

c Termide emulsion contains 0.5% chlordane and 0.25% heptachlor.

d Heptachlor fraction not calculated.

Table V. Chlordane and Heptachlor Residues in Sandy Soils and Air from Houses with Crawl Spaces[a]

No	Termiticide applied	Year treated	Amount applied (L)	Soil depth (cm)	Chlordane (ppm)	Heptachlor (ppm)	Crawl Space Chlordane ($\mu g/m^3$)	Crawl Space Heptachlor ($\mu g/m^3$)	Kitchen Chlordane ($\mu g/m^3$)	Kitchen Heptachlor ($\mu g/m^3$)	Bedroom Chlordane ($\mu g/m^3$)	Bedroom Heptachlor ($\mu g/m^3$)
31	Termide[b]	1978	927	0-10	156	28	4.6	0.3	<0.05	<0.05	<0.05	<0.05
32	Termide[c]	1983	757	0-10	278	14	3.2	1.1	2.6		3.5	0.2
33	Chlordane	1979	757	0-10	1567		18.8		1.8		3.3	
				10-20	<0.05							
34	Chlordane	1982	492	0-10	395		7.5		2.2		3.3	
				10-20	131							
35	Chlordane	1980	378	0-10	238		3.6		3.1		4.0	
				10-20	55							
36	Chlordane	1980	378	0-10	352		10.5		2.3		3.2	
				10-20	584							
37	Chlordane	1980	587	0-10	504		24.8		5.7		2.8	
				10-20	42							
38	Chlordane	1978	378	0-10	526		28.7		1.6		1.2	
				10-20	70							
39	Chlordane	1979	416	0-10	155		17.7		2.0		3.5	
				10-20	94							
40	Chlordane	1982	681	0-10	385		13.3		1.9		4.6	
41	Termide	1980	757	0-10	352	39	11.5	2.6	4.5	1.4	6.0	1.5
				10-20	584	82						
42	Termide	1983	322	0-10	4885	393	22.9	8.9	2.6	1.4	4.0	2.0
				10-20	68	<0.001						
43	Termide	1980	681	0-10	1035	154	2.1	0.4	0.6	0.1	0.8	0.1
44	Termide	1983	681	0-10	3532	1453	28.4	1.8	1.4	0.3	3.0	0.3
				10-20	ND	ND						
45	Termide	1983	416	0-10	1406	819	7.6	2.3	5.3	1.6	7.2	2.0

a Houses sampled between June and October, 1983.
b Termide emulsion contains 0.5% chlordane and 0.25% heptachlor.
c Chlordane applied as a 1.0% emulsion.
d Heptachlor fraction not calculated.

Table VI.   Chlordane and Heptachlor Residues in Air from Houses
Constructed on Concrete Slabs[a]

No	Termiticide applied	Year treated	Amount applied (L)	Chlordane ($\mu g/m^3$)	Heptachlord,e ($\mu g/m^3$)	Chlordane ($\mu g/m^3$)	Heptachlord,c ($\mu g/m^3$)
46	Termide[b]	1980	568	ND	ND	ND	ND
47	Termide	1980	738	ND	ND	ND	ND
48	Termide	1979	700	ND	ND	ND	ND
49	Chlordane[c]	1982	1230	4.3		1.4	
50	Chlordane	1982	590	ND		ND	
51	Chlordane	1983	757	ND		ND	
52	Chlordane	1983	624	0.7		1.0	
53	Termide	1982	568	2.0	0.9	1.3	0.4
54	Termide	1980	435	0.6	0.3	0.8	0.2
55	Termide	1982	416	3.0	0.6	4.2	0.2
56	Termide	1981	378	2.4	1.0	3.0	0.7
57	Chlordane	1983	624	3.0		1.6	
58	Chlordane	1983	624	1.6		5.7	
59	Chlordane	1981	605	1.4		ND	
60	Termide	1983	341	3.9	0.7	4.7	0.8

[a] Samples taken between June and October, 1983 from houses located on sandy soils; no crawl space.

[b] Termide emulsion contains 0.5% chlordane and 0.25% heptachlor.

[c] Chlordane applied as a 1.0% emulsion.

[d] None detected.

[e] Heptachlor fraction not calculated.

of slab-constructed dwellings, residues were lower in the latter. There could be much less volatilization from soil under a concrete slab than from soil without the slab and as was mentioned previously, five of these houses had no detectable residues.

Ninety-three percent of the 120 rooms sampled for chlordane had airborne concentrations below the 5.0 $\mu g/m^3$ limit, and none of the rooms had heptachlor concentrations above the 2.0 $\mu g/m^3$ proposed limit. When chlordane concentrations in the air of the two rooms sampled per house were averaged, only three houses (5%) had levels above the suggested limit. If samples were taken again, it is probable that the distribution would be different.

The interim guidelines proposed by the National Academy of Sciences are to be applied to long-term continuous exposure (of at least one year) (14). Thus, additional sampling of these houses at regular intervals for at least a one-year period would be necessary in order to determine if the residues of chlordane and heptachlor were above the interim guidelines. The results suggest that the houses were treated following label directions, because the residue concentrations in the air of 95% of the houses were below the interim guidelines.

Nontechnical Summary

Chlordane, a material composed of a number of chlorine-containing compounds, is used widely by pest-control firms to protect homes and

businesses from subterranean termites. Large quantities (i.e. 100
to 200 gal) of this termiticide are applied in trenches dug into
soil around crawl-space walls and chimney bases and into pilasters
and wall voids. Since chlordane remains unchanged for long periods
of time, a study was conducted to determine what quantities might
be present in both soils and the air inside houses. The Committee
on Toxicology of the National Academy of Sciences recommended that
a level no greater than 5.0 micrograms/cubic meter of air (5.0 $\mu g/m^3$)
of chlordane and 2.0 $\mu g/m^3$ of heptachlor, a component of technical
chlordane and a termiticide sometimes used in combination with chlordane, be allowed in the air of homes. Sixty houses, treated by
commercial pest-control firms between 1978 and 1983, were selected
based on construction type and the type of soil (predominately clay
or sandy) and the air in a bedroom and kitchen were analyzed. In
addition soil samples were collected from 45 of the houses (15 were
slab-type construction and soils could not be taken) and analyzed
for chlordane and heptachlor. Chlordane residues averaged 1051 and
1485 parts per million (ppm) in the first 4 inches (in) of sandy
and clay soils, respectively. Concentrations of heptachlor averaged
414 ppm in both soils from 0 to 4 inches. In all rooms sampled, the
average concentrations of chlordane and heptachlor were 2.9 and
0.7 $\mu g/m^3$, well under the guidelines recommended by the National
Academy of Sciences Committee on Toxicology. Of the 120 rooms
sampled, 93 percent (112) of the rooms sampled had airborne concentrations below the 5.0 $\mu g/m^3$ level and none of the rooms had residues
above 2.0 $\mu g/m^3$ of heptachlor. The results suggest that houses
treated according to label directions would fall within the recommended guidelines.

Acknowledgments

This study was supported by a grant from the Pesticide Impact
Assessment Comittee, U.S. Department of Agriculture. Thanks is
extended to W. L. Jones who assisted in the preparation of the soil
samples.

Literature Cited

1. Johnson, H. R. _Pest Control_. 1958, 11, 9-16.
2. Bess, H. A.; Ota, A. K.; Kawanishi, C. _J. Econ. Entomol._. 1966,
    59, 911-915.
3. Malina, M.A.; Kearny, J. M.; Dolen, P. B. _J. Agri. Food Chem._.
    1959, 7, 30-33.
4. "Chlordane Contamination of Government Quarters and Personal
    Property," USAF EHL Tech. Report 70-7, 1970.
5. Livingston, J. M.; Jones, C. R. _Bull. Environ. Contam. Toxicol._.
    1981, 27, 406-411.
6. "Chlordane in Air Force Family Housing: A Study of Houses
    Treated After Construction," USAF OEHL Report 81-45, 1981.
7. Wright, C. G.; Leidy, R. B. _Bull. Environ. Contam. Toxicol._.
    1982, 28, 617-623.
8. "Chlordane in Military Family Housing," National Academy of
    Sciences, 1979.

9. "Threshold Limit Values for Chemical Substances in the Workroom Environment with Intended Changes for 1983-84," American Conference of Governmental Industrial Hygienists, 1983.
10. Wright, C. G.; Leidy, R. B.; Dupree, H. E., Jr. Bull. Environ. Contam. Toxicol. 1981, 26, 548-553.
11. Weber, J. B. In "Research Methods in Weed Science, 2nd Edition"; Truelove, B., Ed.; Southern Weed Science Society: Auburn, AL 1977; Chap. 6.
12. Bennett, G. W.; Ballee, D. L.; Hall, R. C.; Fahey, J. E.; Butts, W. L.; Osmum, J. V. Bull. Environ. Contam. Toxicol. 1974, 11, 64-69.
13. Leidy, R. B.; Wright, C. G.; Dupree, H. E., Jr. J. Environ. Sci. Health. 1982, B17, 311-316.
14. "Analysis of the Risks and Benefits of Seven Chemicals Used for Subterranean Termite Control," U.S. EPA Report EPA-540/9-83-005, 1983, 75 pp.

RECEIVED September 14, 1984

Paraquat: A Model for Measuring Exposure

J. M. R. S. BANDARA, P. C. KEARNEY, P. G. VINCENT, and W. A. GENTNER

Pesticide Degradation Laboratory and Weed Science Laboratory, Agricultural Environmental Quality Institute, Beltsville Agricultural Research Center, Agriculture Research Service, U.S. Department of Agriculture, Beltsville, MD 20705

Residues on gloves and plastic boots were used as surrogates to measure herbicide transfer from treated plants. No human exposure occurred since harvesters wore protective clothing. The model was paraquat (1,1'-dimethyl-4,4'-bipyridinium ion) residues on Cannabis sativa (marihuana). The use of paraquat on Cannabis to reduce marihuana production presents a unique model situation when the grower attempts to salvage the treated plant. Marihuana plants were grown in a greenhouse, moved to a field and ground-sprayed with a solution of paraquat (0.6 kg/ha) plus 100 uCi (methyl ^{14}C) paraquat. Leaves of sprayed plants were harvested at 0, 1, 2, 4, 8 and 29 h after spraying. Time 0 was 10 min after spraying. Leather gloves, worn over rubber gloves, and boots were analyzed for residues. The highest residues were measured at time 0 (0.95 mg right glove, 0.50 mg left glove) and declined rapidly during the first 4 h after spraying. Residues on boot covers were lower than glove residues and also exhibited a rapid decline with time of picking. The mean plant paraquat residue, measured by combustion analysis, based on leaves harvested at time 0, was 4.65 mg per 10.41 g dry matter per plant and remained fairly constant during the first 8 h, but showed a loss of 64% (based on ^{14}C) at 29 h.

The herbicide paraquat (1,1'-dimethyl-4,4'-bipyridinium ion) is used widely in vegetation control programs. It is estimated that paraquat has been used in the United States on 10-12 million acres annually and is registered on 63 crops. Recommended rates vary from 0.25 to 1.5 lb/acre. Human exposure should be limited during application, due to the toxic nature of paraquat. Most worker exposure studies (1-3) have addressed the issue of occupational body burden when engaged in paraquat application with conventional spray equipment. Precautions taken to reduce respiratory and dermal routes of entry substantially lower the risk of potential adverse health effects.

The decision to use paraquat on Cannabis to control illegal
marihuana production in the United States and Mexico provides another
route of human exposure. This exposure results from residues accumulated at harvest, immediately after, and at subsequent times,
following a spray application. This occurs when the grower attempts
to salvage treated Cannabis plants after an authorized spray operation is conducted to destroy the crop. The herbicide's rapid desiccation renders the treated Cannabis unusable as a harvestable
commodity within hours of treatment. Plants are usually hand-
harvested by stripping the leaves to remove the vegetation. Depending on climatic conditions and either the awareness or lack of
awareness of the harvester, protective body cover may be minimal.
Much remains to be known about the concentration, stability and
possible transfer of residues of paraquat in and on treated Cannabis.
We are engaged in a number of studies to learn more about the fate of
paraquat on marihuana.

The objective of the present experiment was to estimate the possible transfer of paraquat residues from Cannabis and soil to humans
engaged in harvesting treated plants. Residues on gloves and plastic
boots were used as surrogates to measure transfer from treated plants
and soil. No human exposure occurred in these experiments since the
harvesters were completely covered with protective clothing.

Methods and Materials

Chemicals. A commercial preparation of paraquat containing 29.1
percent w/w of active ingredient (1,1'-dimethyl-4,4'-bipyridinium
dichloride) was obtained from Ortho Agricultural Chemical Division
of Chevron Chemical Company, San Francisco, California 94804.
(Methyl-^{14}C) paraquat, specific activity 7.91 mCi/mmol, was purchased from the Pathfinder Laboratories, Inc., 11542 Fort Mims
Drive, St. Louis, Missouri 63141.

Protective Clothing. Disposable nuclear coveralls made of 100
percent spunbonded olefin, Cat. #118-125 or 126 (Durafab, Cleburne,
Texas 76031), liquid proof poly-D disposable boots, Cat. #038-300,
reusable rubber gloves, Cat. #034-005 or 010 (Atomic Products
Corporation, P.O. Box 1157, Center Moriches, New York 11934), leather
gloves (Wells, Lamont, Sears, Roebuck & Co.), 28x30 cm, 100 percent
cotton white cloth patches; and Model #8714 Acid Gas Respirators
(220-7W, 3M Center, St. Paul, Minnesota 55101) were used as protective clothing by harvesters and the applicator.

Field Application. Cannabis sativa L. (marihuana) plants grown in
12.7-cm pots under greenhouse conditions for 5 months were used in
the study. The plants were about 60 cm in height. A guarded, secure
treatment area enclosed by an 8-foot woven wire fence topped
with a double barbed wire standoff, located at the Beltsville
Agricultural Research Center, BARC-West, Beltsville, Maryland, was
selected for the experimental site. Cannabis plants grown in the
greenhouse were moved to the experimental site just prior to treatment. The experiment contained 96 plants in 4 replications. Each
replication contained 6 plots (183x92 cm), arranged in the field
in a randomized block design, with 4 plants per plot. Blocks were
separated by a 92-cm alley.

A paraquat (5700 ml) solution containing 1,198 ppm paraquat and 100 uCi of (methyl-^{14}C) paraquat was sprayed onto Cannabis plants at 8:30 a.m. on August 11, 1983 with an experimental plot sprayer.

Harvesting. Four participants were used as harvesters, and leaves from four plants per plot were collected from each replication at each harvest. Each harvester was accompanied by an assistant who helped in the suiting up, sample collection, and sample cataloging. A practice run was held prior to the day of treatment. Leaves of plants were harvested at 0, 1, 2, 4, 8, and 29 h after spraying. Time 0 was 10 min after spraying. All harvesters were right-handed and were dressed with coveralls, respirators, rubber gloves, and disposable plastic boots. Cloth patches were used to cover the arms and legs.

Leather gloves were worn over the rubber gloves by all personnel to eliminate dermal hand exposure. Preliminary analyses of filter paper placed inside the rubber gloves indicated no penetration of ^{14}C paraquat. Leaves of each plant in a plot were stripped toward the plant base with the right hand while the tip of the stem was held in the left hand. The leaves were then stored in a plastic bag, which was sealed afterwards.

All protective clothing and harvested leaf samples were then transported to the laboratory within 30 min after each harvest and stored at -5°C. There was ample sunlight during the late morning and afternoon on harvest day. Midday temperatures were greater than 30°C, which did limit more extensive afternoon sampling due to the extreme heat buildup in the protective coveralls.

Residues. Each leather glove was cut into small pieces (ca. 3x3 cm) with a razor blade and then refluxed with 100 ml of 18N sulfuric acid in a wide-mouthed 1000 ml boiling flask fitted with a water-cooled condenser for 3 h. Separate razor blades were used for each glove to minimize contamination. Gloves from the left and right hand were refluxed separately.

Acid extracts were combusted for 2 min in a Packard, Tricarb Model 306 sample oxidizer. Three 0.5-ml aliquots of each of the cooled sulfuric acid extracts were transferred into combustion cones containing a paper absorbent. About 0.1 g of Combust Aid was added immediately prior to placement in the combustion basket of the oxidizer. Labeled $^{14}CO_2$ was trapped in Carbo-Sorb (approx. 7 ml) and scintillation cocktail containing Permafluor V (about 13 ml). Radioactivity was measured by liquid scintillation analysis in a Beckman LS 6800 counter and corrected for efficiency and recovery. Data collected as dpm's were converted to mg based on the amount of paraquat ion in the original spray solution.

Disposable plastic boots were refluxed in 50 ml of 18N H_2SO_4 and combusted as above.

Plant Samples. Air-dried plant samples were ground in a Wiley mill. Care was taken to avoid cross contamination between samples through the mill. Five hundred mg each of dried leaf sample were combusted to trap the $^{14}CO_2$ as above. Five 1-gram samples were selected at random from each time interval, pooled and extracted with methanol or ethyl acetate (150 ml) for 4 h in a soxhlet apparatus.

Volumes were reduced to 10 ml and an aliquot (0.1 ml) was analyzed
by combustion as outlined above.

Results

Glove Residues. Based on field observation and previous worker
exposure data (1), the hands of the harvesters would appear to be
the primary site of exposure. The ^{14}C residues on gloves expressed in mg paraquat, measured individually and collectively with
time, are shown in Figure 1. These residues resulted from a spray
concentration of 0.6 kg/ha (0.5 lb/acre). The effect of harvesting
method, i.e., where the right glove was used to strip the leaves
toward the stem while holding the distal end firmly in the left hand,
clearly resulted in higher residues on the right glove. Residues on
gloves declined rapidly during the first 4 h after spraying, which
may reflect a loss due to increased binding of the bipyridinium ion
to some plant constituent and(or) some change in the bipyridinium
ion due to photodecomposition or metabolism in the Cannabis plant.
Previous studies indicate a rapid decomposition of dilute aqueous
solutions of paraquat due to UV irradiation from a mercury-vapor lamp
(4), whereas natural sunlight caused little degradation. Paraquat
has a sharp absorption band at 257 nm, which is absent in the solar
spectrum. Based on studies in tomato, bean, and corn (5), and
alligatorweed and bean (6), it was concluded that paraquat is not
metabolically degraded in plants. A literature search revealed no
plant metabolism studies on paraquat in Cannabis.

After 8 h the treated Cannabis plants showed signs of substantial desiccation and browning, which probably further reduced the
transfer of paraquat to the gloves of harvesters. The cumulative
residues for both hands after 0, 1, 2, 4, 8, and 29 h was 1.45, 2.42,
3.07, 3.60, 4.01, and 4.24 mg, respectively. These cumulative
residues would appear to be higher than those reported by Forbess et
al. (1) on hands of either sprayer (0.081-1.324 mg) or mixers
(nd-0.231 mg) engaged in paraquat applications to grape vineyards.

Boot Residues. The possible exposure of the harvester through foot
contact with soil residues of paraquat may be academic in the more
temperate zones where Cannabis can be grown. It is a possible route
where the grower does not normally wear shoes, particularly in remote
tropic areas of cultivation. The data for residues on boot covers
proved more difficult to interpret, and consequently the values shown
in Figure 2 represent the extremes, i.e., the highest and lowest
residues, and the mean values. The highest residues were measured in
a harvester whose body weight was 90 kg, as opposed to the lowest
residues in the lightest harvester, whose body weight was 56.6 kg.
Traffic patterns in the plots, distance to the plot, time required
to harvest the plant material, soil moisture, plus other unaccounted
for variables, probably contributed to foot residues. The levels
of exposure through boots were considerably less than through
gloves, but the pattern of declining residues with time was similar.
The lower transfer of paraquat residues in soil to boots probably
reflects the strong binding of the bipyridinium cations to the negative charges on certain clay minerals (7), and to a lesser extent
the binding to soil organic matter.

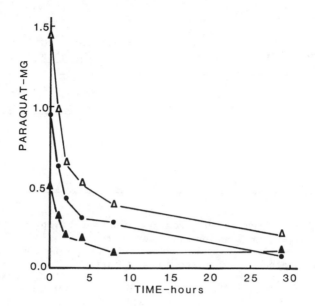

Figure 1. Paraquat residues measured on leather gloves used to harvest sprayed <u>Cannabis</u> plants at various time intervals after the initial application. Each point represents the average of residues on 4 gloves. Key: △, both gloves; ▲, left glove; and ●, right glove.

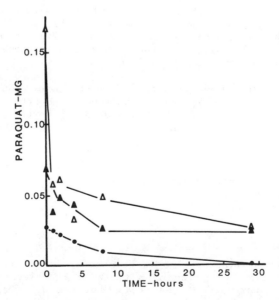

Figure 2. Paraquat residues measured on boot covers from soils in plots sprayed with the herbicide. Key: ▲, rep mean; △, highest; and ●, lowest.

Table I.   Paraquat Residues and Extractable ^{14}C from
[^{14}C-Methyl] Paraquat Measured in Air-dry <u>Cannabis</u> Plants

Time of Harvest (hours)	Plant Residues (ppm)	Percent ^{14}C Extracted EtAc	MeOH
0	446	0.0	19.0
1	467	0.0	15.5
2	398	1.0	18.4
4	433	0.0	16.8
8	433	0.2	14.6
29	138	0.0	6.5

<u>Plant Residues</u>.   The paraquat residues in <u>Cannabis</u> plants at differ-
ent times after application and the percent of ^{14}C extract with
ethyl acetate and methanol are shown in Table I.   Combustion of plant
material harvested at 29 h showed a significant loss of ^{14}C (69%)
when compared to time 0.   The amount of ^{14}C extracted with
methanol also exhibited a decline with time, particularly at 29 h.
Vincent et al. (8) have also observed a similar loss of paraquat
residues on the same collection of <u>Cannabis,</u> using a residue method
based on sodium dithioate reduction of the extracted paraquat,
followed by spectrophotometric analysis.   Attempts to examine the
possible production of labeled products by thin-layer chromatography
on cellulose-coated plates with several solvent systems have been
unsuccessful to date due to the high ratio of plant material to
labeled paraquat in the samples.   The plant residues measured in
the present study would appear to be consistent with mean values
(331 ppm) found in 20 confiscated marihuana samples reported by
Turner et al. (9), although there was considerable variation
(2-2264 ppm) in the confiscated samples.

<u>Summary</u> – The herbicide paraquat is used in marihuana control
programs.   Growers are exposed to paraquat when they attempt to
harvest sprayed plants.   Residues measured on leather gloves and
plastic boots were used as models to measure paraquat transfer from
plant and soil residues.   The highest residues were measured on
gloves immediately after spraying and declined rapidly during the
next 4 h.   Boot residues were lower than those on gloves.   Plant
residues remained fairly constant during the first day but exhibited
a sharp decline after 29 h.

Acknowledgments

Use of a company or product name in this paper is solely to provide
specific information.   Mention of a trade or proprietary name does
not constitute a warranty of the product by the U.S. Department of
Agriculture or an endorsement by the Department over other products
that may also be suitable.

Literature Cited

1. Forbess, R.C.; Morris, J.R.; Lavy, T.L.; Talbert, R.E.; Flynn,
    R.R. Hortscience 1982, 17, 955-6.
2. Staiff, D.C.; Comer, S.W.; Armstrong, J.F.; Wolfe, H.K. Environ.
    Contam. Toxicol. 1975, 14, 334-9.
3. Swan, A.A.B. Br. J. Ind. Med. 1969, 26, 322-9.
4. Slade, P. Nature 1965, 207, 515.
5. Slade, P. Weed Res. 1966, 6, 158.
6. Funderburk, H.H.; Lawrence, J.M. Weeds 1964, 12, 259.
7. Knight, B.A.G.; Tomlinson, T.E. J. Soil Sci. 1967, 18, 233.
8. Vincent, P.G.; Lydon, J.; Gentner, W.A. Proc. Weed Sci. Soc. Am.
    1984, Abstr. 219, 85.
9. Turner, C.E.; Cheng, P.C.; Torres, L.M.; Elsohly, M.A. Bull.
    Narcotics 1978, 30, 47-56.

RECEIVED October 10, 1984

Applicator Exposure to Pesticides Applied to Turfgrass

R. P. FREEBORG[1], W. H. DANIEL[1], and V. J. KONOPINSKI[2]

[1] Department of Agronomy, Purdue University, West Lafayette, IN 47906
[2] Indiana State Board of Health, Indianapolis, IN 46202

Applicators for lawn care companies can encounter long
term exposure periods while making required applications of pesticides to turf. Studies have shown that
inhalation of a pesticide was minimal as were dermal
exposures on the body and lower leg area. Wrist exposures were generally low in most cases. When higher
wrist concentrations were measured they appeared to be
related to whether the right or left hand was used by
the applicator. Highest concentrations were recorded
in the thigh-scrotal area and were also related to application techniques. Design of clothing to protect
the scrotal area may be advisable. For example, a
waterproof apron or properly designed non-absorbent
pants could reduce exposure and add protection.

Within recent years the commercial lawn care industry has developed
into a major business employing thousands of applicators who treat
millions of residential and industrial lawns with pesticides. The
rapid development of the custom-type lawn care reflects the demand
for such a service.

In 1976 it was estimated that Americans spent $9 billion on
home lawn and garden supplies. Although home lawn accounts comprise the largest number of customers for the lawn service companies, they also care for many of the grounds surrounding office
buildings, hotels, motels, churches, schools, apartments, condo-
miniums, cemeteries, industrial plants, shopping centers and banks.

The telephone directories of many cities have more than 100
listings under 'lawn maintenance' in the yellow pages. In Chicago
there are approximately 200. More than 4,790 professionally
trained employees treat less than 5% of the 80 million lawns in the
USA. Of these lawn care companies, 84% are independently owned;
only 7% are franchised operations. (1)

Lawn owners who avail themselves of the outdoor maintenance

0097-6156/85/0273-0287$06.00/0

services expect qualified people with professional equipment to
apply the correct materials, including pesticides, at the proper
time to obtain desirable results.

The period of daily exposure to one specific pesticide can
be up to six to eight weeks with the applicator working eight to
ten hours per day up to six days each week to meet acreage goals
established by the company. Spray volume worked with in one day
may amount to 1,000 gallons of water plus pesticide which, applied
at the rate of 4 gallons per 1,000 sq. ft., would require treatment of approximately 5.7 acres, or 31 residential lawns.

There are usually four eight-week treatment schedules offered
to the home owners. Pesticides are generally included in the first
and second, and sometimes in the third and fourth spray period.
Use will vary based on geography and pest control needs.

There is currently a trend to reduce use of pesticides as
much as possible. Cost is one factor that has influenced this
trend. Also, because insecticides currently available have a short
active life when applied to the soil, applications must be made
when insects are active to get full benefit of the insecticides.
Applications of insecticides to each customer's lawn are often
made only when insect activity is evident or past history in a
community has shown continual insect infestations. These factors
help to explain a decrease in the use of insecticides in recent
years.

Diazinon and trichlorfon (Dylox 50% WP or Proxol 80 SP) are
two insecticides frequently used by the commercial lawn industry
because of their relatively low level of acute toxicity. Recommended rates for insect control may vary. Diazinon may be applied
at 1 to 3 oz. active ingredient per 1,000 sq. ft. Trichlorfon is
also used for control of insects at 2 to 3 oz. active ingredient
per 1,000 sq. ft. Lawn insects controlled include chinch bugs,
sod webworms, cut worms, army worms, and grubs.

In this report tests of operator exposure were conducted
with the Nice N'Green Company and ChemLawn Corporation. Studies
to evaluate potential applicator exposure to diazinon (0,0-diethyl
0-[methyl-2-(1-methyl ethyl)-4-primidinyl]phosphorothioate) insecticide were made on 3 August, 18 and 28 September, 1979; and for
the insecticide trichlorfon (dimethyl 2,2,2, trichloro-1-hydroxy-
ethyl) phosphonate) on 5 September, 1979.

Trichlorfon was on the Rebuttal Presumption Against Registration (RPAR) list, however diazinon was not at the time exposure
studies were made. It was selected for measurement because of
its widespread use in the industry.

Materials and Methods

It was the intent of this study to determine both inhalation as well as dermal exposure. Concentrations of pesticides encountered through inhalation were measured using a Bendix model BDX44 personal air sampling pump. Air flow rates were established in the laboratory and frequent checks of the rotometer flow rate and adjustments in rates were made as needed to maintain a constant air flow volume throughout the field study.

The field monitor used to collect inhalation samples was a three-piece Gelman No. 4336 cassette with cellulose support pad and NG4, 37 mm (0.8 pore size) Gelman membrane filter. DHEW (NIOSH) Pub. No. 77-159 #21.01.

Dermal exposures were determined by adhering absorbent pads to the body under clothing at up to ten lcoations on the body. Wrist, ankle and thigh pads were 11.7 x 22.8 (289 cm^2) Johnson & Johnson sterile 'Surgipads' (HR1 8137-002145). All other body pads were Johnson & Johnson cotton gauze sponges (HR1 8137-007-623). Gauze pads were folded, 10.2 x 10.2 cm (104 cm^2) 12 ply. Total gauze area was 1238.8 cm^2. These were made from type VII (20 x 12) gauze.

Inhalation measurements included exposure during insecticide addition to the tank, travel time throughout the day, time involved in spray application, and truck and equipment cleanup time at the end of the day for Tests 1 and 2. Test 3 was a granular application which required individual separate handling procedures at each site. Test 4 required addition of a wettable powder to the tank. Because of greater potential exposure from the powder as the insecticide was added to the tank a separate inhalation measurement was made during tank mixture preparation (Table I).

Field monitor cassettes and absorbent pads were collected immediately after completion of the work schedule and placed in sterile 'Zwirl Pak' plastic bags and sealed. Samples were then placed in 10° F. temperature prior to analysis.

Analytical Procedures

The Association of Agricultural Chemists (2) analytical method 6.431-6.435 was used for the following changes:

1. For diazinon an additional step was added to 6.432. After shaking, the samples were placed in a sonic bath for 15 minutes. Samples were then extracted and standards were prepared in methylene chloride instead of acetone.

2. In the analytical procedure for trichlorfon, dermal pad samples were extracted with acetone, concentrated and diluted to 10 ml in acteone for trichlorfon analysis for gas chromatography.

The filters used to determine inhalation exposure could not be desorbed with acetone because the Gelman filters used in the cassette to determine inhalation exposure would not dissolve, so they were treated with methanol as above. One ml of this solution was concentrated to dryness and the residue was dissolved in 1 ml acetone.

The following data were collected from each of four exposure studies. Three were for diazinon and one for trichlorfon exposure. All studies were made under actual conditions normal for the application procedure.

Table I. Custom Lawn Applicator Exposure to Insecticides, 1979

App.Date	Pesticide	Flow rate l/min.	Exposure Total/[1] minutes	App./2	Air Volume App. liters	Filter Analy. μg	Concentration Total μg/m³	App.
3 AU	trichlorfon	1.4	300	113	158	9.6	.023	.061
18 SE	"	1.9	400	106	201	9.6	.013	.048
28 SE	"	1.9	326	34	65	13.3	.021	.204
5 SE	trichlorfon	1.9	456	161	306	2.	.002	.007
5 SE	"	2.0	(mixing)[3]	24)	(46)			.109

1. Total time is based on time from initial morning operation procedures until spray truck is returned to garage.

2. Application time is that which was devoted to spray application only.

3. Mixing time is that required to prepare the tank mix for application.

Diazinon Exposure

Test 1
    Location: Downers Grove, Illinois
    Applicator: Mike Oatis
    Date of application: 3 August 1979
    Insecticide: Diazinon AG500, liquid
    Application equipment: 1,000 gallon tank and Meyer centri-
        fugal pump and spray equipment was mounted on a truck bed.
        The tank contained 800 gals. total volume water plus
        insecticide and fertilizer. A ChemLawn spray gun with 40
        psi at the nozzle applied 4 gallons of insecticide and
        water per minute per 1,000 sq.ft.
    Weather: 11:00 am to 4:00 pm - 77-84°, R. H. 77-63%,
        wind speed, 13-8 mph
    Total work time: 300 minutes
    Total application time: 113 minutes

Sample identification Surgipad	Concentration of Diazinon $\mu g/100$ cm^2
front upper	6.9
back upper	6.9
right wrist	3.9
left wrist	19.9
right ankle	6.9
left ankle	6.9

Test 2
    Location: Indianapolis, Indiana
    Date of application: 18 September 1979
    Insecticide: Diazinon AG500, liquid
    Application equipment: 1,200 gallon tank with John Bean
        piston pump with ChemLawn spray gun. Application rate
        4 gpm insecticide and water per 1,000 sq. ft.
    Weather: 6:55 am to 1:35 pm - 61-77° F, R. H. 93-62%
        wind speed, SW 6 NW 9 mph
    Total work time: 400 minutes
    Total application time: 106 minutes

Sample identification Cotton gauze pads	Concentration of Diazinon $\mu g/100$ cm^2
front upper	12.8
back upper	12.8
front lower	12.8
back lower	12.8
Surgipads	
right wrist	5.9
left wrist	5.9
right ankle	23.7
left ankle	5.9
right thigh	29.6
left thigh	189.4

Test 3
    Location: Indianapolis, Indiana
    Date of application: 29 September 1979
    Insecticide: Diazinon (granular) 5% GR
    Application rate: 5.5 lbs. ai/acre
    Application equipment: Cyclone model B1 rotary spreader
    Weather: 6:51 am to 12:17 pm - 63-66° F., R. H. 87-84%
        wind W 7 mph
    Total work time: 326 minutes
    Total applicatin time: 34 minutes

Sample identification	Concentration of Diazinon
Cotton gauze pads	$\mu g/100$ cm^2
front upper	12.8
front lower	38.3
back upper	9.2
back lower	12.8
Surgipads	
right wrist	43.4
left wrist	130.2
right ankle	17.8
left ankle	5.9
right thigh	592.
left thigh	237.

Test 4
    Location: Indianapolis, Indiana
    Date of application: 5 September 1979
    Insecticide: Dylox (trichlorfon) wettable powder
    Application rate: 8 lbs. ai/acre
    Weather: 7:30 am to 3:06 pm - 68-86° F., R. H. 93-48%
        wind, NE 8 NE 10 mph
    Total work time: 456 minutes
    Total application time: 161 minutes, application
                  24 minutes, transportation-mising

Sample identification	Concentration of trichlorfon
Cotton gauze pads	$\mu g/100$ cm^2
front upper	n.d.*
front lower	n.d.
back upper	n.d.
back lower	n.d.
Surgipads	
right wrist	n.d.
left wrist	0.35
right ankle	3.5
left ankle	2.1
right thigh	1.0
left thigh	1.4

* not detectable

Results

Inhalation exposure, diazinon
The amount of diazinon to which operators were exposed via inhalation during the three tests was 0.023, 0.013, and 0.021 µg/m³ for the total work day of 67, 300, 400 and 625 minutes. The amounts applicators were exposed to if the measurements were based entirely on application time were 0.061, 0.048, and 0.025 µg/m³. The amount of time committed to actual spray applications was 6, 113, 106 and 34 minutes. Table I.
When inhalation concentrations were determined based on a TWA (Time Weighted Average) work day, the total exposure concentrations were less than 0.1 µg/m³ TWA established (DHEW, NIOSH 77-159,#11.01). When determined based on actual application time, exposure on 29 September of 0.205 µg/m³ was the largest recorded. The Threshold Limit Value-Short Term Exposure Limit (TLV-STEL) (3) for diazinon is reported as 0.3 µg/m³. Thus, based on the STEL, the exposure levels were below the 0.3 µg/m³.
According to the ACGIH publication (4) the STEL should be considered a maximal allowable concentration, or ceiling, not to be exceeded at any time during a 15-minute excursion period. The average time spent treating any one residential site was approximately six minutes.

Inhalation exposure, Trichlorfon
There appears to be no available TWA or TLV-STEL for trichlorfon. However, based on the organophosphate level as established for diazinon, the concentrations of 0.002 for the total work day and 0.007 µg/m³ for the application time were low. A concentration of 0.109 µg/m³ was measured during tank preparation. The TWA limit is 0.1 µg/m³.

Dermal exposure, Diazinon
Dermal concentrations were determined by adhering absorbent pads without backing to the body and then extracting the insecticide adhering to the pads.
Front and back body pads as well as ankle pads generally showed only traces or low levels of diazinon. Body pads with the greatest amount of exposure contamination were those on the wrist and on the inner thigh just below the scrotal area. Table II includes a list of wrist dermal exposure.

Table II. Wrist Dermal Exposure

	Wrist	
Date	Right	Left
	µg/cu²	
3 August	3.9	19.9
18 September	5.9	5.9
28 September	43.4	130.2

Concentrations above the lower detectable limit were found on 3 August, left wrist 19.9 µg/100 cm² pad, and on 28 September, right wrist 43.4 and leftwrist 130.2 µg/289 cm². It should be noted that

on 18 and 28 September the applicator used his left hand to hold
and guide the spray application. This may partially account for the
greater exposure concentration on the left wrist.

The highest exposure levels were found on the 289 cm² pads
taken from the upper thigh, scrotal area (Table III).

Table III. Thigh-Scrotal Dermal Exposure

	Thigh	
Date	Right	Left
µg/200 cm²		
18 September 1979	39	189
28 September 1979	592	347

Samples to determine exposure in the thigh-scrotal area were
collected on 18 and 28 September. The application on 18 September
was a liquid spray, that on 28 September was a dry granule applied
with a rotary type spreader. In practice, when applying the liquid
spray, the applicator normally walks at a brisk pace and the hand
held nozzle releasing the spray is swinging from side to side in a
rhythmical motion. It appears that exposure levels are highest on
the left or right thigh, depending on whether the applicator is left
or right handed. Exposure during the granular application on 28
September was greater than that experienced from the liquid spray
application.

Dermal exposure, Trichlorfon
Dermal exposure levels for trichlorfon were not detectable on the
front or back of the upper body. Also all wrist and ankle pad exposures were low. The thigh exposure levels did not reflect those
high concentrations for diazinon.

Conclusion
In conclusion, it would appear that inhalation exposure levels based
on total work day time are below the TWA for organophosphates diazinon and trichlorfon. However, in some instances, the STEL may be
approached or exceeded. For these situations, care should be taken
with the application spray pattern and existing wind speed and direction to minimize exposure. Dermal exposure levels were generally low, the exception being that for the wrist and thigh-scrotal
area. Frequent washing of hands and wrists would tend to reduce the
potential for a build-up in the wrist area. Thigh-scrotal area concentrations, which were high on two occasions, may need additional
confirmation. To reduce the exposure a non-absorbent apron could
shield the applicator using hand held spray nozz and protect
this part of the body from potentially hazardous exposure levels.

Nontechnical Summary
Estimates are that 5,000 employees of lawn care companies treated 5%
of the 80 million lawns in the USA in 1980. Pesticides most used
include preemergent grass weed, broadleaf weed and insect control
pesticides. Applicators applying these pesticides are exposed for
periods of six to eight weeks. Measurements made to determine exposure showed long term exposure resulted in very low levels of
pesticide inhalation. Also, pesticide concentrations reaching the

skin under the clothing were very low to non-detectable. Only wrist
and thighs had measurable concentrations. Occasional cleansing of
the hands and wrist should protect this exposure site. Clothing
that would protect the crotch area such as a waterproof apron or
properly designed non-absorbent pants could reduce exposure and add
protection.

Acknowledgments

This study was made possible through funding provided by the North
Central Region Impact Assessment Program.

Literature Cited

1. Daniel, W. H. and R. P. Freeborg. Turf Managers' Handbook.
West Lafayette, Indiana, 1979, p. 376-77.

2. Triazines And Other Pesticides, Association of Agricultural
Chemists, 1980, 13th ed.

3. National Institute For Occupational Safety And Health, 77-159,
No. 11.01. U. S. Department of Health,Education and Welfare. 1977.

4. Threshold Limit Values For Chemical And Physical Agents In
Workroom Environments. 1978.

RECEIVED September 11, 1984

Potential Exposure in the Application of Pesticides to Orchard and Field Crops

TERRY D. SPITTLER and JOHN B. BOURKE

Pesticide Residue Laboratory, New York State Agricultural Experiment Station, Cornell University, Geneva, NY 14456

Dermal exposure to pesticides in the cultivation of apples, green beans, onions, and cabbage was measured for a variety of defined tasks including mixing, application, and harvesting. Exposures resulting from applications using a variety of sprayer types were compared. Enclosed spray cabs on tractors reduced exposure to applicators using airblast sprayers for orchard work by a factor of four, but no effect was evident for low-boom field crop uses. Spray cabs might reduce the exposure noted for drop nozzle applications, however, no rigs so fitted were available for comparison. Instances were observed where the use of a spray cab in field crop application led to relatively higher potential exposure than that experienced by an adequately clothed operator on an open tractor. A significant percentage of exposure was shown to be received during mix-fill operations which were independent of crop and spray protection equipment. Little significant exposure was registered for scouts or harvesters.

Our participation in the surge of interest in worker exposure to pesticides that took place within the last five years was predicated on the premise that· worker exposure assessments should be auxiliary studies of ongoing operations. This preference for monitoring actual practice unquestionably had its roots in the prevailing economic realities, i.e. there was not enough research money available in this area to conduct full scale simulated applications. But, there were also the following advantages to assessing exposure in an existing operation:

A. The operation was probably already funded, and, therefore, only supplementary support for the monitoring needed to be obtained.

B. An operation conducted for a real purpose, and not just for the sake of doing an exposure study, was more likely to reflect true situations and conditions, and be conducted by persons experienced in those procedures who, are less likely to commit routine errors resulting in misleading exposure determinations.

C. Because such projects usually were attempting to make a specific point or to answer a specific question, a concurrent exposure assessment with the same parameters yielded useful exposure data on current or proposed practices.

D. The significance (and funding potential) of a project was enhanced by the addition of an exposure phase when care was taken in its proposal and implementation. Utilization of an existing resource, in this case a "host project", also helped obtain independent support for the exposure work.

Certain limitations were also inherent to these studies. Care had to be taken that measuring devices did not interfere with, or in any way compromise the safety equipment or protective devices that would otherwise be utilized, and field technicians had to remain passive observers who neither advised nor assisted in any of the tasks under study. Because time, itself, is a valuable commodity, manipulations involving the monitoring devices could not unduly interfere with the normal flow of operations on the projects.

The determination of absolute or "total exposure" has long been established as being beyond the scope of our studies of volunteer agricultural workers in ongoing operations. Instead, we focused our attention on isolating specific tasks or practices within the production scheme that allowed us to obtain the relative worker exposure associated with the various operations pertaining to each job and/or function. Once defined, variables such as time, lbs applied, gallonage, and acres treated could be normalized, and the consequences of independent variables such as sprayer type, formulation, protective devices, or application techniques could be intelligently gauged.

Throughout all three of the seasons that this work was carried out, we endeavored to maintain these comparative studies, while simultaneously keeping the measuring techniques as consistent as possible from year to year. Topical, or dermal exposure, one of the more important general routes for pesticide entry, was measured using gauze patches placed according to tenets developed for these general operations (1,2).

Experimental

In practice, three 4" x 4" sixteen-layered gauze patches, with foil-backing, were pinned on the subjects; F(over the heart), B(on the center of the back), and L(on the outside of the left leg at knee level). At the end of a defined task or time interval -- the particulars of which were recorded and frequently photographed -- the patches were removed and a 26 cm^2 circle was cut from the center and analyzed for the chemicals of interest. It has been generally recognized that mixers register high potential exposure on gloves or other hand monitoring devices(3). However, because the usual practice is for mixers to wear their own "pesticide resistant" gloves, the employment of our absorbent cotton monitoring gloves might have compromised prudent practice and was accordingly not done. Whole body suits (disposable coveralls) were employed for certain specific tasks, and air monitors were utilized in one field study.

Four basic cultivation programs were investigated during the course of our worker exposure studies. Each of these and the unique variables for which comparative potential exposure levels could be determined are listed below.

A. APPLE ORCHARDS, AIRBLAST APPLICATION (1980)

    1. Chemical Control Centers
    2. Spray Cabs

B. GREEN BEANS, DRY FIELD (1981)

    1. Spray Cabs
    2. High Pressure Low Boom vs Low Pressure Low Boom Sprayers
    3. Integrated planting/herbicide treatments vs separate operations

C. CABBAGE, DRY FIELD (1982)

    1. Low Pressure Low Boom vs Drop Nozzle Sprayers

D. ONIONS, MUCKLAND (1982)

    1. Low Pressure Low Boom vs High Pressure Low Boom vs High Pressure High Boom vs Drop Nozzle Sprayers.

In addition, the 1981 and 1982 studies looked at the exposure received by IPM scouts who frequented the treated fields to make damage assessments. Harvesters were also addressed in the 81-82 work. Tables I-III give an outline of each years monitoring by chemical and devices. Extensive photodocumentation of our programs, particularly of the mixing operations in all four studies, proved invaluable in identifying exposure mechanisms. Since reproduction of this media is not practical here, conceptual observations from this source will be interjected into the discussion of the four individual programs.

Table I.   Pesticide Exposure Samples Analyzed in Apple Orchard
                              Operations, 1980

Pesticide	Task[1]	#Patches (Sets)
Guthion	M+A	36 (12)
Benlate	M+A	9 (3)
Methyl Parathion	M+A	12 (4)
Plictran	M+A	21 (7)
Imidan	M+A	75 (25)

[1]   M = Mixer, A = Applicator

     All chemical analyses, except those for Manex, where
performed using standard pesticide analytical methods such as
those contained in the Pesticide Analytical Manual, and utilized
equipment and supplies available through numerous commercial
laboratory sources(4).   Dermal patches were constructed in our
laboratory by taping four, four-ply surgical dressings (4" x 4")
to a 4" x 4" square of aluminum foil with masking tape.   The
gauze was preextracted with acetone.   Gloves were ordinary, 100%
cotton, white gardening gloves and were not preextracted.
Estimations for Manex were performed by digesting the sample in
nitric   acid,   diluting   with   water,   and determining total
manganese by atomic absorbtion spectrometry (A.A.).   The Mn
background from the patches or gloves was negligible, but some
contamination by windblown soil occasionally may have increased
the levels found.

Apple Production (1980)

Chemical Control Centers were the driving force for this
investigation, with the primary concern being the environmental
impact and the changes in worker exposure patterns, if any,
consequential to their establishment and use.   They consist of a
secure chemical storage room, a water supply, a concrete pad for
mixing, filling and cleaning, and a catch basin with leach lines
for disposal of dilute spillage and rinse water.   This facet has
already been published(5).   Incidental to this, we were also
able to directly compare two operations that differed only in
that one used spray cab-equipped tractors to pull their airblast
sprayers, and the other did not.
     Table IV and V give results obtained for Imidan, one of the
few materials having a significant number of observations from
which to draw comparative conclusions. Data are given in μg
chemical/cm^2 at each body location, along with application
parameters useable for normalization of these numbers for
comparative purposes.   All materials were applied in mature
fruit tree protection programs using airblast sprayers of 500
gal/load capacity with 3 X low-volume nozzles.   The only viable
comparison to be made is that between Farm X having no spray
cabs on their tractors, and Farm Y having spray cabs with
charcoal air filters for their tractors.   All persons monitored
both mixed and applied their own materials, thus each fill-spray
batch is defined as a cycle (Cy).   Since the subjects within an

Table II. Pesticide Exposure Samples Analyzed in Green Bean Operations, 1981

Pesticide	Task[1]	#Patches(Sets)	#Other(Type)
Premerge	M	3 (1)	
Premerge	A	6 (2)	
Premerge	M+A	12 (4)	2(Coveralls)
Parathion	M	12 (4)	
Parathion	A	15 (5)	
Parathion	M+A	3 (1)	
Parathion	H	12 (4)	
Benlate	M	30 (10)	
Benlate	A	42 (14)	
Benlate	M+A	3 (1)	
Benlate	H	21 (7)	
Benlate	S	33 (11)	
Orthene	M	9 (3)	
Orthene	A	12 (4)	4(Air Tubes)
Orthene	M+A	3 (1)	
Orthene	H	15 (5)	
Orthene	S	33 (11)	
Sevin	H	12 (4)	
Sevin	S	9 (3)	
Treflan	H	42 (14)	
Lorsban	M	3 (1)	
Lorsban	A	6 (2)	
Lorsban	M+A	6 (2)	

1   M = Mixer; A = Applicator; H = Harvester; S = Scout

Table III. Pesticide Exposure Samples Analyzed In Onion and
                         Cabbage Operations, 1982

Pesticide	Task[1]	#Patches(Sets)	#Gloves (Pairs)
Parathion	M-C	39 (13)	
Parathion	M+A-C	3 (1)	
Parathion	A-C	42 (14)	
Parathion	H-C	12 (4)	
Parathion	S-C	33 (11)	24 (12)
Parathion	M-O	30 (10)	
Parathion	M+A-O	21 (7)	
Parathion	A-O	39 (13)	
Parathion	H-O	24 (8)	
Parathion	S-O	27 (9)	
Manex	M-O	30 (10)	
Manex	M+A-O	21 (7)	
Manex	A-O	39 (13)	
Manex	H-O	24 (8)	
Manex	S-O	15 (5)	
Manex	S-C	15 (5)	6 (3)
Bravo	M-C	6 (2)	
Bravo	A-C	6 (2)	
Bravo	S-C	18 (6)	6 (3)
Bravo	M-O	9 (3)	
Bravo	M+A-O	21 (7)	
Bravo	M-O	18 (6)	
Bravo	H-O	15 (5)	
Bravo	S-O	15 (5)	
Thiodan	M-C	30 (10)	
Thiodan	A-C	39 (13)	
Thiodan	S-C	30 (10)	16 (8)
Randox	M-O	9 (3)	
Randox	M+A-O	3 (1)	
Randox	A-O	12 (4)	
Randox	S-O	3 (1)	
Randox	S-C	15 (5)	8 (4)
Systox	H-C	6 (2)	
Systox	S-C	15 (5)	6 (3)
Pydrin	M-C	9 (3)	
Pydrin	A-C	9 (3)	
Pydrin	S-C	15 (5)	6 (3)

1   M = Mixer, A = Applicator, H = Harvester, S = Scout,
     C = Cabbage, O = Onions

orchard operation switched back and forth on equivalent rigs, no distinction was made between subjects at a given farm.

Simple treatment of these results allowed us to formulated some simple conclusions; this was the intent of the program, to make straight-forward observations leading to practical suggestions that could minimize mixer/applicator exposure.

When the total Imidan exposure results are compared on normalized bases (/Hr, /Cy, /Lb), the obvious point is that the use of a spray cab reduces the potential dermal exposure to about 1/3 or 1/4 of that shown for an open tractor. Similar results were obtained for Guthion, where exposure ratios ranged from 5.7 to 3.1.

In fact, these ratio, would be much higher if only the application step were being considered, but, because of the short time span, at dawn, when the winds were still and these spraying operations could be conducted, we were not able to routinely delay the operators by changing patches between the mixing and application stages. Mixing exposure is, of course, not influenced by spray cabs and is known to be generally high (6). Here it was considered to be equal for both operations -- the variation in exposure was attributed to the spray cabs. Our photodocumentation of filling operations in all four studies showed clouds and eddies of dry formulated pesticides around the mixers as they emptied bags of material into the filling hatches.

Table IV. Imidan Patch Exposures and Mix/Apply Productivity for Two Orchard Operations

	Patch Location[1] ($\mu g/cm^2$)			Parameter Totals			
	F	B	L =	Total Exp	Hours	Cycles	Pounds
Farm X	27.6	8.8	19.9	56.3	14.0	18	185
Farm Y	13.2	11.1	16.0	40.3	31.3	41	615

[1] F = Front, B = Back, L = Leg

Table V. Total Imidan Patch Exposure[1] for Two Orchard Operations Normalized for Mix/Apply Productivity Parameters

Farm	Exp/Hr	Exp/Cy	Exp/10 lbs
X	4.0	3.1	3.0
Y	1.3	1.0	0.67
X/Y	3.1	3.0	4.5

[1] Exp = $\mu g/cm^2$

In summary, there is a 3- to 5-fold decrease associated with the use of a spray cab in airblast operations, when the mixings and fillings are done under similar conditions. There is no evidence that a Chemical Control Center influences the potential dermal exposure resulting from spray operations as defined in this study. Patches worn by our technicians in the Chemical Control Centers during the course of the study gave no evidence of pesticide exposure to casual frequenters of the area.

Green Bean Production (1981)

The 1981 growing season provided a unique opportunity for assessing the impact of a new chemical pesticide use pattern on the ecosystems in and surrounding the target plots. For the first time the widespread use of insecticides in green bean production, to combat infestations of the European corn borer, was being recommended. Prior to this season only herbicide and fungicide treatments were utilized in commercial production; few insect pests bothered the relatively fast-growing crop enough to require regular control. In addition, an Integrated Pest Management (IPM) pilot program was already in place in bean cultivation and field personnel could be shared. This program also had the professional staff required to conduct the species population studies on contiguous areas and within the subject fields.

The second objective, however, was to assess the potential exposure to pesticides of all personnel involved in green (snap) bean production. Ground preparation, planting, maintenance spraying, IPM scouting, and harvesting were monitored throughout the 1981 season, using several appropriate collection devices designed to measure potential exposure via certain routes during the performance of specific tasks. In addition to patches, disposable coveralls were worn for certain tasks, then collected and analyzed. Patch sets placed under the Tyvex coveralls measured any chemical penetrating the material. For direct comparison, a set of patches was also pinned to the outside, offset, of course, so as not to interfere with those under the garment. Air monitors were also utilized in one phase of the program.

Because much of the equipment encountered in field crop production is farm built and/or multipurpose, we were not able to obtain large numbers of comparative runs with only one independent variable as had been the case in the orchard work. Most of the data support only semiquantitative evaluations of alternative devices and practices utilized at specific steps in production(7).

Analysis of whole body suits (by extraction of the quartered garment) showed that almost twice as much chemical/hour (Premerge) was deposited over the entire body when Premerge alone was applied from an open tractor using low pressure sprayers as compared to the situation where a combination rig for planting, fertilizer incorporation, and preemergent spraying was employed (11 mg/hr vs 6.5 mg/hr). However, because of the more rapid coverage and greater payload of the former equipment, the actual exposure/acre treated was considerably less when the single purpose unit was used. The high toxicity of Premerge required that gloves, a hat, coveralls and a respirator be worn during all stages of the operation, regardless of equipment type. One accident was documentated in which a pressure hose split and sprayed the subject applicator with Premerge. Repairs were effected with patches still in place on the clothing; the whole incident resulting in a very high potential exposure to an unprotected worker. No penetration of the suit was detected.

Some exposure to chest patches was registered for Lorsban seed treatment during the planting/application operation. This presumably came about from lifting seedbags to fill the planter hoppers. The amounts were small and because of the presence of Premerge in the vicinity, the workers were (or should have been) generally well protected.

There appeared to be little, if any, dermal exposure measured under normal application conditions when low pressure low boom sprayers (LPLB) were used on open tractors: likewise for our measurements of a similar truck-mounted device in which the subject applicators worked in a cab with the windows down. In situations where the subjects were required to dismount in the field to clear nozzles or move booms or obstacles, the leg patches invariably received material from the newly treated foliage. Chest patches were occasionally contaminated at this stage also. Both truck and tractor mounted sprayers showed similar exposure patterns for applicators.

Applicator exposure with high pressure low boom sprayers was found to be even less than that recorded for LPLB devices. Tractors with and without spray cabs were tested, and there was seen no overriding advantage to the spray cab under normal conditions. Under severe conditions, like gusting winds or line ruptures, a cab would logically afford more protection. However, winds should generally cause reconsideration of the days operations.

Again, extra-vehicular activity to remove obstacles or adjust booms resulted in some contact exposure. The chemicals studied were Benlate, Orthene and Parathion, with no preferential transfer being evident for the freshly applied material (i.e., contamination ratios on patches were roughly equal to the stated ratio in the tank mixes).

An attempt was made to measure the concentration of Orthene in air both within and outside of a spray cab. Air was drawn through two different glass tubes, each containing 400 mg of silica gel, by MDA Model 808 Air Inhalation Pumps (MDA Scientific, Glenview, IL) operating at 100 cm^3/min. and placed as described above. Duplicate experiments lasting 0.40 and 0.45 hr, and sampling 2400 cm^3 and 2700 cm^3 of air, respectively, were conducted. Although recovery was shown to be 100% for extraction of Orthene from the tubes, no measureable amount of chemical (<0.5 μg/2L) was detected. These data imply, and the patch data support, that there is very little airborne pesticide in the vicinity of the spray cab during the proper operation of this equipment.

Interestingly, applicators on open vehicles wore protective devices and thus were still protected when events caused them to dismount. However, the apparent security afforded by spray cabs caused several subjects to work without coveralls, shirts, gloves, hats and respirators, and they were very vulnerable when they had to leave their protected environment to deal with minor problems. Spray cabs usage was, in fact, increasing the risk of potential exposure under certain circumstances by abetting their neglect of personal protection.

In most instances we were able to isolate the mixing phase from the application phase of the protection cycle by changing patches. Almost all high exposures during mixing were recorded on the chest patches, except when the subject was squatting on a truck bed to add chemicals or fill the tank. In these instances, the leg patch was also subject to contamination. Our photodocumentation shows that the use of gloves in all phases of the mixing operations is essential.

Variations in formulation caused different exposure problems; the most severe being Benlate 50 WP which forms dust clouds when emptied in the filling hole and when the "empty" bag is handled. Orthene SP caused fewer airborne particles. Parathion 8E (and Premerge 3EC), being liquids, caused problems only when poor technique resulted in splashing or spilling. However, the high toxicity of both of these materials makes their careful handling imperative.

Full protection should be worn for the filling operations (coveralls, gloves, mask, hat). Mixing time was only about 20% of the application cycle, but usually caused about 75% of the potential dermal exposure as measured in our study.

Scouting has become a regular and important crop maintenance procedure. Although frequently conducted by contract or public program personnel, it nonetheless involves having persons enter treated or soon to be retreated fields for purposes of assessing pest populations or damage thresholds. Slight residues were found on some scout leg patches when reentry had been within several days of application. One chest patch also picked up some Benlate during these operations. Except for the incident where a scout was sprayed by an aerial applicator, this vocation entailed negligible dermal exposure as measured by our techniques.

Since most of a scout's time is spent handling foliage, it became apparent that we should have included glove analyses in the scout monitoring protocol. While recognized too late for this study, this parameter was incorporated into subsequent surveys.

Hand picking, the traditional method of green bean harvesting, had not been employed on the subject farms for several years, and no monitorable hand operations could be found in the area. While the topic might still be viable with regard to family plots or U-Pick enterprises, it is, for all practical purposes, obsolete as far as serious commercial growers are concerned. Accordingly, our study was confined to mechanical picker operators and an occasional truck driver frequenting the field being harvested.

There was no appreciable exposure to Benlate, Orthene, Parathion, Treflan, or Sevin detected on any harvest personnel patches. Enclosed cabs on the harvesters thus do not have any bearing on pesticide exposure, and should be designed and selected from the point of view of operator comfort and mechanical safety. Orthene, the material frequently used closest to crop picking, was analyzed for in a field sampled on harvest day. Although measurable residues of 0.25 ppm for beans, 0.45 ppm for plant trash (leaves & stems), and <0.02 ppm for surface soil were present, mechanical harvesting essentially eliminated any significant contact with treated commodities.

Onion and Cabbage Production (1982)

As was encountered in our earlier assessment of field crop production of green beans, the data allow only semiquantitative evaluations of exposure trends due to the large variation in equipment and practices encountered. This situation is not unusual when one considers that the small size and mixed cropping practices of the typical farms in this area require that equipment be adaptable to multiple functions. Full data from these studies are contained in our 1982 NEPIAP Report (8).

Applications to the early growth stages of cabbage using LPLB equipment resulted in no measurable exposure during both calm weather and in moderate winds. Seven application cycles using a LPLB sprayer to treat onions yielded no measurable amounts of Parathion or Bravo on the patches, but calculated values ca. 5 μg/cm^2 were observed for Manex. However, since this chemical was determined by measuring Mn, manganese present in soil dust could have caused these readings. The occurrence of similar readings for onion harvesters supports this assertion.

Contradictory evidence is presented for HPLB equipment if sprayer type is taken as the independent variable. One subject treated onions with Bravo, Manex, and Parathion, and received potential dermal exposure to Manex in the neighborhood of 4 μg/cm^2 (average of F, B & L locations) for three application cycles and two mix and apply cycles. Identical levels were also found for two intervening mix cycles. A second subject, on the other hand, conducted three application cycles using similar equipment and only one leg patch registered exposure to Manex and none were positive for Parathion. Three mixing cycles were likewise shown to be free of potential exposure. Soil moisture conditions were not recorded so we could not determine conclusively if airborne dust was a factor in this discrepancy. However, the absence of Mn in both the mixing and application phases of this operation points in that direction.

Only one onion operation was observed using high pressure high boom (HPHB) equipment: the materials being applied were Parathion and Manex. No Parathion was found in four application cycles, but Manex was present at levels between 2 and 6 μg/cm^2 for the first three out of four cycles. Both the last mix and the last application of the day were exposure-free.

The application of Parathion and Thiodan mixtures to cabbages using drop nozzle (DN) rigs revealed a positive relationship between these rear mounted (or trailed) spray rigs and potential applicator exposure, particularly on the legs and back. The potential exposure for application cycles measured on three different subjects decreased in the order L>B>F, with the chest area frequently being residue free. This is consistent with a situation when the "overspray" is eddying behind and below an applicator on an open tractor. Taking a typical run and averaging the three exposures measured for Parathion, $(0+2.5+7.1)/3 = 3.2$ $\mu g/cm^2$, then multiply this times the area determined for a set of full body disposable coveralls (17,700 cm^2) produces a total potential dermal exposure of 57 mg. Performing this same calculation for the Thiodan measured on the same patches yields 27 mg Thiodan total dermal exposure. Normalization to one hour gives exposure rates of 122 and 58 mg/hr total exposure, respectively. Both of these figures are similar to values previously reported and point out the approximate amounts potentially available for dermal assimilation (6). Protective clothing shields the body from much of this, of course, but more could (should) be done to further reduce these levels.

Other materials applied with drop nozzle sprayers showed lesser levels of exposure, and as the level of analytical sensitivity was reached, the L>B>F relationship deteriorated.

Drop nozzle application is a situation in field crop maintenance where the addition of a spray cab might be expected to significantly reduce potential applicator exposure. Alternatively, the use of other boom sprayers (HPHB, HPLB, LPLB) appear to give less exposure than the drop nozzle rigs.

The harvesting operation is heavily mechanized for both commodities, so in this study human subjects are best described as either drivers or crew. Only one cabbage harvester registered any exposure, and that was limited to Systox on one chest patch for a crewman who stood on a platform and culled out small or rotten heads with a pitch fork. Cabbages were harvested from mineral soil fields in our study and there was little airborne dust during the operations.

Conditions were very dusty during the onion harvest on muckland soil, particularly for the harvester driver and crewmen who followed in the wake of the undercutter that severed the roots, removed loose dirt, and dropped the onions on the soil surface. The driver of that machine showed only leg patch exposure to Manex, whereas the other drivers and crewmen exposed to the dust tail registered Manex exposure of approximately 2- and 4- $\mu g/cm^2$, respectively, on all patches.

It was not determined if the dustborne Mn was from residual Manex or merely a trace element in the soil, as this question was not evident until after the selected analytical method had yield these results. Soil samples from that operation had not been taken and were thus unavailable for subsequent investigation.

In general, harvesters in these situations are going to be exposed to soil residues, but not necessarily to dislodgeable residues from plants, as the latter are not frequently handled. The question of exposure during subsequent packing, processing, and distribution of the crops was not addressed. Protective clothing for harvesters is a difficult topic to evaluate because of both the comfort demands of the tasks and the transient nature of the personnel.

Scouts showed occasional dermal patch exposure, results that would be not unexpected for personnel whose function it is to walk, kneel, and crawl throughout treated acreage. This year's scout monitoring protocol also included gloves, and the high levels of dislodgeable residue obtained for Thiodan, in particular, augurs well for making their use mandatory. Risks attendant to scouting did not appear to be unduly high, however.

Nontechnical Summary

Spray cabs were shown to be of benefit in reducing potential dermal exposure to pesticides in airblast (apple orchards) and drop nozzle spraying (cabbages). Certain combinations of circumstances existed where applicators were more at risk because of their leaving the cabs unprotected than if they worked with prudent, personal, protection on an open vehicle. Other types of normal boom applications to field crops (green beans, cabbage, onions) revealed little potential dermal exposure as measured by our topical patches. Only potential dermal exposure was addressed in this study, and no assessment or recommendations concerning respired or ingested materials were made. Subjective inferences may be drawn by recognizing that the conditions that promote body deposition can also place pesticide materials in the vicinity of the nose and mouth. Therefore, the use of a dust mask, or preferably a respirator, is encouraged under all suspect conditions.

Mixers receive most of their exposure as a result of splashes, powder spills, contact with encrusted equipment, overflows, and other random events. None of these are predictable, yet the magnitude of these potential exposures obliterates the long term contribution of vapors, low level dust clouds, etc., when statistical correlations are made. Consequently, the most practical approach would be to revamp the mixing process so that the opportunities for accidents are minimized, recognizing that this short time-span operation should be conducted under strict protective conditions.

Acknowledgments

The assistance of J. Andaloro, K. Rose, C. Hoy, D. Harrison, C. Eckel and numerous volunteer subjects was appreciated. Funding for these projects was through the Northeast Pesticide Impact Assessment Program.

Literature Cited

1. Davis, J. E.; "Materials and Methods Used by FDA, Field Studies Section, Wenatchee, WA, for Assessment of Pesticide Exposure" Environmental Protection Agency, 1978, 11p.
2. Bourke, J. B.; Spittler, T. D.; Baker, P. B.; Dewey, J. E.; DeRue, T. K.; Winkler, F. "Analysis of Potential Pesticide Exposure to Workers by Chemical Control Centers" Under Contract USDA-TPSU NYSAES-0-195; 1980.
3. Davis, J. E.; Residue Reviews 1980, 75, 34.
4. "Pesticide Analytical Manual" II; Food and Drug Administration: Washington, D.C. 1982.
5. Spittler, T.D.; Bourke, J. B.; Baker, P. B.; Dewey, J. E.; DeRue, T.K.; Winkler, F., in "Treatment and Disposal of Pesticide Wastes"; Seiber, J. N., Ed.; ACS SYMPOSIUM SERIES, American Chemical Society; Washington, D.C., 1984.
6. Jegier, Z.; Archives of Environmental Health 1964, 8, 670.
7. Bourke, J. B.; Spittler, T.D.; Andaloro, J. T.; Baker, P.B.; Eckenrode, C. J.; Shelton, A. M. "Economic and Environmental Impact of Insecticide Use in Northeastern Vegetable Production: II Worker Exposure and Environmental Stress" Under Contract USDA-TPSU NYSAES-1-221; 1981.
8. Bourke, J. B.; Spittler, T.D.; Andaloro, J. T.; Eckenrode, C. J.; Shelton, A. M. "Worker Exposure and Environmental Considerations of Pesticide Usage in Commercial Onion and Cabbage Production in the Northeast" Under Contract USDA-TPSU NYSAES-0511-2400; 1982.

RECEIVED August 28, 1984

The Potential for Applicator–Worker Exposure to Pesticides in Greenhouse Operations

ACIE C. WALDRON

North Central Region Pesticide Impact Assessment Program, Department of Entomology, Ohio State University, Columbus, OH 43210

Airborne and surface foliar measurements of pesticide residues following high and low volume spray and fog applications to greenhouses showed that the potential hazard to workers is initially much greater than from similar outdoor operations. Airborne residues dissipated within a 2-4 hour period when the greenhouse was vented and/or there was considerable air movement, but were evident for several hours in unvented greenhouses. Climatic-atmospheric conditions directly affected the persistence of pesticide residues. Although airborne residue dissipation from high volume application was faster than that from low volume, the former may involve the greatest hazard because such applications are made during the daytime when workers may be present in other locations in the greenhouse in contrast to low volume applications made at night in closed greenhouses after workers have vacated the premises. Surface foliar pesticide residues are also of concern to the greenhouse worker.

Vegetable and flower crop production in greenhouses are beset with unique situations and problems in pest control. The confined, enclosed area makes any registered pesticide applied as a fumigant, or that may volatilize after surface application, potentially very effective against pests. On the other hand, the health hazard associated with airborne pesticides is considerably greater indoors than similar operations outdoors. Pesticide levels in the ambient out-of-door air are usually in the nanograms-per-cubic meter range, but indoor levels may be in the microgram to milligram-per-cubic meter range and may persist for a longer period of time.

Many greenhouse operations are labor-intensive and require frequent worker exposure to the greenhouse atmosphere and the treated plant foliage. Pesticides may be applied to greenhouse crops throughout the year, generally on a 3-day schedule. High volume (HV) applications are usually made with other workers present in adjacent areas of the greenhouse. Low volume (LV) applications are usually in

0097-6156/85/0273-0311$06.00/0
© 1985 American Chemical Society

the evening or early night when only the applicator is present.
Factors which affect worker exposure to pesticides include the type
of activity, pesticide particle size, formulation, climatic conditions, duration of exposure and attitude of the worker in relation
to avoiding conditions conducive to exposure. Protective clothing
of some kind plus respirators or gas masks are usually worn by the
applicator during treatment, but the degree of protection offered
may be limited, depending on the type of equipment used to apply the
pesticide. Thus, pesticide use in greenhouses may present a particular problem for applicator and worker exposure to pesticide residues, both in the air and on treated foliage.

Research on pesticide exposure experienced by applicators and
workers in greenhouses is very limited, and consequently, was noted
as a data gap in the Rebuttable Presumption Against Registration
(RPAR) process of reviewing pesticide registrations early in the
Pesticide Impact Assessment Program (PIAP). Multiyear studies on
pesticide/greenhouse relationships for the North Central Region
Pesticide Impact Assessment Program (NCRPIAP) were initiated by Drs.
Richard K. Lindquist, Harvey R. Krueger and Charles C. Powell, Jr.
at the Ohio Agricultural Research and Development Center (OARDC) in
1979 (1) and by Dr. Delbert D. Hemphill at the University of Missouri
in 1980 (2). The major objectives of the research were (a) to
develop procedures for sampling and measuring pesticide residues in
the greenhouse atmosphere; (b) to measure airborne and surface residue of selected pesticides in greenhouses at intervals after application to determine the exposure potential to applicators and
workers; (c) to determine the effects of time, temperature, light
intensity, and air movement on the atmospheric concentration of
pesticides; and (d) to develop procedures to reduce human hazards
associated with greenhouse pesticide applications. This paper constitutes a brief summarization of public information data currently
held in PIAP files.

Procedures

Initial efforts in greenhouse-pesticide-exposure research were to
develop procedures for measuring the volatility and hence airborne
concentration of pesticides in the greenhouse atmosphere over a
period of time. This was followed by analysis for surface residues
on foliage and structural surfaces and finally determining the degree
of protection provided to the applicator and worker through the wearing of appropriate protective clothing and devices. Studies were
conducted in both commercially and university operated greenhouses
utilizing both the grower and technical personnel as applicators. HV
applications were made using standard power spraying equipment (1)
and the knapsack sprayer (2). LV applications were made with thermal
pulse jet foggers, mechanical aerosol generators and spinning disc
(controlled droplet) equipment as related to the availability and the
type of formulation (1). The particulars on the various application
procedures for pesticide fogs, foliar sprays and granules are included in the research publications and reports by the principal investigators (1,2). Greenhouse crops in the studies conducted by Lindquist
included tomatoes, chrysanthemums and roses while Hemphill used leaf
lettuce. Such crops are quite labor intensive requiring workers to
spend considerable time in the greenhouse and, consequently, provide

a maximum potential for exposure to airborne and surface pesticide
residues. Hemphill applied wettable powder formulations of carbaryl,
captan and folpet, whereas Lindquist evaluated various formulations
of aldicarb, dichlorvos, benomyl, chlorothalonil, permethrin,
methomyl, oxamyl and triadimeform at some time during the study.

Greenhouse air was sampled by drawing the air through sequential
samplers calibrated to measure air volume filtered per unit of time;
i.e. 1.8 cubic meters per hour for Hemphill's research and 4 cubic
feet per hour for Lindquist's. The air was drawn through 0.5 inch
diameter collection tubes containing 20 cubic centimeters of purified
amberlite and glass wool plugs (Lindquist). Hemphill used samplers
containing activated charcoal with glass fiber filters and glass
fiber filters with polyurethane foam plugs. Samplers were capable of
providing hourly samples over the 24 hour period although the length
of time for collection and the interval between sampling was altered
according to the individual design of the particular study. The
greenhouse environment, which included the variables of temperature,
relative humidity, light intensity, air movement and ventilation, was
recorded for the sampling intervals. After the collection of samples
the residues were extracted with acetone or hexane-acetone and
analyzed by gas chromatography using suitable detection systems. In
calculating respiratory exposure Hemphill used the formula:

$$\text{Exposure} = \frac{\text{Air concentration} \times 1.8 \text{ M}^3/\text{hr}}{70 \text{ kg}} \times 100\%$$

in which the air concentration is the residue determined in the
collection column per unit of time, 1.8 M^3/hr is the average ventilation rate, 70 kg is the weight of an average man and the absorption
factor is assumed to be 100%. Lindquist calculated inhalation exposure potential by determining the pesticide residue collected in the
column per hour and multiplying by a factor of 7.5 which is the ratio
of the average human air intake of 30 cubic feet per hour to the air
flow through the samplers of 4 cubic feet per hour.

Surface pesticide residues were determined by Lindquist, et al,
by the strategic placement of glass plates throughout the greenhouse
and the subsequent measurement of residue collected thereon following the pesticide application. Residue measurements from glass
plates were preferred over analysis of foliage because of the ease in
conducting several experiments over a period of time in replacing the
plates rather than waiting for the pesticide to completely dissipate
from the treated foliage. Also measurement of residue from the upper
and under surfaces of the glass plate provide a means of determining
the plant coverage from different application methods. Glass slides
coated with magnesium oxide provided a means of determining pesticide
droplet deposition from LV application, but was not practical for use
with HV because the spray washed the coating from the slides.

The measurement of dermal exposure to applicators and greenhouse
workers was conducted by attaching gauze pads to the inside and outside surfaces of the clothing, extracting the pesticide residue from
the pads and determining concentrations by gas chromatography. Greenhouse workers were not required to wear special clothing - only that
normally worn for the work involved.

Results and Discussion

Sequential sampling systems, with the absorbent materials indicated,

were effective in collecting airborne pesticide residues from greenhouse atmospheres. However, as one would expect, the environmental
conditions, the nature of the greenhouse, pesticide formulation, and
methods of application are determinant factors in the potential for
applicator/worker exposure. Airborne pesticide residues are the
"highest" immediately after spraying, as expected, but dissipate
rapidly with time. The rate of dissipation is enhanced greatly when
the greenhouse is vented to the outside atmosphere or there is considerable air movement due to the design of the greenhouse. Lindquist
found residues of dichlorvos applied as a thermal fog decreased from
exposure concentrations of 200-400 ug/hr during the first one or two
hour sampling period to approximately the 1-3 ug/hr range at 10 hours
and then remained relatively the same over the next 12 hours (Figure
1). Permethrin applied as a thermal fog showed the initial sharp
decline in residue level during the 1 and 2 hour sampling periods
and the rapid drop after opening the vents. Applications of permethrin made in the evening to a closed greenhouse resulted in fairly
persistent airborne residue levels after the first 2 hour interval
and until the vents were opened in the morning 8-10 hours after
application. HV applications of permethrin dissipated much faster
than LV applications, and for LV application the dissipation rate for
the pulse jet applicator was several magnitudes slower than the
mechanical aerosol generator. Typical dissipation curves for
dichlorvos and permethrin are shown in Figure 1. The curves represent the means of residue measurement of from 3-5 different applications of the particular pesticide. Indications are that applicators and workers would be subject to significant concentrations of
airborne residues of these insecticides during the initial hours
after application until the greenhouse was effectively vented.

Aldicarb granules applied to greenhouse chrysanthemums did not
produce any airborne residue concentrations. Likewise, triadimeform
applied by volatilization and low volume spray applications resulted
in essentially non-detectable residues. The application of oxamyl
resulted in considerable fluctuation in the amounts detected, but the
airborne concentrations were very low throughout the sampling period.
Consequently, further investigations with these pesticides were dis-
continued.

The results of Hemphill's research with carbaryl showed a relatively rapid decline with a drop to non-quantitatively detectable
levels 4 hours after application (Table I). The decline in residue
levels for captan and folpet was not significant during the first 2
hour interval but reached non measurable levels 4 hours after application. Carbaryl and captan concentrations in air were lower than
the Threshold Limit Value (TLV) of 5 mg/M^3 established by the American Conference of Governmental Industrial Hygienists in 1974. There
is not an established TLV level for folpet. The estimated respiratory exposure for the three pesticides, based upon the assumption of
100 percent absorption, is shown in Table II for the 0 and 2 hour
sampling periods. Comparison of the data with the no observable
effect level (NOEL) for carbaryl of 0.06 mg/kg body weight and captan
and folpet at 0.01 mg/kg established by the International Agency of
Research on Cancer (IARC) committee of the World Health Organization
(WHO) in 1979, indicates that unprotected inhalation exposure, although very low based upon the LD_{50}, exceeded the NOEL for the first
two hours after spraying.

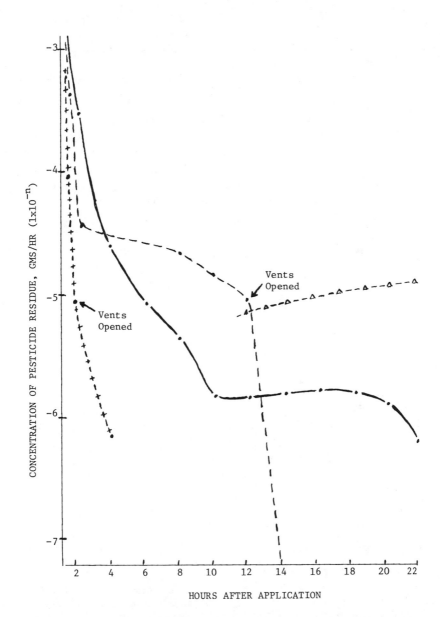

Figure 1. Residues of typical pesticides in greenhouse air. (Means of 3-5 applications and samplings for each chemical.) Key: ———, dichlorvos (fog); -----, permethrin (fog--greenhouse closed overnight); +-+-+, permethrin (fog--greenhouse closed 1½-2 hours); and △--△--, methomyl (spray).

Table I. Mean Concentration of Pesticide Chemicals in a Greenhouse
Atmosphere

Pesticide	Concentration at Time Interval[a]				Condition at Time Interval			
	(Conc. ug/M^3)				Temp (°C)		Rel Hum (%)	
Hours =	0	2	4	24	0	2	0	2
Carbaryl	53.0	38.3	b	b	13.5	13.1	58.0	58.8
Captan	18.7	13.3	b	b	19.4	19.9	49.5	52.6
Folpet	15.7	13.3	b	b	18.6	17.7	71.5	69.3

a   Mean value for six experiments.
b   Trace concentrations either too low to quantify based on minimum
    detectable level of 5 ug/M^3 or non measurable.

Table II. Mean Estimated Respiratory Exposure for Three Pesticides

Pesticide	Estimated Exposure at Time Interval[a]	
	0 hrs	2 hrs
	$(mg/kg\text{-}hr^{-1})$	
Carbaryl	1.36×10^{-1}	9.82×10^{-2}
Captan	4.81×10^{-2}	3.4×10^{-2}
Folpet	4.04×10^{-2}	3.4×10^{-2}

a   Based on the assumption of 100% respiratory exposure over a 60
    minute period.

The effects of sunlight on the concentration of airborne carbaryl, captan and folpet residues in the greenhouse atmosphere is
shown in Table III. The figures given are the mean of 3 replicate
determinations by Hemphill. There were significant differences in
residue concentrations between sunny and cloudy days for carbaryl
and captan, but not for folpet, with sunlight effecting a lower
residue concentration. The effects of temperature and relative humidity on airborne concentrations were not readily interpretable in
either Hemphill's or Lindquist's studies. However the effects of air
movement were easily observable in that methomyl residues were not
detectable at the 12 hour interval in a plastic bubble greenhouse
with air movement of 150 ft/min in contrast to measurable residues
(Figure 1) that appeared to slightly increase over a 12 to 48 hour
time interval in a glasshouse with air movement at 33 ft/min. (1).
Surface residues from HV pesticide applications measured at 20
designated locations in the greenhouse were generally more uniformly
distributed throughout the greenhouse than were those of LV application (Figure 2). This may have been partially due to the procedures whereby HV applications were made by spraying while retreat-
ing out of the greenhouse and LV applications were made at night from

Table III. The Effect of Sunlight on Airborne Residues of Pesticides in the Greenhouse

Pesticide	Mean Concentration of Residues (ug/M^3) [a]			
	Bright		Cloudy	
	0 hrs	2 hrs	0 hrs	2 hrs
Carbaryl	32.39	20.61	73.61[b]	55.95[b]
Captan	11.78	8.83	25.52[b]	17.67[b]
Folpet	11.12	6.87	19.63[c]	19.63[c]

a   The means of three measurements.
b   Significant differences at the 5% level from measurements under sunny conditions.
c   No significant differences from measurements under sunny conditions.

a single point at the end of the greenhouse. Although permethrin applications were made at the same rate, surface residues varied according to application method. LV application with a microgen applicator on three different dates resulted in the highest average deposition but also the greatest variation in range, whereas the HV application averaged about 1/2 that of the microgen but was approximately 9-10 fold greater than the residue from the LV application with a pulsfog. The average residue deposition with the microgen for each of three applications was 95, 237 and 327 ng/cm^2, but with extremes of 17-288, 44-417 and 35-812 ng/cm^2, respectively; for the HV application 177, 167, 151 ng/cm^2 with extremes of 148-258, 92-245 and 43-341 ng/cm^2, respectively; and for the pulsfog 17.5, 28.8 and 20.4 ng/cm^2 with extremes of 4-97, 6-64 and 8-81 ng/cm^2, respectively. In most cases the majority of the residue values for the HV and the pulsfog applications were clustered fairly close to the average. However, because comparative applications were not made on the same day nor under the same temperature and relative humidity, a valid comparison and evaluation of the data is impractical at present other than the indication of potential exposure to workers from surface residues following pesticide application.

Pesticide formulation and volatility of the chemical greatly affects the ratio of airborne to surface residues. Wettable powder formulation of permethrin resulted in an airborne concentration of 0.39 ug/1 during the first 2 hours after application, whereas the emulsifiable concentrate of the same pesticide resulted in a concentration of 2.82 ug/1. The surface deposition of benomyl averaged approximately 750 ng/cm^2 from a HV application and 632 from an LV application (Figure 2) and airborne residues were not measurable 1 hour after application. Approximately 33 percent of the benomyl deposition from the HV application was on the under surface of the glass plate, whereas only 1 percent from the LV application was so deposited.

Data relative to the effect of greenhouse structure on airborne and surface pesticide residues and the reduction of the exposure potential due to the use of protective clothing and equipment and

Greenhouse length = 175 feet

206[a]	206	184	149	196
23[b]	9	16	20	17
69[c]	220	133	101	160
860[d]	830	650	900	450
370[e]	860	840	860	230

140[a]	156	257	183	164
13[b]	18	25	21	15
297[c]	204	205	392	285
690[d]	1160	510	850	480
530[e]	930	1030	1200	770

137[a]	186	135	166	161
15[b]	66	17	15	30
294[c]	319	311	328	220
830[d]	510	520	840	790
360[e]	450	900	610	240

102[a]	149	173	131	120
39[b]	19	14	30	20
309[c]	58	273	91	119
640[d]	960	920	830	850
240[e]	540	700	560	420

Greenhouse width = 22.5 feet

a = Average of HV application of permethrin from 3 dates.
b = Average of LV pulsfog application of permethrin from 3 dates.
c = Average of LV microgen application of permethrin from 3 dates.
d = HV application of benomyl.
e = LV pulsfog application of benomyl.

a,b,c,d,e notes apply to all numbers horizontally across the figure.

Figure 2. Pesticide surface residues (ng/cm^2) measured at 20 designated locations in the greenhouse after HV and LV applications of permethrin or benomyl.

personal safety practices exercised by greenhouse workers has not yet been reported.

Summary

Studies conducted under the sponsorship of the NCRPIAP in Ohio and Missouri have provided satisfactory methods for determining airborne and surface pesticide residues from greenhouse applications and have indicated the potential exposure to applicators and workers. Although airborne residues quickly dissipate when the vents are opened at time intervals after the spraying operation, the initial exposure to the applicator and to any worker who enters the greenhouse soon after application is evident and requires proper attention to personal protection. Pesticides are applied as high volume (HV) and low volume (LV) sprays and fogs to greenhouse crops throughout the year often on a 3-day schedule. HV applications are usually made with other workers present in adjacent areas of the greenhouse, whereas LV applications are made during the evening when only the applicator is present. Protective clothing of some kind, plus respirators or gas masks, are usually worn by the applicators during treatments, but the degree of protection offered may be limited and depends upon the type of equipment used to apply the pesticide.

There is potential for exposure from all application methods, but the actual amount of exposure may vary tremendously. Low volume applications generally result in higher residues than high volume. It could thus be concluded that LV applications will result in greater worker exposure to the pesticide. However, the opposite may be true and LV applications could be less hazardous because they are generally made in the evening, require a relatively short period of time with no workers present, the applicator moves away from the pesticide application and out of the area and the greenhouse is usually vented in the morning before anyone enters. The additional data to separate actual worker exposure from potential exposure should be a valuable contribution to the study.

Literature Cited

1. Lindquist, R.K., H.R. Krueger and C.C. Powell, Jr. "Measurement of Pesticide Concentrations in Air Inside Greenhouses" NCRPIAP Project #67 (30-NC-OH-0) FY-1979 and "Measurement of Airborne Concentrations and Dislodgeable Residues of Selected Pesticides in Greenhouse Crop Production" NCRPIAP Project #97 (52-NC-OH-0) FY-1980. The Ohio Agricultural Research and Development Center, The Ohio State University. Unpublished Final Research Reports submitted to the NCRPIAP Regional Office, Columbus, Ohio and to USDA-CSRS-S&E.
2. Hemphill, D.D. "Concentrations of Selected Agricultural Chemicals in the Greenhouse Atmosphere" NCRPIAP Project #105 (48-NC-MO-0), FY-1980. University of Missouri. Unpublished Final Research Report submitted to the NCRPIAP Regional Office, Columbus, Ohio and to USDA-CSRS-S&E.

RECEIVED August 28, 1984

TRENDS IN EXPOSURE ASSESSMENT AND PROTECTION

Advances in the Unified Field Model for Reentry Hazards

WILLIAM J. POPENDORF

Agricultural Medical Research Facility, University of Iowa, Iowa City, IA 52242

This paper summarizes the development and application of both a philosophic and quantitative framework for unifying research approaches and findings in residue decay, exposure assessment, and cholinesterase response (Popendorf & Leffingwell, Res. Rev. 82:125, 1982). Examples are provided for using this model to interpret the potential cholinesterase response from a known foliar residue and to establish reentry intervals to prevent excessive cholinesterase inhibition. The potential and limitations of extrapolating this approach to other settings is also discussed, as are the needs for future research to support a comprehensive approach to pesticide use, residues, and exposure controls.

Exposure of harvesters to pesticide residues on crops and their foliage has been discussed as a hazard for 35 years (1). This hazard has come to be called the "reentry problem". Two years ago Leffingwell and I published a comprehensive review of the research and regulatory approaches surrounding the "reentry problem" in an effort to synthesize a unifying framework to the otherwise diverse aspects of this field worker problem (2). Borrowing from Einstein and viewing this framework as a semi-empirical model rather than a theory, I called this synthesis the "unified field model". This paper will discuss (a) how to use this model in practice, (b) some recent research relating to this model, and (c) new research suggested by this model.

Using the Unified Field Model

The concepts comprised within the "unified field model" are embodied in Figure 1. The 1982 report (2) discussed each of the measurable conditions of residue, dose, and response (the boxes in Figure 1) and the processes or mechanisms (arrows) which connect them. The unified field model went beyond a concept to a sequence

0097–6156/85/0273–0323$06.00/0

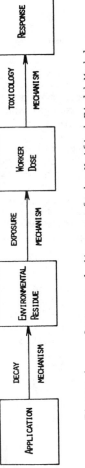

Figure 1. Conceptual diagram of the Unified Field Model. (Reproduced with premission from Ref. 15. Copyright 1980, American Industrial Hygiene Association.)

of formulae which characterize the mechanisms relating the original residue (R_q) to the residue at reentry (R), the deposited dose (D'), the dose per tissue mass (D), and the acetyl cholinesterase response (ΔAChE). Thus, the unified field model for organophosphate (OP) pesticides was also postulated as Equations 1-4, Table I. The form of the residue decay Equation 1 is simplified from decay patterns in the real world, but it is characteristic (2,3). Among the various residue exposure assessment studies, an empirical linear relationship between residue and dose has been found (2). At least for OP pesticides, cholinesterase inhibition (ΔAChE) is well established and accepted as a response criterion (2,4,5), although not without exception (2 p. 133).

Table I. Quantitative Form of Unified Field Model

$$R = R_o \exp(-k_r T) \quad (1)$$
$$D' = k_d \, t \, R \quad (2)$$
$$D = k_a \, D'/m \quad (3)$$
$$\Delta AChE = 1 - \exp(-k_e D/LD_{50}) \quad (4)$$

where
R = the residue at any point in time after application

R_o = the initial deposited residue, e.g. $\mu g/cm^2$

k_r = pesticide specific residue decay coefficient

T = reentry interval, days

D' = deposited dose (mg) on harvester's skin

k_d = crop specific residue transfer coefficient, cm^2/hr

t = work (exposure) period, hr

D = adsorbed or absorbed dose per body mass, mg/kg

k_a = absorption coefficient for fraction absorbed

m = body mass (nominal 70 kg)

ΔAChE = fraction of RBC cholinesterase inhibited

k_e = enzyme coefficient (use 6.0 when using topical dermal dose and k_a = 1.0)

LD_{50} = dermal dose to kill half of a group of test rats

The temporal sequence of events in the real world progresses through Figure 1 from left-to-right; and if one were to make real-time decisions based on a known residue, then one would use Equations 1 to 4 in the same order as shown. However, from the point of view of a reentry policy and setting reentry intervals, one must proceed from right-to-left, and from Equation 4 to 1. In either case, one of the basic elements in an occupational health decision is establishing an acceptable level of response; in this case, an acceptable ΔAChE.

Acceptable levels of cholinesterase inhibition have been discussed before (2,5) and have been adopted into at least one governmental standard (6). The concept of regulating occupational work practices on the basis of a biologic response is tenuous at

best, especially if the level of exposures is highly variable and the
time-frame and potential for disabling or lethal doses is great. For
instance in California, medical surveillance of pesticide manufacturers, formulators, and applicators is legally required, and RBC
AChE inhibition is restricted to 40% of an individual's baseline
activity (6). Using Equation 4 and data compiled in the original
review (2), one can calculate that a single dose sufficient to inhibit 40% AChE is only a factor of 2 less than would begin to cause
disabling clinical symptoms (60%) and 3x less than the LD_1 (lethal
to 1% of exposed group of rats)(7). On the other hand elaborating
on Equation 4 and depending upon the biokinetics of enzyme reversion
(reversible inhibition) for a given OP, 2 to 3 consecutive daily
doses each sufficient to inhibit 40% of the AChE will also produce
60 to 80% inhibition and similar clinical symptoms. And finally it
will be shown in Figure 3, that consecutive daily inhibitions of less
than 2% may result in a progressive depletion of 40% AChE after 8
weeks. Based on a general knowledge of the frequency of medically
monitored workers being administratively removed from further exposure and a cursory review of the few fatalities reported in
California, one might conclude that cholinesterase inhibition can
occur both progressively and from acute over-exposures.

     Routine cholinesterase monitoring among harvesters would suffer
the same limitations and require such extensive administrative
procedures as to be as poorly received by labor as by farm managers.
It is, in fact, the goal of a reentry interval policy to provide
equivalent field worker protection without requiring blood
monitoring. Establishing a control criterion should include a
consideration of the same range of exposure patterns: from variable
exposures with intermittent high peaks to consistent but low daily
exposures. There is reason to believe that both acute and
progressive inhibition has occurred among California harvesters,
that progressive inhibition can occur nationwide, and that conditions for both probably exist worldwide.

     Examples of reentry-response calculations for several reported
residues were provided in my 1982 paper (2). A more generalized and
practical set of examples will be followed here. To begin with, let
us first discuss issues related to R_o. Some general limits and
guidelines can be constructed based on plane geometry and mass
balance. For instance, a 1 pound pesticide application distributed
uniformly onto a flat 1 acre field (1 lb AIA) would result in an
average initial residue of 11 $\mu g/cm^2$. The amount of foliage per
acre varies by crop, size of plants, and plant spacing; for
instance, data by Turrell (8) indicate citrus foliage can comprise
roughly 1.5 to 4 times the land surface area upon which the trees
are planted. Thus, such initial deposits on citrus foliage might
ideally range from 7 to 3 $\mu g/cm^2$. Other mechanisms such as drift,
foliar versus ground deposition, gallonage of water and runoff,
evaporation while drying, foliar absorption, etc will further reduce
initial residues. Reported field measurements vary from near the
ideal to well below: an application of 1 lb AIA captan on
strawberries (9) is likely to result in an initial residue of 6 to
10 $\mu g/cm^2$ of projected leaf area (or 3 to 5 $\mu g/cm^2$ counting both
sides); for parathion on citrus (3), 1 $\mu g/cm^2$ (or 0.5 counting both
sides); and some more closely planted, tall crops such as tobacco
(10,11) may range from 1.0 to 0.1.

Hazard assessments can be made of this initial residue using the unified field model with decay time, T, set equal to zero days. Figure 2 provides an overview of the anticholinesterase potential calculated from known residues as follows:

(1) Find R from Equation 1 or equivalent tables or figures. In our case, T=0, therefore $R=R_o=1.0$ µg/cm^2, corresponding to citrus.

(2) Find the skin dose, D', from Equation 2. The dosing coefficient k_d is crop (and work practice) specific, and may also be affected by residue penetration through clothing worn in different regions. Table II provides a summary of known and extrapolated values of k_d. For practical purposes in our example, let k_d=5000 cm^2/hr and t=8 hours, the nominal U.S. customary workday, even though in any given situation it may be more or less.

(3) Find the tissue dose, D. The use of Equations 3 and 4 depends upon the chemical, its target organ, and the effect. For OPs when using dermal LD_{50} in Equation 4, the absorption coefficient (k_a) must be assumed to be 1.0 since fractional dermal absorption rates are accounted for within the dermal LD_{50} versus say intraperitoneal or intravenous LD_{50}. The use of an oral LD_{50} adds even more confounding differences and should be avoided within this setting. For other non-cholinergic effects, a known fractional absorption coefficient could be incorporated (2, pp 157). A nominal 70 kg (154 lb) average man should be assumed if dosing calculations are to be based on one of the nominal 1.9 m^2 skin area models (2, pp 155).

(4) Find the cholinesterase response using k_e=6. This response is a change from whatever pre-exposure activity was present (possibly already depressed from previous exposures). For multiple, simultaneous OP exposures the sum of the individual doses over their respective LD_{50}s is calculated (e.g. $-k_e \quad D_i/LD_{50,i}$) before taking the exponent (2).

Table II. Summary of K_d dosing coefficient values (cm^2/hr) to predict harvester dose mg/hr from residue µg/cm^2 based on projected leaf area (ref. 2,8) or total leaf area (ref. 13)

Crop	via projected A	via total area	(ref.)
citrus	5,000[a]	10,000[a]	(2,18)
peach	1,900[b]	3,800[b]	(2)
grape	1,600[b]	3,200[b]	
strawberry	4,000[c]	8,000[c]	(9)
tomato (mechanical)	33[d]	67[d]	

a) dose adjusted for knit glove penetration
b) value extrapolated from foliar versus airborne dust correlations (32)
c) dose not adjusted for wet glove effect (14,19)
d) dose to operators normally wearing vinyl-rubber gloves

Thus, the ΔAChE can be predicted either by using Equations 1-4 in sequence or by combining them into Equation 5; this can be further simplified to Equation 6 in our assumed citrus situation where R_o=1 $\mu g/cm^2$ (one sided), T=0, k_d=5000 cm^2/hr, and t=8 hr.

$$\Delta AChE = 1 - \exp\ (-k_e k_a k_d\ t\ R_o\ \exp\ (-k_r T)\ /m\ LD_{50}) \quad (5)$$
$$\Delta AChE = 1 - \exp\ (-3.437 LD_{50}) \quad (6)$$

The results of this equation are plotted along the Y axis of Figure 2 for various LD_{50}s from 0.1 to 300 mg/kg. One can see that under these assumed "day zero" conditions, OP pesticides with LD_{50}s greater than 100 mg/kg present a minimal reentry hazard. For more toxic residues down toward 10 mg/kg, the hazard is not likely to be acute (in the sense that one or a very few days exposure will not produce symptoms), but progressive depletion of cholinesterase becomes an increasing hazard. Below 10 mg/kg the time-frame for progressive depletion to clinical symptoms is going to be 3 days or less.

For other conditions of application, R_o will usually be less than linearly proportional to application rate because of increased runoff at higher rates and especially at higher gallonages. On the other hand by examining Equation 5, an equivalent anticholinesterase potential can be expected for equal ratios of R or D to LD_{50}; that is to say, an initial residue of 1 $\mu g/cm^2$ with a toxicity of 30 mg/kg is equivalent to a 3 $\mu g/cm^2$ residue with an LD_{50} of 90 mg/kg (both R/LD_{50} ratios of 1:30 in their respective units). Different ratios of residue-to-toxicity are exponentially related to both the reference anticholinesterase effect and the difference in the R/LD_{50} ratios.

If one finds that the initial residue is too hazardous (as determined by potential cholinesterase response along the Y axis), then one can wait a sufficient number of half lifes (N) for the concentration of residue to decay to acceptable levels. Moving right from the Y axis, Figure 2 shows the relationship between residue hazard and time assuming no increase in the residue's inherent toxicity as from oxon formation. As can be seen in Equation 5, the change in ΔAChE versus T is related by an exponent of an exponent, a situation most simply described by example.

For instance, take the case of Systox (demeton) residues with an LD_{50} of 11 mg/kg [7]. It is clear from Equation 6 and Figure 2 that the 27% response predictable for residues of 1 $\mu g/cm^2$ on day 0 would be unacceptable. The next question is, what reentry interval would be required to reach an acceptable residue? The question of "an acceptable single day AChE response" cannot be answered without knowing or assuming a temporal pattern of exposure, e.g. daily, weekly, or once in a "blue moon". Figure 3 provides some idea of the progressive cholinesterase inhibition trend expected over a harvest season given various consecutive daily inhibitions. Not shown in this figure is that intermittent, high exposures could have the same long-term effect, e.g. an 8% inhibition every 4 days would result in the same "pseudoequilibrium" of 40% inhibition as 2% every day. Very little data exist to guide us in characterizing the temporal pattern to which real-world harvesters are exposed. A moderate assumption might permit 4% inhibition per day, while a conservative (worst case) assumption might permit only 1%.

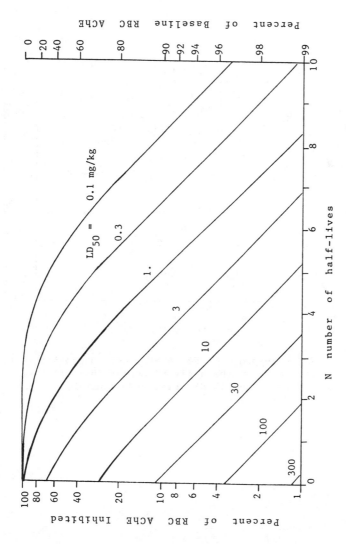

Figure 2. Response of RBC AChE based on an R_O = 1 μg/cm², k_d = 5000 cm²/hr, a single working day t = 8 hours, and m = 70kg.

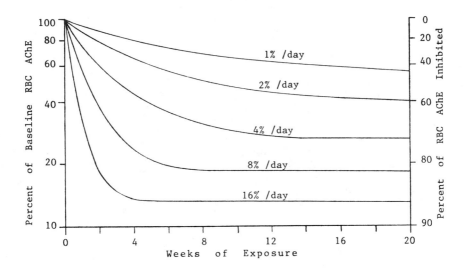

Figure 3. Cumulative response of RBC AChE based on repetitive OP exposure sufficient to cause the daily responses indicated followed by 10% reversion and 1% RBC replacement/day.

Given a 4% response criterion, a corresponding reentry interval
can then be calculated using either Figure 2 (yielding the interval
in terms of 3 half-lives), Equations 4 through 1 in reverse order,
or again combining them or rearranging Equation 5 to form Equation
7. Unfortunately, I could find no reported foliar residue data for
Systox. Nigg and Stamper (12) reported half-lives for Metasystox-R
on citrus foliage of 17 and 2 days during dry and wet weather,
respectively. Assuming a Systox half-life of 6 days (corresponding
to a k_r=.12) yields Equation 8:

$$T = \frac{-1}{k_r} \ln \frac{-mLD_{50} \ln (1- \Delta AChE)}{k_e k_a k_d t R_o} \tag{7}$$

$$T = \frac{-1}{k_r} \ln \frac{-LD_{50} \ln (1- \Delta AChE)}{3.43} = 17 \text{ days} \tag{8}$$

It is clear that many assumptions were needed to calculate this
reentry value. If these assumptions are reasonable, the calculated
T=17 days contrasts sharply with the current EPA required reentry
interval for Systox of 2 days. These assumptions provide some clues
to the kinds of further research necessary to implement this model
more broadly. These topics for further research will be reviewed
shortly. But first by way of summarizing the current uses of the
unified field model, I will review recent research related to each
mechanism.

Recent Related Research
Residue decay has been perhaps one of the better researched aspects
of the reentry problem, especially by the residue chemists
represented here. However, there has been no significant progress
in the past 2 to 3 years concerning decay mechanisms and the many
gaps in the residue decay data banks. Existing data has been
generated by a variety of residue extraction methods (2), but the
most common is the dislodgeable or punch sample in which the residue
is "extracted" from the foliage in an aqueous media, then back
extracted into an organic solvent for analysis (13). The continuing
production of such data is necessary and deserves three comments:
   (1) There have in the past been three ways of calculating
       foliar residue results. One calculates ppm by weight;
       and there are two ways to calculate $\mu g/cm^2$ by area.
       Either of the latter two calculations are preferred
       because the foliage is not ingested or otherwise contacted
       "by weight", and the residue transferred to harvesters is
       from the leaf surface. The leaf area can be calculated on
       the basis of either its projected area (one-sided) or
       total surface area (two-sided). Residues calculated on
       the basis of the former can be converted to the latter by
       dividing by 2; alternatively, the k_d value can be adjusted
       for the method used to calculate the residue as shown in
       Table II. The former "per area" method has the historic
       precedent (8), but the latter is probably in more
       common use today (13).
   (2) There continues to be the possibility for repartitioning,
       particularly during the aqueous extraction phase, between

residues unbound to the leaf surface, those bound to or under the leaf surface, those on surface dust or other detritous, and the water. This repartitioning could be exhibited in various ways. In some unpublished work with Leffingwell with a fungicide on tomatoes, we found the presence of foliar dust to greatly increase recovery efficiencies. As mentioned in the previous paper, Zweig et al (14) seem to have found the k_d for vinclozoline on strawberries to be much higher than for carbaryl, etc. And we previously reported a k_d for supracide oxon on citrus to be 4 times that for other residues (2,15).

(3)   Finally, there is considerable variability in reporting temporal trends in residue data. The exponential model presented in Equation 1 has been used for many years as a matter of convenience as much as a matter of fit (16). Any alternative equation could be used provided it yields values in appropriate units, $\mu g/cm^2$. Some decay patterns can get quite complex (2,3,17), and some of these have not yet been characterized mathematically (17). Tabular or graphical solutions are also possible except somewhat more cumbersome.

In regards to exposure mechanisms, the residue dosing coefficient has recently shown both continuing promise as well as limitations. One of the limits concerns the measurement of dermal dose, especially to hands. Ethanol hand rinsing was recently shown by Davis et al (18) to measure roughly 20% as much hand exposure to apple-thinners as measurements using cotton gloves (2,15). Some preliminary results of our comparisons between the use of gloves versus washing was presented by Noel and Zweig a year ago at Seattle (19). Our findings for short term exposures (1/2 hour) were similar to those by Davis (19) but in our studies the two methods appeared to converge over longer work-exposure intervals. Analyses of more extensive studies conducted along these lines are currently being completed.

On the bright side is the finding by Nigg et al of k_d values for Florida citrus (20) harvesters to equal those in California (15). In some ways this is as much a surprise as a validation given some differences in methodologies such as the use in Florida of ethanol hand rinses and the placement of lower body pads outside the clothing. "On the other hand", California citrus harvesters doses were calculated by reducing the exposure retained in the glove to that 7% of material which penetrated the gloves; and all other dosimeter pads except those on the head were placed under the clothing (2). It would seem that these methodological differences "balanced out" to yield equal k_d values (Table II).

Other recent studies in strawberries have also found a reasonably linear dose-rate/residue ratio; however, it is unexpected that the resulting k_d transfer coefficient for strawberries should be equal to that for citrus because the distribution of the dermal doses are different as are the major mechanisms of exposure, being largely contaminated dry "airborne" dust deposition onto the whole-body in the tree crops and hand contact often with wet foliage in strawberries (14).

The units of k_d probably have more of a direct relevance where direct contact predominates. If the mass of residue and dose were expressed in the same units, e.g. mg, then the units of k_d are cm^2/hr. For example, the k_d for citrus residues based on both sides of the leaf is 10,000 cm^2/hr (18). In the abstract, this could represent the equivalent amount of foliage per hour either directly contacted or otherwise disturbed during harvest from which all residue would be removed and deposited onto the harvester. In reality, neither is all the residue removed from the foliage being harvested nor is all the residue removed from the leaves deposited onto the picker. The resulting k_d will therefore be considerably less than the actual foliage involved depending upon the relative values of removal and deposition. The k_d value of 10,000 noted above is only 0.5% of the actual 2×10^6 cm^2/hr (both sides of foliage) (9) passed over by harvesting one orange tree per hour (21). If roughly 50% of the citrus foliar residue is removed during harvest (22), roughly 1% of the removed residue is deposited upon the citrus harvester. Intuitively it seems likely that deposition (if not foliar removal) is more quantitative for low, wet foliage like strawberries than for high, dry foliage like citrus.

The basis for the toxicological relationship, Equation 4, was laid nearly 30 years ago by research on both rats and humans by Grob and Harvey (4). This same relationship held true during the more recent rat dermal dose-response studies by Knaak et al, 1980 (2, 23), and in fact the enzyme coefficient (k_e) they found in the laboratory was not statistically significantly different from that found in our field harvester studies (2). The use of the value $k_e=6$ for any organophosphate seems reasonably reliable given the consistency among the LD_1/LD_{50} ratios reported by Gaines (7) with 95% confidence limits of $\pm 61\%$ (2).

The uses of Equation 4 seems relatively straight-forward for acute single exposures but it also has application to multiple exposures. A simplified application of Equation 4 to multiple doses would predict that the cumulative effect of N multiple doses would be calculated by Equation 9:

$$\text{Approximate Cumulative } \Delta AChE = 1 - (\exp(-k_e D/LD_{50}))^N \quad (9)$$

Thus for example, 5 consecutive daily doses each inhibiting 10% of the existing enzymes might produce a 40% cumulative response, sufficient to require administrative removal of the worker from further exposure (6). In point of fact, several biochemical and physiologic processes require considerable modification of Equation 9 to accurately predict cumulative responses especially for daily inhibitions less than 10%. These processes and their implications were discussed in the 1982 review (2) and include:

a)   The reversion of a fraction of the recently inhibited enzymes to their active or uninhibited state (5),

b)   The continual replacement of RBC with their associated fresh AChE, and

c)   The undefined effect of induced plasma ChE or pseudo-cholinesterase production which can have a buffering effect upon further OP responses.

Each of these will have a somewhat moderating effect on cumulative responses, contributing to the reestablishment of a biochemical equilibrium in cholinesterase activity within the blood at a

partially inhibited state determined by the daily dose, dose
frequency, and the above biochemical parameters. This equilibrium
effect was demonstrated 25 years ago by Grob and Harvey (4,2).

Historically, attempts to demonstrate cumulative affects among
harvesters or other field workers have been frought with difficulty.
For instance an analysis of data generated by a 1970 EPA survey of
822 individuals in one California county found that farm workers had
lower blood cholinesterase than similar non-field individuals, that
low blood enzyme levels were associated with symptoms of headache
and enteric disturbances, and that at least some individuals
exhibited seasonal inhibition; but no clear seasonal trend was found
for the group (24). In retrospect, this latter finding is not
unexpected given not only the variability in pesticide use patterns
both between and within crops, but even the variability within
residues of a single pesticide-crop combination (2,3).

A more focused study of two east-coast migrant harvest crews
was recently completed by Owens and Owens (25). Although their
study has not yet been published, they found substantial seasonal
cholinesterase responses over 5 months within both crews, e.g.
Figure 4. The range of crops was broad, only general pesticide use
histories and no residues within these fields could be obtained, and
certain logistic constraints in cholinesterase monitoring place some
limits on the precision of the data; but the clear trend and
substantial response make the conclusion of cumulative effects
unmistakable.

Needed Research

The dual intent for the unified field model was both to provide
relationships among past research projects as well as to illuminate
future research needs. One of these needs is exemplified by Figure
4. The example of Systox (demeton) described earlier was among the
reported pesticides to which the crews studied by Owens and Owens
were exposed. Its toxicity clearly has the potential to induce both
rapid cholinesterase inhibition from infrequent reentries soon after
application and cumulative inhibition from frequent reentries after
several half-lives. There are in fact a wide range of combinations
of residue-dosing levels and frequencies which could account for the
responses reported by these east-coast harvesters. There are no
data published on pesticide use patterns, residue decay, levels at
harvest, or migrant work patterns from this region. The lengths to
which the Owenses had to go to track a given population attest that
not only to the difficulty in obtaining large scale epidemiologic data
from a migrant work force, but also to the potential utility of the
unified field model in designing, interpreting, and extrapolating
such studies.

What is clearly needed along these lines is first more complete
residue data for those pesticides which can contribute to either
acute or chronic ChE inhibition based on toxicity and application
rates (cf. Figure 2). Second, we need more information about the
use patterns for these pesticides (lbs applied, acres treated,
number of treatments) for the crops on which they are registered in
each region if not each state. And third, representative surveys of
migrant work patterns (crops harvested, duration, sequence)
preferably including prior pesticide use histories in each field

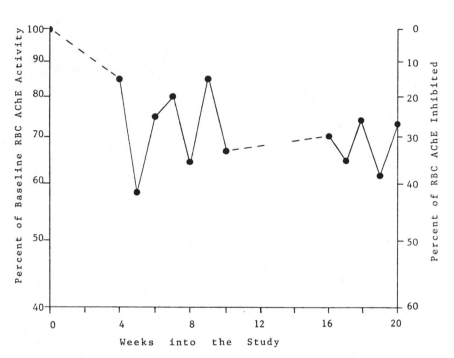

Figure 4. Unadjusted "Crew I" mean RBC AChE activity referenced to the group mean baseline (pre-exposure) activity. (Adapted from Ref. 25.)

and/or residues in each field would greatly help to establish the pattern of residue-dosing levels and frequency upon which sound reentry requirements should be based.

Coincident with the need for residue data is further knowledge about the mechanisms of pesticide decay and in particular about the variability in the residue of the parent OP and its oxon. It was described in the 1982 review how infrequent, acute, harvester poisonings can occur with little or no seasonal cumulative inhibition (2). There is currently no way to anticipate either which chemical residues can be highly variable nor to anticipate the factors or conditions causing unexpectedly high residues either in California or anywhere else. California has responded to this problem by increasing reentry intervals only in response to recurring poisonings. My current group is now working on a computer program to simulate the effect on cohort cholinesterase caused by variability in residue, residue decay, and each subsequent step in the unified field model, but that study will not tell us when we can expect such variability.

Progressing from residue decay to exposure, the research picture is only slightly better. The range of k_d (dosing coefficient) values thus far developed (Table II) does not cover a long list of crops, but those developed do present a fairly broad spectrum of harvest practices from which educated guesses can be made to many other crops. The expansion of the crop list to other crops is a less critical although useful research need, especially for some of those crops with potentially hazardous combinations of pesticide toxicity and application rate. Leffingwell and Zweig have recently completed the chemical analyses of more professional citrus residue-dose samples collected in 1982 to bolster the data base of a crop of long-standing interest.

The issues of how or whether to measure dermal dose versus urinary excretion is another important research need which also leads into the absorption submodel. The external dose measurement has two potential advantages over urinary excretion:

    a)   it can not only tell how much exposure, but also where on the body it occurs (and presumably how),

    b)   it can be used for pesticides without a measurable urinary metabolite.

The internal excretion measurement has two potential advantages over skin testing:

    a)   it reflects absorbed dose (which is especially important for non-OPs).

    b)   it integrates pesticide exposures both before, during, and after the study period (a mixed blessing).

Unresolved issues include how many samples of each are required and how can one relate dose to absorption, excretion to ΔAChE, or (of academic interest) dose to excretion. The difficulty in correlating dermal dose and excretion (2,26,27) is related in part to the differences mentioned earlier between measuring dose with pads-and-gloves and washing the skin (2,18). The correlation difficulty is most severe with the skin wash technique because it measures the dose that isn't absorbed. Depending upon the time-history of exposure and the kinetics of absorption, it should be equally expected that dermal dose by washing and urinary excretion will even

be negatively correlated. Dermal hand dose measured by gloves would
have the same zero or negative relationship unless only that dose
expected to penetrate the glove were considered (2). Dermal dose
measured by gauze pads of approximately 3x3 inches (60 cm^2) should
not significantly affect either dermal exposure or absorbed dose
because even if a dozen locations were monitored they will only
cover approximately 4% of the body; on the other hand, this 4%
coverage is an intrinsic limitation to the precision of pad
assessments if the dose were spacially nonuniform. Although the
video dermal scanning for a fluorescent surrogate powder discussed
by Fenske (28) is yet another alternative with some potential, from
a practical viewpoint, I have found at least during application
studies that the inherent variability between pads on the right and
left sides of the body was statistically insignificant compared to
the variability in exposure levels among study participants.

The issue of the accuracy of the hand measurement as suggested
by Davis et al (19) is a closely related but somewhat separate
issue. We too have found when the gloves (and hands) were wetted
with dew (as in strawberry harvest), they appeared to retain more
residue than could be washed from the hands (14). Another hand
dosing phenomenon reported 10 years ago (21) described the "...
caking of dust and debris to build up on the hands [of peach
or similar fruit harvesters] within about an hour." The proportion
of the pesticide content of this cake actually in contact with or
transferable to the skin is no doubt smaller than that which can be
washed off and possibly much smaller than that retained by the
gloves. In fact the use of absorbent gloves evolved as much from
their routine use by California citrus harvesters (21) as by earlier
example (29), and estimating actual hand dose while wearing them
required the measurement of an adjustment for glove penetration
(2,30). Appropriately designed studies could usefully explore
either (or a combination) of these dose related issues.

The steps of absorption (k_a) and response can assume either
concurrent or separate research implications. The basic unified
field model conveniently jumps over these separate steps by
assigning k_a=1 and k_e=6 to be used with human field dermal dose
measurements and rat dermal LD_{50}. Although this value is very
similar to the k_e based on rat laboratory dermal dose and LD_{50}, it
was based on a very small number of field conditions. The
justification for further research to refine or validate k_e=6 will
come in part from the previously mentioned computer simulation
project.

The use of k_e=6 is clearly applicable only to OPs and AChE as
the response variable of interest. For noncholinergic effects,
another dose-response submodel must be considered. The purpose of
k_a was to suggest the utilization of a dermal absorption coefficient
to project a measured topical dermal dose into an internal dose
which could be compared to the internal doses associated with other
dose-response studies such as chronic feeding studies. K_a values
have been derived from radioactive tracer studies (31) although
these seem to have limited application to field conditions, and do
not necessarily relate to the chemical structure of either the
absorbed moiety or the excreted urinary metabolite (2). K_a

values can also be generated from concurrent field dose and excretion measurements provided the previous methodological precautions are taken and some parallel controlled-dose versus excretion data is available (2).

Summary

It cannot be said that the "unified field model" has all the answers to the reentry problem. It was developed to address a defined and somewhat limited range of hazards relating to overexposure to cholinesterase inhibiting OP's. At this point it can be used to identify a range of residue and work practices which are likely to present acute and/or progressive reentry hazards. Although it can predict the response from a known residue or residue decay scanario, the historic voids of such data for certain regions, pesticides, and/or crops, and the current lack of a generalizable and quantifiable submodel for chronic hazards prevents its universal application.

I do not wish to imply that only the more acutely toxic OP pesticides are a reentry (or even application) hazard. To the contrary, I feel that many of these materials if used properly, have a minimal long-term health risk from noncholinergic effects. But I am concerned about the lack of a comprehensive view of pesticide use, residues, and exposure patterns (33). Beginning 15 years ago, we as a national society began a move from reliance on pesticides of low acute toxicity but with unacceptable long-term health and environmental hazards toward more labile chemicals, especially the OPs. As a rule, most of the more toxic OPs are less stable, and the more stable OPs (and non-OPs) have a longer opportunity for adverse noncholinergic health effects. Thus, not only would unwarranted and inflexible restrictions on the more toxic OPs potentially increase less detectable health risks but such restrictions would further frustrate current progress in integrated pest management. The current focus of the unified field model on toxic OPs stemmed primarily from nonfatal, temporarily disabling harvester poisonings in California. The quantitative model clearly has application there and elsewhere to inhibitions which can produce nondisabling AChE effects, and I believe the concept has application to reentry hazards from any pesticide.

Nontechnical Summary

The Unified Field Model comprises both a concept and a quantitative method for integrating the aspects of residue decay, harvester exposure, and cholinesterase (enzyme) response to organophosphate pesticide residues on foliage. Examples are provided for using this model to anticipate residues capable of causing unacceptable changes in cholinesterase activity (potentially leading to temporarily disabling health effects) and for calculating the time needed for these residues to decay to acceptable levels (the "Reentry Interval"). While this model is consistent with past and current research findings, future research is needed: (1) to expand residue decay data and knowledge of environmental effects on residue decay, (2) to estimate the potential frequency with which harvesters are exposed to recent residues, (3) to expand the range of crops for which residue:dose-rate ratios are known and to clarify some technical ambiquities in measuring hand dermal doses, and (4) to validate some methods for expanding the dermal absorption-response phases of this model to other classes of pesticides.

Literature Cited

1. Abrams, H.K.; Leonard, A.R. Calif. Med., 1950, 73, 183-186.
2. Popendorf, W.J.; Leffingwell, J.T. Residue Reviews, 1982, 82, 125-201.
3. Popendorf, W.J.; Leffingwell, J.T. J. Agr. Food Chem., 1978, 26, 437-441.
4. Grob, D.; Harvey, A.M. J. Clin. Inv., 1958, 37, 350-368.
5. Wills, J.H.; Dubois, K.P. CRC Critical Reviews in Toxicol., 1972, 1, 153-202.
6. "Safety of Employed Persons" Title 3, Chap. 4, Part 2 477, California Administrative Code, 1979.
7. Gaines, T.B. Toxicol. Applied Pharmacol., 1969, 14, 515-534.
8. Turrell, F.M. Bot. Gaz., 1961, 122, 284-298.
9. Popendorf, W.J.; Leffingwell, J.T.; McLean, H.R.; Zweig, G. "Pesticide Exposure to Strawberry Pickers, 1981 Studies" California project report to Pesticide Hazard Assessment Program, U.S. Environmental Protection Agency, 1982.
10. Keil, J.E.; Loadholt, C.B.; Brown, B.L.; Sandifer, S.H.; Sitterly, W.R. Pest. Monit. J., 1972, 6, 73-75.
11. Sheets, T.J.; Silluttamabucha, N.; Jackson, M.D.; Smith, F.D. Arch. Envir. Contam. Toxicol., 1974, 2, 75-85.
12. Nigg, H.N.; Stamper, J.H. Arch. Environ. Contam. Toxicol., 1981, 10, 497-504.
13. Iwata, Y.; Spear, R.C.; Knaak, J.B.; Foster R.J. Bull. Environ. Contam. Toxicol., 1977, 18, 649-653.
14. Zweig, G.; Gao, R.; Witt, J.M.; Popendorf, W.; Bogen, K. ACS Symposium Series, Chapter , in this book.
15. Popendorf, W.J. Amer. Ind. Hyg. Assoc. J., 1980, 41, 652-659.
16. Sutherland, G.L.; Polen, P.B.; Widmark, G. J. Assoc. Offic. Anal. Chem., 1971, 54, 1316-1317.
17. Iwata, Y. Residue Reviews, 1980, 75, 127-147.
18. Davis, J.E.; Stevens, E.R.; Staiff, D.C. Bull. Environ. Contam. Toxicol., 1983, 31, 631-638.
19. Noel, M.E.; Zweig, G.; Popendorf, W. Presentation at A.C.S. National Meeting, 1983.
20. Nigg, H.N.; Stamper, J.H.; Queen, R.M. Amer. Ind. Hyg. Assoc. J., 1984, 45, 182-186.
21. Popendorf, W.J.; Spear, R.C. Amer. Ind. Hyg. Assoc. J., 1974, 35, 374-380.
22. Spear, R.C.; Popendorf, W.J.; Spencer, W.F.; Milby, T.H. J. Occup. Med., 1977, 19, 411-414.
23. Knaak, J.B.; Schlocker, P.; Ackerman, C.R.; Seiber, J.N. Bull. Environ. Contam. Toxicol., 1980, 24, 796-804.
24. Ray, R. M.S. Thesis, University of California, Berkeley, 1974.
25. Owens, E.W.; Owens, S.Y. Science, 1984 submitted.
26. Franklin, C.A.; Fenske, R.A.; Greenhalgh, R.; Mathieu, L.; Denley, H.U.; Leffingwell, J.T.; Spear, R.C. J. Toxicol. Environ. Health, 1981, 7, 715-732.
27. Lavy, T.L.; Shepard, J.S.; Mattice, J.D. J. Agric. Food Chem., 1980, 28, 626-630.

28. Fenske, R.; Leffingwell, J.T.; Spear, R.C. ACS Symposium
     Series, Chapter   , in this book.
29. Quinby, G.E.; Walker, K.C.; Durham, W.F. J. Econ. Entom.,
     1958, 51, 831.
30. Popendorf, W.J. Ph.D. Thesis, University of California,
     Berkeley, 1976.
31. Maibach, H.I.; Feldman, R.J.; Milby, T.H.; Serat, W.F. Arch.
     Environ. Health, 1971, 23, 208-218.
32. Popendorf, W.J.; Pryor, A.; Wenk, H.R. Ann. Ann. Amer. Conf.
     Gov. Ind. Hyg., 1982, 2, 101-115.
33. Guest Editorial "Solomon's Baby and the Farmer" Am. Ind.
     Hyg. Assoc. J., 1980, 41, A-4.

RECEIVED December 3, 1984

Data-Base Proposal for Use in Predicting Mixer-Loader–Applicator Exposure

DAVID R. HACKATHORN and DELMONT C. EBERHART

Corporate Industrial Hygiene, Environmental Health Research Department, Mobay Chemical Corporation, Stilwell, KS 66085

Data obtained through a search of the published literature on mixer/loader and applicator exposure studies
were evaluated and summarized by application technique
and chemical class. As a result of this work, it was
clear that the data in the open literature as they currently exist are insufficient to produce a data base
capable of predicting exposure for risk assessment purposes. However, it was encouraging that where acceptable data of sufficient volume were available the
correlations were quite good.
This review of the literature revealed that incomplete reporting of data was a bigger factor in making
data incomparable than was sampling technique. Differences in exposure evaluation technique were less important for comparing data than the way in which the
exposures were reported. In response to this problem, a
reporting format for field exposure data is proposed
which would allow the development of a generic field
exposure data base. If existing unpublished data were
made available on a generic basis then the resulting
data base could be used to develop exposure models for
risk assessment.

Worker exposure data is a major component of risk assessment
for the use of agricultural chemicals. It has become a routine part
of the product review and registration process for new chemicals.
Of special interest recently is the exposure to workers who mix,
load and apply pesticides in the field. These work tasks are done
by one, two or sometimes even three persons in a work crew. There
have been numerous studies conducted and reported in the literature
which characterize the exposure of this group under various application conditions. It is this body of data which we have reviewed as
a possible data base.

There are two purposes for the work presented here: first, to
report on the suitability of the data available in the literature
for predicting mixer-loader/applicator exposure; and secondly, to
propose a plan to accomplish development of a predictive model for
this exposure group. The idea of assembling a data base using existing data is not new but, in fact, has been discussed for many
years. The principle has also been used on a limited basis by the
Environmental Protection Agency and the California Department of
Food and Agriculture. However, no systematic review of the literature or definition of criteria for a data base could be found.
Therefore, an in-house study to investigate these needs was begun.

Before we can talk about a data base, we should first identify
what data we are talking about. For this purpose we have defined
the worker exposure value as the amount of compound available for
inhalation, dermal absorption or ingestion in the work environment
under consideration. Various measurement techniques including sampling the air in the breathing zone of the worker, recovering pesticide contamination from the skin, or collecting the pesticide
impacting on a patch used to simulate skin contact have been used to
estimate mixer/loader-applicator exposure. All of these methods
attempt to measure the amount of chemical available for inhalation
or dermal absorption in the immediate environment of the worker.
These exposure estimates are not sufficient of themselves to define
the amount of chemical inhaled, absorbed or ingested by the worker.
The dose received by the worker is also dependent on intake and
absorption factors such as breathing rate and dermal absorption
rate. All of these factors must be considered for comparison of the
estimated dose to the toxicity data in a risk assessment. Although
these factors are often chemical specific, the exposure value, as we
have defined it, is not. We are therefore limiting our proposal to
include only worker exposure values which are free of chemical
specific biases.

Recently some emphasis has been placed on obtaining exposure
data on each individual compound under consideration. These studies
can be costly in both time and money. In some cases they are not
even a major factor in the judgement of risk simply because the toxicity and/or dermal absorption values are very low. In other cases
the uncertainty of using exposure estimates from small sample groups
compromises the risk assessment. Addressing these problems requires
some form of data management.

So we began by looking at the possibility of developing a
generic exposure data base for at least the limited group,
mixer-loader/applicators. This group was a good candidate because
the exposure values as defined above are primarily dependent on the
physical parameters involved in the application process such as:

> Application Technique
> Application Rate
> Type of Crop
> Formulation Type
> Class of Compound
> Climatic Conditions
> Protective Equipment
> Work Practices

In fact, in order for the generic data base to be a viable approach, the following assumptions must be accepted.

1. For most pesticides the distribution of compound in the work environment is defined by the physical application parameters rather than the chemical properties.

2. The major factor affecting exposure during application is the physical distribution of the compound in the work environment.

3. The major factors affecting exposure during mixing and loading are the formulation type, packaging type and mixing equipment.

While these assumptions appear to be valid from our knowledge of exposure data, the actual proof can only be accomplished by compilation and review of a data base which identifies these parameters for each study.

Our first task was to conduct a thorough search of the published literature for mixer-loader/applicator studies. Each study was then reviewed critically for content and documentation of exposure parameters. Those studies found to be acceptable were catalogued for use in the data base, and those studies found to be inadequate were listed with the reasons for rejection. A short form summarizing the data was then completed for each accepted study, and the data was segregated according to application technique, rate and compound class. Data summaries were then prepared for these groups. Further segregation of data was not possible due to the small number of acceptable studies and inconsistent reporting formats which limit the comparability of data between studies.

Of the 82 mixer-loader/applicator studies found in the literature, only 41 were determined to be acceptable. Some studies reported on more than one application technique and some application techniques were studied with several compound classes at more than one application rate. There were 12 exposure groups compared by application technique, application rate and compound class (See Table I). Some groups, such as airblast spraying, contain more data than others. Tables II, III, IV and V are examples of the type of summaries that can be prepared from data in the literature.

The major advantage to grouping the data and combining studies is in the vastly increased number of samples used to characterize the exposure range. In the case of airblast spraying (Tables II, III and IV) insufficient detail was available on individual samples to establish a group mean. Therefore, the range of means was used as a conservative representation of the data. Even so, this approach produces a more dependable estimate of exposure distribution because of the large number of samples and exposure situations than can be obtained from a single study no matter how well the study is done.

The value of the data base model would be further improved if the data were reported uniformly and in sufficient detail that a group mean could be calculated from all the data points. The aerial application data in Table V shows a mean calculated from all the data points. The geometric mean and standard deviation are used

Table I. Applicator Exposure Subgroups

Application Type	Compound Class	Rate	No. of Dermal Samples
Airblast Spraying	Organophosphates	0.5–3 lb AI/acre	131
	Organophosphates	3–4 lb AI/acre	90
	Chlorinated Insecticides	1–3 lb AI/acre	85
	Chlorinated Hydrocarbon Insecticides	4–8 lb AI/acre	40
	Fungicides	2 lb AI/acre	30
Ground–Rig Boom	Organophosphates	0.5–3 lb AI/acre	28
	Herbicides	1–1.3 lb AI/acre	26
Power Hand Gun	Organophosphates	0.25–.67 lb AI/100 gal	36
	Chlorinated Hydrocarbon Insecticides	0.13–.42 lb AI/100 gal	29
Backpack Sprayer	Organophosphates	0.1–0.4% Spray	16
Aerial Application	Organophosphates	0.6–1.5 lb AI/acre	18
	Phenoxy Herbicides	2 lb AI/acre	9

Table II. Applicator Exposure During Airblast Spraying of Organophosphates in Orchards
Application Rate: 0.5–3 lb AI/acre

| Airborne Exposure (mg/hr)[a] | | | Dermal Exposure (mg/hr)[b] | | | Ref. |
Mean[c]	# Samples	Range	Mean[c]	# Samples	Range	Number
0.26(±.34)	20	0.07–1.60	12.5(±18.9)	20	1.1–69.7	(1)
0.08(–)	4	0.03–0.13	2.5(–)	4	1.5–4.9	(2)
0.03(–)	10	0.01–0.05	2.4(–)	10	0.7–5.8	(2)
0.03(–)	8	0.01–0.07	18(–)	4	1.3–38	(3)
0.02(–)	12	–	19.4(–)	63	–	(4)
0.06(–)	25	–	27.9(–)	30	–	(4)
0.02–0.26	79	0.01–1.60	2.4–27.9	131	0.7–69.7	

a Respiratory exposure determined from respirator pads
b Dermal exposure calculated according to Durham and Wolfe (1962) (5)
c Arithmetic mean and standard deviation

Table III. Applicator Exposure During Airblast Spraying of Chlorinated Hydrocarbon Insecticides in Orchards Application Rate: 1-3 lb AI/acre

| Airborne Exposure (mg/hr)[a] | | | Dermal Exposure (mg/hr)[b] | | | Ref. |
Range	Mean[c]	# Samples	Range	Mean[c]	# Samples	Number
0.02-0.04	0.01(-)	2	6.3-31.1	15.5(-)	4	(3)
0.001-0.02	0.01(-)	12	1.3-6.1	2.5(-)	7	(3)
0.03-0.07	0.05(-)	8	0.4-150.6	30.5(-)	10	(6)
0.01-0.05	0.02(-)	15	0.6-95.3	24.7(-)	17	(6)
0.01-0.17	0.07(-)	5	2.0-149.9	36.4(-)	12	(6)
-	0.01(±.002)	34	-	7.7(-)	35	(7)
0.001-0.17	0.01-0.07	76	0.4-150.6	2.5-36.4	85	

a Respiratory exposure determined from respirator pads (except #7 in which personal air samplers were used)
b Dermal exposure calculated according to Durham and Wolfe (1962) (5)
c Arithmetic mean and standard deviation

Table IV. Applicator Exposure During Airblast Spraying of Organophosphates in Orchards
Application Rate: 3-4 lb AI/acre

Airborne Exposure (mg/hr)[a]			Dermal Exposure (mg/hr)[b]			Ref.
Range	Mean[c]	# Samples	Range	Mean[c]	# Samples	Number
0.02-0.08	0.04(-)	8	1.1-146	27(-)	21	(3)
0.02-0.24	0.11(-)	7	5.9-59	30(-)	4	(3)
0.02-0.29	0.11(-)	5	9.6-87.1	41.3(-)	4	(6)
0.01-0.08	0.06(-)	15	0.3-157.5	23.4(-)	20	(6)
0.01-0.14	0.04(-)	14	0.6-250.1	44.2(-)	20	(6)
0.003-0.009	0.005(±0.002)	18	1.8-136.8	35.7(±49.5)	21	(8)
0.003-0.29	0.005-0.11	67	0.3-250.1	23.4-44.2	90	

a Respiratory exposure determined from respirator pads
b Dermal exposure calculated according to Durham and Wolfe (1962) (5)
c Arithmetic mean and standard deviation

Table V. Exposure During Aerial Application of Organophosphates, 1978–Present
Application Rate: 0.6–1.5 lb AI/acre

	Airborne Exposure (mg/hr)[a]			Dermal Exposure (mg/hr)[b]			Ref.
	Range	Mean[c]	# Samples	Range	Mean[c]	# Samples	Number
Pilots							
	0.001–0.002	0.001(±24%)	5	0.06–0.64	0.19(±152%)	5	(9)
	0.007–0.199	0.040(±233%)	11	0.24–2.30	0.88(±82%)	11	(10)
	0.007–0.009	0.008(±19%)	2	0.53–1.22	0.80(±80%)	2	(11)
	0.001–0.199	0.015(±530%)	18	0.06–2.30	0.57(±162%)	18	---
Mixer/Loaders							
	0.001–0.002	0.002(±36%)	3	0.10–1.84	0.43(±321%)	3	(9)
	0.013–0.214	0.068(±116%)	9	0.31–2.82	1.12(±83%)	10	(10)
	0.001–0.214	0.028(±483%)	12	0.10–2.82	0.90(±144%)	13	---

Flaggers

0.002–1.44	0.057(±2830%)	3	3.8–28.1	9.7(±173%)	3	(9)
0.023–1.35	0.090(±243%)	11	0.18–3.34	0.92(±118%)	11	(10)
0.03–0.07[d]	0.048(±35%)	6	3.09–26.65	7.63(±106%)	6	(11)
0.002–1.44	0.069(±328%)	20	0.18–28.1	2.47(±286%)	20	

[a] Respiratory exposures based on 1.25–1.5 m^3/hr Respiratory Volume
[b] Dermal exposure calculated for head, neck and hands only
[c] Geometric mean and standard deviation
[d] Work also included mixing and loading

because they are believed to best represent the distribution of exposure data (12). As in any statistical evaluation, an increased number of data points will provide a sample mean and standard deviation
that more accurately approaches the true mean and standard deviation
of the population. Thus, compiling the data from several studies
will reduce the uncertainty associated with small data sets and consequently provide a better definition of the expected exposure for
risk assessments.

Another point which can be made from the example summaries
shown here is the indication of comparability of exposures to application rates. In Table II, for example, the range of dermal exposures for Organophosphates applied at .5 - 3 lbs AI/acre is quite
similar to the range of dermal exposures for Chlorinated Hydrocarbon
Insecticides applied at 1 - 3 lb AI/acre shown in Table III. And
the general relationship is further indicated by the proportional
increase in the range of dermal exposures noted for Organophosphates
applied at 3 - 4 lb AI/acre shown in Table IV. These examples, however, only serve to encourage us to believe in the viability of a
data base for mixer-loader/applicator exposures if more data were
available that could be compared on an equal basis.

Unfortunately, however, we must conclude that the field exposure data in the open literature, as they currently exist, are insufficient to produce a data base capable of accurately predicting
exposure distributions for risk assessment purposes. The main reasons for this conclusion are that only 50% of the studies available
are documented sufficiently to use, and of those adequately documented, the reporting formats are often incomparable. The encouraging note, of course, is that where the exposure data were
comparable, the correlation between studies was very good. It is,
however, the overall lack of studies which makes the data in the
literature inadequate for risk assessment.

There are many more exposure studies done in private industry
and by government agencies than the number available in the published literature. It is the data in these studies which offers the
best hope for constructing a viable data base for predicting
mixer-loader/applicator exposures. The benefits are clear in cost
and time savings. There is a limit in any society to the amount of
resources that can be spent on risk assessment. It would be far
better to jointly apply those resources to areas where data is inadequate or where the data will provide more usable information for
risk assessment. Mixer-loader/applicator data offers a special
opportunity to test this premise because it can be reported and used
on a generic basis which would improve the quality of risk assessments while at the same time minimize the potential loss of
proprietary information and cost to companies.

We are, therefore, proposing that a generic field exposure data
base be developed using all of the data available which meets the
scientific criteria for adequacy whether it be from the literature,
the government, government contracts, universities or private industry. However, in order to accomplish this, two primary needs must
be met.

1) Internal data from studies conducted by individual companies
    must be made available on a generic basis.

2) A uniform reporting system must be adopted to allow all data to
    be evaluated, entered and compared on an equal basis.

In order to meet the second requirement we are proposing that
exposure data be reported on forms such as those shown in Examples 1
and 2.   From our experience in reviewing the literature, it is
clear that the data must be reported in a format similar to this in
order to achieve comparability.

The proposal is being supported and pushed forward by the Field
Exposure Assessment Subcommittee of the Toxicology Committee of the
National Agricultural Chemicals Association. The subcommittee is
working through the member companies to get cooperation and agreement on a way to implement the data base. There is still a long way
to go to resolve all of the potential problems, although the benefits from better use of resources and improved risk assessments
would appear to be worth the cost.

There is one additional point we would like to make which shows
one of the potential benefits of the data base from a regulatory
viewpoint. Certainly one of the main reasons field exposure studies
are carried out whether they provide new information or not is to
meet a registration requirement. The objective is to provide adequate information for a risk assessment, and as we pointed out, this
could be accomplished in many instances through a data base if it
were available. But to carry that one step further the data base
could be used as a preliminary screen to determine when a field exposure study would be needed on a specific chemical. The concept is
outlined in Table VI and it is suggested as a logical alternative
to case-by-case negotiation.

Page_____
Reference#_____

APPLICATOR EXPOSURE SURVEY FORM

COMPOUND IDENTIFICATION: SURVEY INFORMATION:
Class_____   Survey Date_____
Action_____   Location_____
Formulation_____   Temperature_____ RH_____
Packaging_____   Wind Speed/Direction_____
                                            Time of Day_____

APPLICATION INFORMATION:
Application Technique_____
Rate(lb AI/acre)_____ Total lb AI Applied_____
Final Mix Concentration (lb AI/gal Carrier)_____ Tank Capacity_____
Number Tank Applications Monitored_____ Average Time/Tank Application_____
Crop_____ Total Acreage Applied_____
Vehicle Make and Model_____
Open Cab_____ Closed Cab/Window Open_____
Closed Cab/Window Closed_____ Closed Cab/Window Closed/Filtered Air_____
Ground Speed (mph)_____
Describe Spray Equipment_____
_____

Number of Nozzles (or Shanks)_____ Disc #_____
Nozzle Pressure (psi)_____ Pump Speed (rpm)_____

Describe Application Procedure:_____
_____

Describe Personal Protective Equipment And Other Clothing Worn During Application:
_____
_____

AIRBORNE EXPOSURE DATA:
TWA (mg/m^3)_____ mg/lb AI (Applied)_____
Sample Volume_____ Sample Time (hr)_____
Type of Sample_____ mg/hr_____

                                            mg/lb
DERMAL EXPOSURE DATA: AI applied   mg/hr
a. Outside Protective Clothing (Excluding Hands) _____ _____
b. Inside Protective Clothing (Excluding Hands) _____ _____
c. Exposed Areas (Excluding Hands)   _____ _____
d. Hand Exposure   _____ _____
e. Total Dermal Exposure (b + c + d)   _____ _____
f. Sample Time (hr)_____
g. Sampling Technique_____

Did Work Involve Potential Exposure Situations Other Than Application?_____
If Yes, Explain (Type of Work, Amount of Time, Spills, Splashes, etc.)_____
_____

Example 1.

Page_____
Reference#_____

MIXER/LOADER EXPOSURE SURVEY FORM

COMPOUND IDENTIFICATION: SURVEY INFORMATION:
Class_____   Survey Date_____
Action_____   Location_____
Formulation_____   Temperature_____ RH_____
Packaging_____   Wind Speed/Direction_____
                                            Time of Day_____

MIXING/LOADING INFORMATION:
Mixing Capabilities: Open_____ or Closed_____
Describe Mixing Procedure and Equipment:_____
_____

Final Mix Concentration: (lb AI/gal Carrier)_____ Type of Carrier_____
Other Tank Additives:_____
Number of Tank Mixes Monitored_____
Average Time/Tank Mix_____
Total lb AI Mixed_____ Tank Capacity (gal)_____
Application Rate: (lb AI/acre)_____ Total Acreage Applied_____

Describe Personal Protective Equipment And Other Clothing Worn During M/L:_____
_____

AIRBORNE EXPOSURE DATA:
TWA (mg/m^3)_____ mg/lb AI (Mixed)_____
Sample Volume_____ Sample Time (hr)_____
Type of Sample_____ mg/hr_____

	mg/lb AI mixed	mg/hr
DERMAL EXPOSURE DATA:		
a. Outside Protective Clothing (excluding hands)		
b. Inside Protective Clothing (excluding hands)		
c. Exposed Areas (excluding hands)		
d. Hand Exposure		
e. Total Dermal Exposure (b + c + d)		

f. Sample Time (hr)_____
g. Sampling Technique_____

Did Work Involve Potential Exposure Situations Other Than Mixing and Loading?____
If Yes, Explain (Type of Work, Amount of Time, Spills, Splashes, etc.)_____
_____

Example 2.

Table VI. Preliminary Evaluation of Exposure Contribution to a
Risk Assessment

Mean Exposure Level $>$ $\dfrac{\text{Lowest NOEL}}{X}$

Field Exposure Testing
of Compound with
Specific Exposure
Control Measures

$\dfrac{\text{Lowest NOEL}}{10X} <$ Mean Exposure Level $\leq \dfrac{\text{Lowest NOEL}}{X}$

Additional Testing
Dependent on Type of
Effect and Margin of
Safety Required

Mean Exposure Level $<$ $\dfrac{\text{Lowest NOEL}}{10X}$

No Additional Field
Exposure Testing
Needed

NOEL = No Effect Level
X = Uncertainty Factor

Literature Cited

1. Jegier, Z. Exposure to GUTHION During Spraying and Formulating. Arch. Environ. Health 1964, 8, 565-69.
2. Jegier, Z. Health Hazards in Insecticide Spraying of Crops. Arch. Environ. Health 1964, 8, 670-74.
3. Wolfe, H. R.; Durham, W. J; Armstrong, J. F. Exposure of Workers to Pesticides. Arch. Environ. Health 1967, 14, 622-33.
4. Wolfe, H. R.; Armstrong, J. F.; Durham, W. F. Pesticide Exposure from Concentrate Spraying. Arch. Environ. Health 1966, 13, 340.
5. Durham, W. F.; Wolfe, H. R. Measurement of the Exposure of Workers to Pesticides. Bull Wld. Hlth. Org. 1962, 26, 75-91.
6. Wolfe, H. R.; Armstrong, J. F.; Staiff, D. C.; Comer, S. W. Exposure of Spraymen to Pesticides. Arch. Environ. Health 1972, 25, 29-31.
7. Nigg, H. N.; Stamper, J. H. Exposure of Spray Applicators and Mixer Loaders to Chlorobenzilate miticide in Florida Citrus. Arch. Environ. Contam. Toxicol. 1983, 12, 477-482.
8. Wojeck, G. A.; Nigg, H. N.; Stamper, J. G.; Bradway, D. E. Worker Exposure to Ethion in Florida Citrus. Arch. Environ. Contam. Toxicol. 1981, 10, 725-35.
9. Attallah, Y. H.; Cahill, W. P.; Whitacre, D. M. Exposure of Pesticide Applicators and Support Personnel to O-ethyl O-(4-nitrophenyl) phenylphosphonothioate (EPN). Arch. Environ. Contam. Toxicol. 1982, 11, 219-25.
10. Peoples, S. A.; Maddy, K.; Datta, P. R.; Johnston, L.; Smith, C.; Conrad, D.; Cooper, C. Monitoring of Potential Exposures of Mixer-Loaders, Pilots, and Flaggers During Application of tributyl phosphorotrithioate (DEF) and tributyl phosphorotrithioite (FOLEX) to Cotton Fields in the San Joaquin Valley of California in 1979. California Department of Food and Agriculture, 1981.
11. Lotti, et al. Occupation Exposure to the Cotton Defoliant DEF and Merphos. J. of Occupational Med. 1983, 25, 517-22.
12. "Exposure Measurement Action Level and Occupational Environmental Variability," HEW Publication No. (NIOSH) 76-131, December, 1975.

RECEIVED August 28, 1984

Dermal Exposure to Pesticides

The Environmental Protection Agency's Viewpoint

JOSEPH C. REINERT and DAVID J. SEVERN

Office of Pesticide Programs, Hazard Evaluation Division, TS-769C, Exposure Assessment Branch, Environmental Protection Agency, Washington, DC 20460

An organizational overview of the risk assessment process in the EPA's Office of Pesticide Programs (OPP) is presented. A review of many field studies of agricultural worker exposure during pesticide application indicates that typically the principal route of exposure is through the skin. Procedures in OPP for estimating dermal exposure from "surrogate" studies are described. A predictive correlation derived for estimating exposure during airblast application to orchards is presented, as are the results of new studies designed to monitor exposure during pesticide application to row crops using ground boom equipment. Methods for estimating dermal absorption and areas where more research is needed are discussed.

Under the aegis of the Federal Insecticide, Fungicide and Rodenticide Act (FIFRA), the Office of Pesticide Programs (OPP) of the Environmental Protection Agency (EPA) registers chemicals for use as pesticides provided that, among other criteria, "when used in accordance with widespread and commonly recognized practice, [they] will not generally cause unreasonable adverse effects on the environment." Protection of agricultural workers involved in the application of pesticides is considered under the umbrella of this risk criterion, and the estimation of human exposure is an integral part of OPP's risk assessment procedures. An organizational overview of this risk assessment process is shown in Figure 1.

Physical scientists in the Exposure Assessment Branch (EAB) of the Hazard Evaluation Division (HED) have the responsibility of estimating actual worker exposure, which is the principal topic of this talk. Agricultural scientists in the Science Support Branch (SSB) of OPP's Benefits and Use Division (BUD) supply pertinent use information along with estimates of the frequency and duration of each application activity for which an exposure assessment is prepared. This frequency and duration information is critical to estimate annualized exposure, used for chronic risk assessments, most frequently oncogenic assessments. The estimated exposure for the required time interval (daily or annually depending on whether the assessment is for an acute or chronic toxicological concern) is given to HED's Toxicology Branch (TB) where it is considered

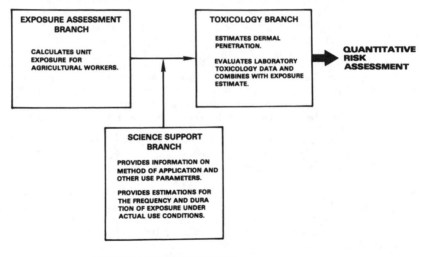

Figure 1. Organizational Overview of the Risk Assessment
Process in the Office of Pesticide Programs.

along with the results of the laboratory effects studies to produce
a quantitative risk assessment. This risk assessment is considered
in the risk/benefit analysis required for regulatory decisions
under FIFRA.

Risk assessments are undertaken when significant adverse
effects are found in laboratory animal studies. Traditionally most
risk assessments have been done for pesticides under RPAR or Rebuttable Presumption Against Registration, now referred to as Special
Review. More recently quantitative risk assessments have been
carried out for pesticides in the Registration Standard or reregis-
tration process or under regular registration review as well.

EAB has reviewed many field studies of pesticide applicator
exposure, and the dermal route is typically the route of highest
potential exposure. For many agricultural work activities, most
of the potential dermal exposure occurs to the hands. In some
instances, field studies have been carried out to assess exposure
for a particular pesticide/application method/crop combination for
which an exposure assessment is required. This primary study is
evaluated, and if judged scientifically acceptable, would be used
directly in the exposure assessment. While it would be highly
desirable to have the results of such a scientifically valid, statistically designed field exposure monitoring study for each assessment we are requested to perform, this is typically not the case.
We therefore rely on available studies for other chemicals, so
called "surrogate studies."

The policy for use of surrogate studies has been published
in the Federal Register (June 25, 1980), and the philosophy and
mechanics of the use of surrogate data have been discussed in
various public fora (1,2).

Considerations involved in choosing whether a study is appropriate to use as a surrogate to estimate exposure are delineated
below:

FACTORS IN CHOOSING APPROPRIATE SURROGATE
STUDIES FOR EXPOSURE ASSESSMENTS

1. Similar Method of Application
2. Similar Use Pattern
3. Similar Type of Formulation (for mixer-loaders)
4. Study Evaluated by EAB
5. Study is Non-proprietary
6. Exposure Measured During Each Separate Application Activity
7. Similar Protective Methods

The key factor is the method of application. Other factors include similarity in use pattern and type of formulation (emulsifiable concentrate, wettable powder, etc.) for mixer-loaders.

In addition, studies used as surrogates must be reviewed and
validated internally, and the studies must be non-proprietary. One
important factor that frequently causes difficulties is that an
otherwise sound exposure study did not separately monitor exposure

during different activities. Even if in actual practice an individual would do both the mixing-loading as well as the application,
it is important to know the proportion of exposure associated with
each activity. A regulatory option such as wearing a face shield,
e.g., might be practical for the relatively short period of time
required for mixing-loading, but might not be acceptable for the
long hours of application in some situations. Also, the magnitude
of potential exposure may be considerably different for each separate activity. In order to properly evaluate exposure reduction
options, the potential exposure in each activity must be calculable.
     In estimating exposure for a pesticide application from a
surrogate study, it has been our experience that the proper (and
logical) conversion factors are amounts of pesticide applied for
applicators and the quantity of chemical handled by mixerloaders.
Unfortunately, these data are not always readily retrievable from
exposure monitoring reports due to the format used for reporting
the data or the insufficiency of experimental details. In such
instances, other factors (e.g., tank concentration for applicators
or time involved in mixing-loading) must be used.
     For certain application methods, OPP does have a considerable
data base. Extensive data exist for monitoring exposure to applicators involved in orchard spraying using airblast equipment. We (3)
have reviewed the available data, discarded studies where exposure
during mixing-loading could not be segregated from exposure during
application, and in an extension of the work of Davis (4), attempted
to examine the exposure to applicators in order to derive statistically valid and useful predictive correlations. A statistically-
significant correlation was found between application rate and
dermal exposure. A Spearman Rank correlation analysis (a test to
determine if an increase in exposure is associated with an increase
in application rate) indicated a statistically significant correlation. Such a significant correlation was not found for another
application parameter, tank concentration. A linear regression
analysis of dermal exposure and application rate also indicated a
significant correlation as is shown in Figure 2. The actual data
points shown are the mean values observed in each study and are
unweighted for the number of replicates in that study. Weighted
values were properly used to generate the regression line and the
95% confidence limits shown with dotted lines. These dermal exposure values assume 3,000 cm^2 of exposed skin, corresponding to
an applicator wearing long pants, a short-sleeved open-necked shirt
and no gloves or facial protection (5). The correlation is quite
remarkable (r=0.7) when you consider that all other application,
climatic, and equipment factors are contained under this umbrella
of uncertainty.
     While we do not presume to understand all the various factors
which contribute to determining dermal exposure during airblast
application, we can with a certain confidence estimate a predicted
value along with an associated range of expected values for this
application technique. While we possess an extensive data base
of laboratory animal studies for oncogenicity (and other acute
and chronic health effects), the bottom line of an overall risk
assessment requires a combination of toxicology data, exposure

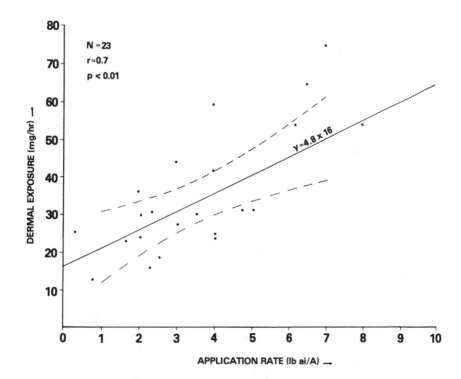

Figure 2. Correlation of Dermal Exposure and Application Rate for Orchard Spraying Using Airblast Equipment. The data points shown are the mean values from the studies. The regression line and 95% confidence limits (dotted lines) were generated using means weighted for the number of replicates in each study. Exposure is normalized for 3,000 cm^2 of exposed skin area.

data, and a procedure for linking the two, i.e. low dose
extrapolation models for quantifying oncogenic risk. Until the
state of the art in this extrapolation procedure becomes more
precise, the present level of sophistication in predicting exposure
for airblast application may be acceptable.

Another method of application for which a great deal of data
is available is ground boom application to row crops. The results
of a series of studies using various pesticides carried out by the
Agency at numerous sites around the country are summarized in Table I.

Table I.   DERMAL EXPOSURE TO APPLICATORS FOR GROUND BOOM
           APPLICATION TO ROW CROPS

	Number of Observations	Mean Level (mg/hr)	Range of Values(mg/hr)
Total dermal exposure	15	24.4	1.0-130
Exposure to hands	15	18.3	0.96-69

These results are contained in a draft report (6) which is
currently undergoing peer review. The final report should be
available by the end of this calendar year. As can been seen,
most of the dermal exposure is to the hands. The reason for this
is uncertain, but very likely results from the applicators hand
contact with the equipment during spraying. Average total exposure
is 18.5 mg/hr. These data were collected under a variety of use
and climatic conditions. Applicator exposure to herbicides, insecticides and fungicides was monitored under actual field conditions
during application to a variety of crops with various types of boom
rigs. Application rates ranged from 0.23 to 3.2 lbs ai/A.

In this same series of ground boom studies, exposure to mixer-
loaders was also measured for two types of formulations. The
liquid formulations ranged in concentration from 0.95 to 5.6 lbs.
active ingredient per gallon, and the wettable powders studied were
either 50 or 80% active ingredient by weight. The results are
summarized in Table II.

Much greater exposure is observed for liquid formulation than
for the wettable powders. The range of exposure observed is very
large for both types of formulations, making the usefulness of a
mean value marginal. This large range is expected since the
individuals are handling the concentrated material, and a small
difference in care can lead to a great difference in exposure. Most
of the potential dermal exposure is to the hands (there was dermal
exposure to areas other than the hands for the liquid formulations,
but this small exposure does not appear when the results are rounded
off to two significant figures).

The data for ground boom applicators and mixer-loaders were
manipulated in various ways in attempts to determine whether useful
predictive correlations of exposure with use parameters can be
found. Some apparently strong, statistically valid correlations
were found. However, even though certain correlations were signif-

Table II.   DERMAL EXPOSURE TO MIXER-LOADERS FOR TWO
             TYPES OF FORMULATIONS

Type of Formulation	Number of Observations	Mean Level (mg/hr)	Range of Values (mg/hr)
WETTABLE POWDER			
Total dermal exposure	11	510	39 - 3,000
Hand exposure	11	500	36 - 3,000
LIQUID FORMULATION			
Total dermal exposure	6	7,800	27 - 32,000
Hand exposure	6	7,800	26 - 32,000

icant, we believe their meaning and usefulness is tenuous. The reason for this is illustrated in the example shown in Figure 3. This graph shows the results of a linear regression analysis of forearm versus hand exposure for all mixer-loaders. This correlation was attempted in hopes of finding a better method for determining hand exposure, which, as discussed in this symposium, is particularly troublesome experimentally. The relationship is apparently significant at the 0.01 level ($r = 0.82$). However, if one data point (point a) is removed from the data set, there is no significant correlation ($r = 0.18$). Because of the small sample size used in all regression analyses, all apparently strong correlations observed were likewise dominated by a single data point. This was not the case for the airblast correlation where the data set was much larger, and removal of any single point did not have a dramatic effect on the correlation. We therefore feel at the present time that it is more appropriate to report just the mean and the range for ground boom applicator exposure, rather than use a derived predictive correlation.

For many other application scenarios, such as backpack spraying and aerial application of oil-based ultra low volume formulations, extensive exposure monitoring studies are unavailable. In such cases, we frequently must rely on a small number of published studies as surrogates. EAB maintains and periodically updates an exposure bibliography that contains all non-proprietary exposure studies of which we are aware. A present goal is to identify and computerize all studies which contain direct exposure data. This project requires a great deal of quality control. The scientific acceptability of the studies which are used in creating the data base must be determined by consistent standards which have been agreed to by all users of the data base. From this data base we

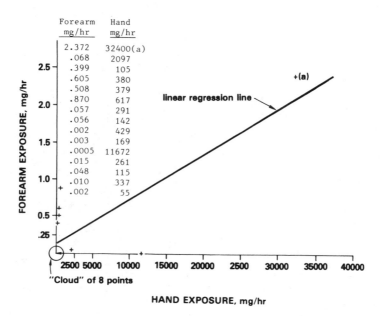

Figure 3. Correlation of Forearm and Hand Exposure for Mixer-Loaders.

could call up all data available for, as an example, aerial application of herbicides. Such an automated system would have
obvious benefits. Some exposure studies which meet the criteria
above and which have been used by EAB are shown below:

GROUND RIG DRIVER   MIXER/LOADER
                                                WP

Wolfe et al, 1967 (7)
Staiff et al, 1975 (8)   Jegier, 1964 (11)
Attallah et al, 1982 (9)   Everhart and Holt, 1982 (19)
Dubelman et al, 1982 (10)
                                                EC

AERIAL
                                           Peoples et al, 1981 (13)
Jegier, 1964 (11)   Attallah et al, 1982 (9)
Lavy et al, 1980 (12)   Dubelman et al, 1982 (10)
Peoples et al, 1981 (13)
Attallah et al, 1982 (9)   DUST

                                           Wolfe and Durham, 1967 (20)

HAND SPRAYING

Wolfe et al, 1967 (7)
Wolfe et al, 1974 (14)
Maddy et al, 1979 (15)
Lavy et al, 1980 (12)

INDOOR HOUSE   SEED TREATMENT

Wolfe et al, 1959 (16)   Stevens and Davis, 1980 (21)
Fletcher et al, 1959 (17)
Haag and Pruggmayer, 1981 (18)

     This list is not intended to be all-inclusive: other scien-
tifically valid studies are available.
     The agency is in the process of writing guidelines for con-
ducting field monitoring studies for agricultural worker exposure.
These guidelines will aid pesticide registrants and others in conducting acceptable field studies. Two issues which will require
extensive discussion and policy resolution are likely to be the
number of replicates and/or number of sites required and the
"when required" section of the guidelines. This latter area will
likely be based on both toxicological factors and a consideration
of the adequacy of the surrogate exposure data base.
     In conclusion, the use of surrogate data for exposure assess-
ments will most certainly continue. The resources required to carry
out field studies for every crop/application method/ pesticide
combination would be overwhelming. EAB's goal is to derive reliable
and useful correlations which will obviate the need for requiring
such extensive studies.
     The preceeding discussion estimates the amount of pesticide
impinging on the skin surface. Estimating actual dose from patch

data requires an estimation of dermal penetration. While formally
a responsibility of TB, HED, I will summarize the procedures
employed to estimate the fraction of pesticide reaching the skin
surface which will actually enter the biological system. These
procedures are as follows:

PROCEDURES FOR ESTIMATING
DERMAL PENETRATION

1.   Assume 100% Dermal Penetration
2.   Compare Biological Endpoints by Oral and Dermal Routes
3.   Estimate on the Basis of Physicochemical Properties
4.   Require Study to Assess Dermal Penetration

Obviously if one assumes that 100% of the pesticide reaching
the surface of the skin penetrates into the body, and there is an
adequate margin of safety or the potential chronic risks are
acceptable, no further machinations are necessary. One can also
compare, when data are available (22), biological effects (usually
LD 50's) for pesticides administered by dermal and oral routes to
estimate dermal penetration. A difficulty with this approach is
that due to differing route-dependent relative metabolism, an
"apparent" dermal penetration of greater than 100% can be calculated
in some cases. Therefore care must be exercised when using this
approach. It is also possible to estimate dermal penetration on the
basis of the physicochemical properties of the pesticide, with a
certain lipophilicity required for significant dermal penetration.
Finally, on a case-by-case basis, TB will require a dermal penetration study.
        TB has distributed outside the agency a draft protocol for
what it considers an acceptable dermal penetration study. The
study is detailed and expensive, but has produced useful results
in the limited number cases where it has been used in close
consultation with TB. The details are delineated below:

HIGHLIGHTS OF A DRAFT PROTOCOL FOR
A DERMAL PENETRATION STUDY

1.   In vivo Rat Study.
2.   Four Doses with 20 Animals per Dose
3.   Radiolabeled Chemical with Field Solvent
4.   Mass Balance Required
5.   Contact Dr. Robert Zendzian (703-557-1511)
     for Protocol and Consultation

The in vivo rat study requires 20 animals at each of four
doses. The doses are chosen to cover the range of exposures likely
to be encountered in the field. The study requires the use of
radiolabeled chemical and an appropriate field solvent. A mass
balance is required to account for deposited pesticide which may
have been lost from the skin surface by a route other than dermal
penetration. The study is expensive and should not be initiated
without consultation with Dr. Robert Zendzian of TB.

Some of the current research needs in OPP in regard to assessing the potential dermal exposure of agricultural workers to pesticides, and regulatory steps that can be taken to mitigate this potential route of exposure are listed below:

RESEARCH NEEDS

1. Further Field Studies for Many Application Scenarios
2. Further Predictive Correlation Development
3. Improved Methods for Measuring Hand Exposure
4. More Dermal Penetration Data
5. More Data of Efficiency of Protective Clothing/Devices

Additional field studies are needed for many application scenarios where data are limited. This will hopefully result in the further development of useful predictive correlations. Improved methodology in the area of estimating hand exposure would be welcome. The data base for estimating dermal penetration also needs to be expanded. Finally, as Dr. Moraski indicated earlier in his presentation, we need to know more about the effectiveness of various items of protective clothing and protective devices. The use of protective clothing has been one of the chief regulatory options used in OPP in many of our recent deliberations.

Nontechnical Summary

The procedures used in the EPA's Office of Pesticide Programs (OPP) to estimate pesticide exposure to agricultural workers are described. Typically, most of exposure occurs through the skin. The level of expected exposure for two types of commonly used pesticide application equipment is discussed. There is also a discussion of the research needed to enable OPP to make more reliable estimates of applicator exposure to pesticides.

Literature Cited

1. Severn, D.J. In "Genetic Toxicology. An Agricultural Perspective"; Fleck R.A. and Hollaender, A., Eds.; Plenum: New York, 1982; pp. 235–242.
2. "Use of Exposure Data for Risk Assessment," Environmental Protection Agency, 1980.
3. Day, H.R. and Reinert, J.C., Manuscript in Preparation.
4. Davis, J.E., unpublised data.
5. Hays, W.J., "Toxicology of Pesticides"; William and Wilkins: Baltimore, 1975.
6. "Applicator and Mixer/Loader Exposure to Pesticides During Ground Boom Spraying Operations," Environmental Protection Agency, 1984.
7. Wolfe, H.R.; Durham W.F.; and Armstrong, J.F. <u>Arch. Environ. Hlth.</u> 1967, 14, 622–33.

8. Staiff, D.C.; Comer, S.W.; Armstrong J.F.; Wolfe, H.R. Bull. Environ. Contam. Toxicol. 1975, 14, 334–40.
9. Atallah, Y.H., Cahill, W.P.; Whitacre, D.M. Arch. Environ. Contam. Toxicol. 1982, 11, 219–25.
10. Dubelman, S.; Lauer, R.; Arras, D.D.; Adams, S.A. J. Ag. Food Chem. 1982, 30, 528–32.
11. Jegier, A. Arch. Environ. Hlth. 1964, 8, 565–69.
12. Lavy T.L.; Shepard, J.S.; Mattice, J.D. J. Ag. Food Chem. 1980, 28, 626–30.
13. "Monitoring of Potential Exposure of Mixer-Loaders, Pilots, and Flaggers During Application of of Tributyl Phosphorothioate (DEF) and Tributyl Phosphorotrithioate (Folex) to Cotton Fields in the San Joaquin Valley of California in 1979," California Department of Food and Agriculture, 1979.
14. Wolfe, H.R.; Armstrong, J.F.; Durham, W.F. Mosquito News 1974, 34, 263–67.
15. "A Study in Southern California in July 1979 of the Potential Dermal and Inhalation Exposure of Applicators and Other Persons Who Might Later Enter or Occupy Areas Treated with Chlordane Used Against Subterranean Termites Under Houses," California Department of Food and Agriculture, 1979.
16. Wolfe, H.R., Walker, K.C.; Elliott, J.W. Bull. Wld. Hlth. Org. 1959, 20, 1–14.
17. Fletcher, T.E.; Press, J.M.; Wilson, D.B. Bull. Wld. Hlth. Org. 1959, 20, 15–25.
18. Haag, F.; Pruggmayer, D., unpublished data.
19. Everhart, L.P.; Holt, R.F. J. Ag. Food Chem. 1982, 30
20. Wolfe, H.R.; Durham, W.F.; Armstrong, J.F. Arch. Environ. Hlth. 1967, 14, 622–33.
21. Stevens, E.R.; Davis, J.E. Bull. Environ. Contam. Toxicol. 1980, in press.
22. Gaines, T.B. Tox. Appl. Pharm. 1969, 14, 515–34.

RECEIVED September 24, 1984

Field Worker Exposure:
The Usefulness of Estimates Based on Generic Data

RICHARD C. HONEYCUTT

Agricultural Division, CIBA-GEIGY Corporation, Greensboro, NC 27419

Generic data derived from existing worker exposure
data are useful for estimating exposure to new
agricultural chemicals. Several methods of using
such data in evaluation of the safety of agrichemi-
cals are discussed. Examples of using generic data
for predicting mixer-loader and applicator exposure
are presented.

The evaluation of the safety of pesticides to farm workers is a
complex endeavor which integrates several types of data such as
metabolism, residue, dissipation, dermal absorption, field worker
exposure, use pattern data, and mammalian toxicology data. One
of the most important elements of such a safety evaluation is the
estimation of exposure of pesticides to field workers. For this
discussion, field workers are defined as mixers, loaders, applicators, cleanup workers, and flaggers. Davis, Wolfe, Popendorf
and others (1-3) have published extensively in this area. With a
considerable volume of data on field worker exposure available,
it is reasonable to consider that it should be possible to summarize these data into a generic form and use them to estimate
actual worker exposure. Dr. Hackathorn's and Dr. Reinert's
papers presented in this symposium series deals extensively with
this concept of using generic data for estimating field worker
exposure.
    Although much data exist to support the concept of using
generic field data to estimate field worker exposure to pesticides, very little has been published to show how such generic
data are actually used to estimate worker exposure. It is the
objective of this paper to demonstrate how laboratory absorption
data, field exposure data and product use data can be integrated
to estimate exposure to pesticides for field workers. These data
when coupled to toxicology data can then be readily used to make
risk assessments for these pesticides to workers. Such exposure
estimates/risk assessments should be favored over actual field
testing since it would obviate the need for involving humans in
such field testing programs. The EPA has strongly recommended

0097–6156/85/0273–0369$06.00/0
© 1985 American Chemical Society

this approach in its March 1982 draft of Subdivision K of the Pesticide Assessment Guidelines for reentry protection (4).

Methods

Obtaining Laboratory and Field Data: The use of the generic approach to estimating field worker exposure can be separated into two distinct methodologies:

1. Obtaining exposure data in the laboratory and field.
2. The Generic Approach, i.e., using these data to extrapolate from one chemical to another.

Laboratory Absorption Studies: Several techniques are available for estimating dermal absorption of pesticides. These techniques are extensively reviewed in an earlier section of this book. For most pesticides, a reasonable estimate of dermal absorption for humans can be made using laboratory data. These data are used to estimate an average dermal absorption rate from which one can calculate the percentage of active ingredient that is absorbed in a typical eight-hour work day.

Field Testing: Historically, field testing has been an important element in determination of exposure levels of pesticides to field workers. These tests have been essential in establishing what factors are important for determination of field exposure. We have done several field tests on worker exposure and have constantly modified our methods to improve the utility and statistical reliability of the data and to lay a data base foundation for developing a generic approach to estimation of exposure levels.

Segmenting Field Tests: Attempts should be made to segment a field worker's daily tasks into four areas - mixer-loader, applicator, cleanup worker, and flaggers (where appropriate). This technique allows one to determine which task produces the most exposure. These data can then be used to write precautionary labels directed at specific tasks. Of course, total exposure for workers carrying out combined tasks can be determined by summation.

Matrices for Field Testing: Patches (4" x 4" - cellulose) are used for determining dermal exposure. Inside versus outside patches are beneficial to determine penetration of protective clothing. Personal air monitors are used for determining respiratory exposure. Cotton gloves can be used for hand exposure estimation. Rubber gloves worn over cotton gloves can be used to determine effectiveness of protective gloves.

Replications: Generally, field studies will be replicated 2-3 times. That is, complete studies are done at 2-3 different dates in the crop season. Each new study consists of two replications of each task, i.e., mixer-loader, applicator, cleanup worker. Each task can be monitored with and without protective clothing.

Calculations: Calculations of dermal exposure are made by extrapolation of patch data to exposed areas of the body. A technique described by Davis (1) is commonly used. The final value
of exposure is in mg/hour. Examples will be used later on to
show how values of mg/hour exposure are converted to lifetime
exposure values.

Use Data: Potential use data for a product is critical for
determination of potential exposure to field workers. There are
four general steps in acquiring adequate data to estimate potential exposure to agricultural workers.

1. Determine total acres to be treated for a particular pest for
   the anticipated market area.
2. Determine number of farms in this area.
3. Determine average acres for a "typical" farm.
4. Determine how many acres treated via commercial application
   versus individual farmer application.

The Generic Approach: Extrapolation of Field Data from One
Chemical to Another: Extrapolation or estimation of exposure of
one chemical Y to field workers using field data from exposure to
chemical X is a complex task in which several factors, as well as
exposure values must be integrated.
      Study of field worker pesticide exposure data has shown that
several factors influence exposure. These factors are mostly
physical in nature. Most of the time the chemical properties of
the pesticide do not come into play as determinants that may have
an impact on exposure levels. The physical factors are:

1. Application Equipment: Examples of application equipment
   are: boom sprayers, airplane, air blast sprayer, backpack
   equipment and high pressure guns. Backpack and air blast
   operations appear to give greatest exposure to applicators.
2. Protective Clothing: Examples of protective clothing are:
   rubber gloves, coveralls, long sleeves, long pants. Hand
   exposure is the major route of dermal exposure to mixer-
   loaders. Rubber gloves reduce mixer-loader dermal exposure
   by as much as 99% if the field worker is careful not to contaminate the inside of the gloves.
3. Formulations: Examples of formulations are: liquid concentrates, wettable powder, prepacks, granules.
4. Use Patterns and Markets: Commercial and individual farm
   operations should be considered. Commercial operations
   result in more lifetime exposure to farm workers. When performing a risk assessment, commercial versus single farm
   operations can be estimated separately using potential market
   data.
5. Weather Factors include rain, wind velocity, wind direction,
   as well as temperature. For most estimates, assumptions are
   made that the weather is sunny and the wind is ≤ 5 mph.
6. Dilution Factors must be considered when estimating exposure
   to field workers. Corrections should be made fo the percentage active ingredient in a concentrate. Corrections should

also be made for concentrations of active ingredient in a
spray solution.

All of the above factors must be considered while implementing
the generic approach to estimating field worker exposure. An
example how field data and several of the above factors are integrated into a generic estimate follow in the results and discussion.

Results and Discussion

Estimates of Field Worker Exposure to Pesticides: An example
will be presented to show how estimates of lifetime field worker
exposure can be made and show how a number of the factors above
come into play during such calculations. These calculations
apply only to chemicals which demonstrate chronic toxicity predominantly. Shorter term estimates must be made for chemicals
showing acute toxicity. For this exercise consider only field
crops such as wheat, corn, and soybeans. The example presented
here will deal with one application type, i.e., ground boom spray
application. Mixer-loaders, cleanup workers and applicators will
be considered. Factors such as effectiveness of protective
clothing will also be considered.   Further, this example will
consider only an individual farm operation scenario.

Example: Estimate exposure of Chemical X (an emulsifiable concentrate) to mixer-loaders-cleanup workers and applicators while
treating a field crop such as wheat using a boom sprayer.

I.   Mixer-Loader - Cleanup Worker Combined Exposure (Individual
     Farm Operation):   Generally mixer-loader people clean equip-
     ment after application is made.

     A.   Field Use Patterns of Chemical X:
          1.   Application rate 1 pound ai/acre in 50 gallons
               water/acre.
          2.   Maximum four applications/year (from label).
          3.   Average wheat field 150 acres (use data).
          4.   System of application = ground boom sprayer. One
               load will treat 10 acres (i.e., spray tank = 500
               gallons).
          5.   Dermal absorption is 50% in eight hours.

     B.   Assumptions:
          1.   Assume mixing-loading-cleanup operation takes 15
               minutes for each load.
          2.   Boom sprayer - one load can treat 10 acres in 100
               minutes (10 minutes/acre).
          3.   Respiratory exposure is insignificant compared to
               dermal exposure.

     C.   Mixer-Loader and Cleanup Worker Boom Spray Operation
          Exposure (Individual Farm Operation):

1. Exposure Time Estimate: Mixer-loader-cleanup worker
    total exposure time – for ground boom spray opera-
    tion.

    a. Loads/farm = 150 acres/farm ÷ 10 acres/load =
        15 loads/farm.
    b. Mixer-loader + cleanup worker time –
        hours/year/farm = 15 loads/farm x 15 minutes
        mixing-loading-cleanup/load x 4 applications/year
        = 900 minutes/year = 15 hours/year.

2. Exposure Estimate: Mixer-loader-cleanup worker –
    individual farm ground boom spray operation.

    a. Exposure to Chemical X can be based on mean
        mixer-loader-cleanup worker exposure from several
        studies on Chemical Y using similar formulation
        (emulsifiable concentrate). Chemical X is 40%
        ai/gallon concentrate. Chemical Y is 80%
        ai/gallon concentrate.
    b. Mean exposure for Chemical Y was 40 mg/hour – no
        gloves; 0.5 mg/hour – rubber gloves.

3. Total Daily Exposure to Chemical X Concentrate –
    Gloves versus No Gloves (Boom Spray – Individual Farm
    Operation):

    a. Mixer-loader-cleanup worker wearing no gloves:

        1) A handling correction factor (HCF) can be
            calculated for active ingredient Chemical X
            versus active ingredient Chemical Y since
            less active ingredient of X will be handled
            versus the amount of Y handled in the actual
            field study.

            $$HCF = \frac{40\% \ ai/gallon \ X}{80\% \ ai/gallon \ Y} = 0.5$$

            Using the HCF and the exposure of mixer-
            loaders to Y without gloves to calculate
            exposure to X: 40 mg/hour x 0.5 =
            20 mg/hour.
        2) Exposure in µg/kg/day = 20 mg/hour x 15
            hours/year ÷ 365 days/year ÷ 70 kg/man x 0.5
            (dermal absorption within 8 hours) x 1,000
            µg/mg = 5.9 µg/kg/day.

    b. Wearing rubber gloves:

        $$5.9 \ µg/kg/day \ x \ \frac{0.5 \ mg/hr}{40 \ mg/hr} = 0.07 \ µg/kg/day$$

II. Applicator Exposure – Boom Spray Operation – Individual Farm
     Operation:

A. Exposure Time Estimate – Applicator Total Exposure
    Time:

    1. Load/farm = 150 acres/farm ÷ 10 acres/load =
        15 loads/farm.
    2. Application hours/year/farm = 15 loads/farm X 100
        minutes/load/application X 4 applications/year X
        1/60 hours/minutes = 100 hours/year.

B. Exposure Estimate – Applicator – Individual Farm Ground
    Boom Spray Operation:

    1. Base exposure to Chemical X can be based on mean
        applicator exposure derived from several studies
        using the same application equipment (i.e., boom
        sprayer) and same concentrations of ai in spray for
        Chemical Y. Chemical Y was 80% ai and applied at 3
        pounds ai/acre in 20 gallons water/acre (0.15 pound
        ai/gallon water). Chemical X is 40% ai and is
        applied at 1 pound ai/50 gallons water/acre (0.02
        pound ai/gallon).
    2. Mean exposure for Chemical Y was 0.2 mg/hour (no
        protective clothing).

C. Applicator Exposure to Chemical X – Boom Sprayer:

    1. A concentration correction factor (CCF) can be cal-
        culated for Chemical X since the concentration of X
        in the spray will be different than Chemical Y:

$$CCF = \frac{0.02 \text{ lb. ai/gallon water/A for X}}{0.15 \text{ lb. ai/gallon water/A for Y}} = 0.13$$

    2. Total dermal exposure to applicators of Chemical Y
        was determined by field tests to be 0.2 mg/hour.
        Using the CCF the exposure of applicators using
        Chemical X versus Y can be determined: 0.2 mg/hour
        x 0.13 = 0.026 mg/hour.
    3. Exposure in µg/kg/day = 0.026 mg/hour x 100
        hours/year ÷ 365 days/year ÷ 70 man/kg x 0.5 (dermal
        absorption) x 1,000 µg/kg = 0.05 µg/kg/day.

There are several advantages of using a generic data approach to
estimating farm worker exposure.

1. Exposure estimates can be used to acquire an EUP without
    field testing and can save up to $50,000/field study.
2. Preferred to field testing where humans involved.
3. Exposure estimates can be used to define areas where further
    research is needed.

4. Such estimates are consistant with previous EPA policy for
    reentry exposure assessment (4).

Nontechnical Summary

The evaluation of risk to agricultural field workers using pesticides involves integrating data from laboratory absorption,
metabolism, field testing, marketing, and toxicity studies. The
generic approach to estimating agricultural worker exposure
attempts to integrate these types of data. Examples demonstrate
how such data can be used to estimate exposure. Several
advantages are given for making such estimates: 1) savings of
time and dollars for registration of a new pesticide, 2) defines
areas where further research is needed, and 3) preferred to field
testing where humans are involved.

Literature Cited

1. Davis, J. E. Residue Reviews, Vol. 75, 1970, P. 33.
2. Wolfe, H. R., W. F. Durham Arch. Environ. Health, Vol. 14,
    1967, p. 622.
3. Popendorf, W. Am. Ind. Hyg. Assoc., Vol. 41, 1980, p. 652.
4. Adams, J. D., Public Draft of Pesticide Assessment Guilde-
    lines, Subdivision K. March 1982.

RECEIVED October 29, 1984

Evaluation of Fluorescent Tracer Methodology for Dermal Exposure Assessment

RICHARD A. FENSKE[1], JOHN T. LEFFINGWELL[2], and ROBERT C. SPEAR[2]

[1]Department of Environmental Science, Cook College, Rutgers University, New Brunswick, NJ 08903
[2]Department of Biomedical and Environmental Health Sciences, University of California, Berkeley, CA 94720

The feasibility of employing fluorescent tracers and video imaging analysis to quantify dermal exposure to pesticide applicators has been demonstrated under realistic field conditions. Six workers loaded a tracer with the organophosphate pesticide, diazinon, into air blast sprayers, and conducted normal dormant spraying in pear orchards. They were examined prior to and immediately after the application. UV-A illumination produced fluorescence on the skin surface, and the pattern of exposure was digitized with a video imaging system. Quantifiable levels of tracer were detected beneath cotton coveralls on five workers. The distribution of exposure over the body surface varied widely due to differences in protective clothing use, work practices and environmental conditions. This assessment method produced exposure values at variance with those calculated by the traditional patch technique.

The need to quantitatively evaluate dermal exposure among pesticide applicators has been recognized since at least 1954 (1). The work outlined here represents a new approach to this problem and provides suggestions for further research in this field of exposure assessment. The tracing of dermal deposition among applicators by means of fluorescent compounds was first undertaken in 1979 (2). Since that time an instrument capable of measuring fluorescence directly on the skin has been developed and tested. The details of the instrumental design and the nature of the fluorescent compound employed as a tracer have been discussed elsewhere (3). This paper reports the results of initial field investigations with the method.

The conceptual basis of this technique is straight-
forward. A non-toxic fluorescent compound is introduced
into a spray apparatus in proportion to the pesticide
being applied. Workers are asked to conduct spray operations normally. Any contamination from mixing and loading, equipment adjustment or spraying is evidenced by the
deposition of tracer on the skin. Immediately following
the spraying episode, the worker is examined under long
wave ultra-violet light in order to visualize the pattern
of exposure on the body surface. The Video Imaging
Technique for Assessing Exposure, or VITAE system, employs a television camera interfaced with a microcomputer
to detect and quantify fluorescence on the skin. A
standard curve relating light intensity to amount of
tracer is used to determine total tracer exposure. The
ratio of tracer to pesticide is established on the basis
of field sampling, and total pesticide exposure reported.

The impetus for this study came from a realization
that the traditional patch technique (4) was inherently
limited in its ability to accurately measure dermal
exposure, and from the great potential which a fluorescent tracer methodology appeared to hold. The ability to
visualize exposure immediately provides valuable qualitative information regarding the exposure process. When
combined with a video image processing system which quantifies fluorescence, the possibility of carefully characterizing dermal exposure seemed well worth the effort
involved.

At the outset it was clear that the development of a
computer-based instrument and the use of a surrogate
compound (tracer) would make the method much more complex
than the traditional approach. Thus, the study has
extended over several years, involving both laboratory
and field tests. Appropriate fluorescent tracers were
first screened, and their chemical and environmental
characteristics studied. Simultaneously, the video image
processing system was designed and tested. Software was
then developed to run the system, and evaluation and
quantification procedures established. Finally, the
system was taken into the field to study applicators
conducting routine spraying operations.

Field Study Conditions

The fluorescent tracer technique was employed in an applicator exposure study in Lake County, CA, in January of
1983. The field trial was based at the offices of the
County Agricultural Commissioner and the University of
California Extension Service, approximately 200 miles
north of San Francisco. The agricultural region surrounding Clear Lake was chosen due to the likelihood of
recruiting owners of small pear orchards as subjects. The
study involved six applicators, and included air
sampling, a modified version of the dermal patch
technique, and the use of a tracer during the spraying of

the organophosphate, diazinon [O,O-diethyl O-(2-isopro-
pyl-6-methyl-4-pyrimidinyl) phosphorothioate]. Field
conditions were standardized as much as possible for the
six subjects, and are summarized in Table I.

Table I. Field Trial Application Parameters

Application Parameter	Worker					
	1	2	3	4	5	6
Tank loadings	3	4	4	4	2	1
Acres sprayed	3.75	4	4	4	2	1
Tank size (gallons)	500	500	500	500	500	500
Gallons sprayed per acre	400	500	500	500	500	500
Total diazinon sprayed (lbs)	20	20	20	20	10	5
Total tracer sprayed (gms)	1200	1200	1200	1200	600	300
Spraying time (minutes)	152	130	102	129	73	48

The major variables were controlled in the following
manner:

Equipment: All subjects employed tractor-powered air
blast sprayers. All of the sprayers were calibrated to
produce a high volume application of either 400 or 500
gallons per acre.

Activity: The subjects were owner-operators and
conducted both their own mixing/loading and spraying.
The monitoring protocol did not distinguish between these
two activities. The pesticide and tracer were added
sequentially to the spray tank, with the worker
instructed to treat both compounds in the same manner.

Pesticide: Subjects were each supplied with four 5 lb.
bags of 50% wettable powder formulation diazinon. The
spray schedule recommended by the University of California Research Entomologist for pear psylla and San Jose
scale was 5 lbs. per acre, and was followed by all subjects except Worker #1. Eight gallons of dormant oil
were also applied to each acre.

Fluorescent Tracer: The Fluorescent Whitening Agent, 4-
methyl-7-diethylaminocoumarin, was employed as a tracer.
This compound is commonly used in commercial products and
has undergone toxicity testing (1)(5). A 300 gm bag of
tracer was added with each 5 lb. bag of diazinon 50% WP

(1134 gms active ingredient), resulting in a tracer tank concentration of 158 ppm, and a ratio of 3.8:1, pesticide:tracer.

Spray Period: Subjects were asked to conduct four complete spray cycles (i.e., four tank loadings and sprayings). Workers #5 and #6 sprayed for a shorter time due to changes in weather, and Worker #1 made only three loadings due to his decision to spray higher concentrations. Spray times ranged from 40-152 minutes.

Protective Clothing: The personal protection employed during the field trial is summarized in Table II. Respirators were used by all subjects. Long sleeve cotton coveralls and short sleeve cotton T-shirts were issued to each subject and were worn throughout the spray period. In some cases extra shirts and work pants were worn beneath this clothing.

Weather: Most of the subjects took a very cautious attitude toward wind conditions. Spraying was not conducted unless the day was calm, and even then one of the workers chose to spray in only one direction to avoid drift. Increasing wind and the threat of rain cut short the spray period of subjects #5 and #6 on the last day of the study.

Materials and Methods: Environmental Sampling

Environmental sampling for the field trial was guided by three aims: 1) establishment of estimates of exposure which allow comparison with other field studies; 2) determination of levels of pesticide and tracer in the environment of the worker; and 3) evaluation of the environmental stability of the tracer.
        The first aim was accomplished by collecting personal air samples and employing a modified version of the traditional patch technique. The second aim required attaching gauze monitors to the spray rig in the vicinity of the worker. The final aim involved spiking gauze monitors with known quantities of the tracer and exposing them to sunlight during the spraying episode. This characterization of the environment of the worker allowed estimation of exposure independent of the video imaging analysis, and provided information necessary for the interpretation of the VITAE system results.

Air Sampling: Personal air samples were collected in the breathing zone of the worker for the entire spray period. A Gilian battery powered pump attached to the belt was connected to an open-faced 37mm cassette with a Millipore filter, and the cassette clipped to the lapel of the coveralls. The pumps were calibrated prior to and immediately after use.

Table II. Personal Protection During Spray

Body Part	Protective Gear worn by Worker #1	#2	#3
Head	baseball cap	baseball cap	hard hat
Face	none	eye glasses	face shield
Hands	rubber gloves	rubber gloves	rubber gloves
Torso	thermal under wear	shirt + T-shirt	shirt + vest
(issued)	coverall	coverall	coverall
(issued)	T-shirt	T-shirt	T-shirt
Legs	thermal	jeans	jeans
(issued)	coverall	coverall	coverall
Feet	rubber boots	rubber boots	rubber boots
Respiratory	MSA dual cartridge	Pesticide dual cartridge	MSA dual cartridge

Body Part	Protective Gear worn by Worker #4	#5	#6
Head	plastic helmet	hard hat	hard hat
Face	face shield	face shield	face shield
Hands	vinyl gloves	polyeth gloves	rubber gloves
Torso	none	none	shirt + T-shirt
(issued)	coverall	coverall	coverall
(issued)	T-shirt	T-shirt	T-shirt
Legs	none	jeans	jeans
(issued)	coverall	coverall	coverall
Feet	plastic boots	rubber boots	leather boots
Respiratory	Pesticide dual cartridge	Pesticide dual cartridge	Pesticide dual cartridge

Personal Sampling: The dermal monitor employed is a modification of the traditional method of Durham and Wolfe (4), and was developed at the University of California, Berkeley. The monitor consists of a solvent-extracted 12-ply surgical gauze pad (3" x 3"), backed by polyethylene, and placed in a paper envelope. The envelope design includes a 6 cm diameter circle cutout. Thus, the exposed gauze sampling surface is 28.27 sq cm. When stapled together this assemblage becomes a sturdy unit, easily attached and removed from a worker's clothing or skin.

Following a protocol similar to Franklin, et al (2), and Davies, et al (6), four dermal monitors were placed on each worker, two on the outside of the coverall, and two on the T-shirt beneath the coverall in order to measure the amount of pesticide and tracer penetrating the outer garment. All outer monitors were placed on the left breast and right shoulder blade; all inner monitors were placed on the right breast and left shoulder blade.

Rig Samples: Three monitors were attached to the top of the spray rig (i.e., parallel to the ground) at the end nearest the tractor, approximately 150 cm from the worker and 150 cm from the tank opening for loading. This distance appeared sufficient to avoid contamination during mixing and loading. These samples indicate the level of pesticide in the environment of the worker, and provide a further measurement of the ratio of pesticide to tracer in the aerosol.

Sun Samples: The fluorescent tracer used in this study can degrade when exposed to direct sunlight (3). The extent of this degradation was measured by placing monitors in the field. Six monitors for each worker were spiked with a measured amount of tracer in acetonitrile just prior to each spray period, and allowed to dry. Three of the monitors were then placed in direct sunlight in an area adjacent to the spraying, but where no exposure to the spray would occur. The other three monitors were not exposed to sunlight and served as controls. The time of sun exposure was noted for the spray period of each worker.

Field Blanks: Two field blanks for each worker were taken to the worksite to monitor potential sample contamination. They were exposed in the area where samples were prepared and collected, and then handled, stored and analyzed in a manner identical to the other environmental samples. All values reported in this study have been adjusted for background levels of diazinon and tracer recovered from these samples.

Analysis: All samples were placed on dry ice upon collection, transported frozen to the laboratory and placed in a deep freeze to await analysis. The air and environmental samples were extracted and analyzed according to the procedures detailed previously (3). Samples were placed in 125 ml Nalgene bottles with 30 ml acetonitrile (Baker "resi-analyzed" grade) and extracted on an oscillating shaker table for 90 minutes. The extraction efficiencies of diazinon and the tracer were 93% and 101%, respectively.

Diazinon samples were analyzed with a Tracor 222 Gas Chromatograph equipped with a flame photometric detector in the phosphorous mode. The diazinon standard employed was obtained from EPA, Research Triangle Park. The limit of detection of the instrument was 0.3 ng with a maximum injection volume of 10 ul. Since all environmental samples were extracted in 30 ml of solvent and were not concentrated, the sensitivity per sample was 900 ng.

The environmental samples were analyzed for tracer with a Turner 430 Spectrofluorometer at fixed wavelengths (excitation = 356 nm; emission = 420 nm). Standards were interspersed with samples, and the amount of tracer present calculated by means of a standard curve. The limit of detection of the instrument for this compound was < 5 ppb, allowing detection of levels as low as 150 ng per sample.

Materials and Methods: Video Imaging Analysis

Evaluation of tracer on the skin surface was conducted with the VITAE system, following a protocol similar to that described elsewhere (3). The system quantifies fluorescence intensity in the following manner: a television camera scans the surface area of a body part 30 times per second. A video digitizer in the computer takes one of these scans, converts the analog camera output to digital values on the basis of a 16 level grey scale, and displays the image on a TV monitor. The data is then stored on disk and is available for later analysis.

The lighting system employed consisted of BLB bulbs (black lights) with filters. The intensity of UV-A light to which subjects were exposed was evaluated prior to examination with a UVX Radiometer (UV Products). With a light-to-subject distance of 90 cm, the maximum long wave UV illumination was 210 uwatts/sq cm. The relative standard deviation of 49 readings taken in a 70 cm x 70 cm region was 4%. Both pre- and post-exposure images were taken of all body regions above the waist for each subject, resulting in a total of 30 pairs of video images per subject (Table III). The legs and the insides of the upper arms were omitted in this trial due to difficulties in subject positioning. The camera-to-subject distance was varied between 70 and 80 cm, and at times the camera was moved up or down to accommodate the location of the body part. A fixed aperture of f/1.4 was employed throughout the study.

A standard target was read at 105 cm (f/1.4) prior to and immediately following each examination period.

Table III. Body Parts for Video Imaging Analysis

Body Part	# Images Recorded	Anatomical Boundaries
Hands (1)	4	up to the wrists
Forearm (2)	8	wrists to the elbow
Upper Arm (2)	6	elbow to the shoulder (excludes insides of arms)
Head (1)	4	includes neck sides and back
Upper Torso (1)	4	neck to breast (includes front of neck)
Lower Torso (1)	4	breast to waist

This measurement served as an indicator of the stability of the system throughout the six day field trial. Readings of these targets are expressed as integrated intensity, or counts. The twelve readings ranged from 6709 to 7414 counts, with a mean value of 6986 counts, and a standard deviation of 157 (RSD = 2.25%). This low variability can be considered negligible for purposes of exposure quantification.

Reduction and analysis of the video imaging data was conducted in the laboratory following the field trial. The steps involved in the calculation of exposure from video images have been detailed elsewhere (3), and are summarized here. A variable background reflectance from the skin is commonly observed with this system. Images of the various body parts must be recorded prior to the worker's exposure to provide baseline data. Thus, the area of interest for quantification on the After image (post-exposure) is outlined and superimposed onto the Before image, and background variability eliminated. Images are then corrected for lens distortions and changes in distance, and adjusted for the nonplanar characterisitics of the various body parts. A standard curve developed in the laboratory serves as the basis for transforming adjusted light intensity to amount of tracer on the skin surface. Ratios of pesticide to tracer based on evironmental samples allow calculation of pesticide exposure. Laboratory studies have demonstrated that pesticides and tracer compounds penetrate cotton coverall fabric at different rates (3). Thus, an empirical penetration factor of 3.4:1 (pesticide to tracer) is employed in the final calculation of exposure for protected regions.

Results and Discussion: Environmental Sampling

Air Samples: Air sampling data provided the most direct means of comparing levels of pesticide in the workplace from this study with those in previous ones. The sampling devices employed are very close to standard, and

the procedures for determining potential exposure expli-
cit and generally uniform.   The results from air samples
in this study are presented in Table IV.   Four of the
workers had similar potential respiratory exposure,
ranging from 8.6 to 30 ug/cu meter.   The sample of
worker #6 had no detectable level of pesticide,
presumably due to his spraying only one tank.   The potential exposure of worker #1 was nearly an order of magnitude greater than the other subjects.   All subjects wore
dual cartridge, half-mask respirators during spraying, so
little if any respiratory exposure actually occurred.

Table IV. Air Sampling Results

Worker #	Time Spraying hrs	diazinon Concentration ug/cu meter	Potential Resp Exposure ug/hr
1	83	202.11	351.7
2	141	30.39	52.9
3	102	8.55	14.9
4	129	23.37	40.7
5	73	14.99	26.1

* Assumes a tidal volume of 1740 liters per hour.
All workers wore respirators.

In a previous applicator study (2), a range of 20-
110 ug/cu meter was observed.   The exposure range of 8.6-
202 ug/cu meter in this study is broader, but of similar
magnitude.   Data from Wolfe et al (7-8) indicate an
exposure range of 6-167 ug/cu meter, quite similar to
levels recorded in this study.   Based on air sampling,
then, exposures appear to be within a normal range for
mixer/loader/applicators employing air blast spraying
equipment.

Sun Samples: The comparison of exposed spiked samples
with controls allows determination of the amount of tracer lost during a typical spray episode, and calculation
of a correction factor for the environmental samples of
each worker.   Variability among three replicate samples
was low, with relative standard deviations less than 5%.
Since sunlight intensity and other environmental factors
varied considerably from day to day and worker to worker,
it was not possible to calculate a rate of degradation.
The loss of tracer ranged from 7% to 22%, with approximately 10-15% lost in two hours.   These results were
quite similar to those observed in controlled studies of
tracer stability (3).   The per cent loss during the spray
episode is employed to correct for loss from the rig and
personal samples of each worker.

Rig Samples: Samples attached to the spray rig during
the application provide an indication of the aerosol
concentration of the two compounds in the vicinity of the
worker.   Results are presented in Table V.   Mean pesticide levels range from 1.3 to 45.23 ug/sq cm, and mean
tracer levels from 0.49 to 17.34 ug/sq cm.   Analysis of

Table V.   Exposure Levels based on Rig Samples
(all values in micrograms/sq cm)

worker	mean diazinon	std dev	mean tracer	std dev	Ratio d:t
1	6.28	0.3	0.97	0.1	6.5
2	45.20	1.7	17.34	2.2	2.6
3	1.29	0.3	0.22	0.05	5.9
4	44.70	1.7	9.70	1.7	4.6
5	19.28	2.6	3.36	0.4	5.7
6	1.86	0.3	0.49	0.1	3.8

Note: N = 3 in all cases

these values by linear regression reveals a highly significant correlation of tracer and pesticide ($r = 0.92$,
$p < .00001$, n = 18).   The relatively high levels of tracer recovered from the samples of Worker #2 tend to
reduce the linearity of this relationship.   If his data
is omitted from the analysis the correlation is improved
($r = 0.984$, $p < .000001$, n = 15).   These same relationships are also evident from the ratios of pesticide to
tracer shown in the table.   The range of ratios is 2.61
to 6.47.   If Worker #2 is excluded, however, the range
narrows markedly (3.80-6.47).   It is not apparent why the
concentration of tracer on the spray rig monitors of
Worker #2 was elevated relative to the other subjects.
It is possible that the samples received disproportionate
tracer exposure during mixing and loading.   It should be
noted from Table V that four of the six calculated standard ratios are higher than the 3.8:1 ratio of the two
compounds when introduced into the spray tank.   These
results indicate a lower water solubility for the tracer
than for the wettable powder formulation of diazinon.
This finding was corroborated by high ratios found in
samples of the tank mix taken prior to spraying.
     The ratio of pesticide to tracer is an essential
calibration factor for the VITAE system's exposure
assessment.   The ratios derived from the rig samples are
mean values of three samples, and are thus the most
statistically reliable indicators of the aerosol ratio
among the measurements taken.   In this study, therefore,
these ratios are employed to transform tracer to pesticide.   Further investigation will be necessary to determine how best to define these values.

<u>Personal   Samples</u>:   Data from the gauze patches on   the
outside of the coveralls,   and on the T-shirt immediately
beneath   the   coveralls are presented in   Table   VI   with
values   expressed as micrograms per sq cm of gauze   monitor.   Consistent   with   the data from the   rig   samples,
Workers   #2,   #4,   and #5 show relatively high levels   of
tracer and pesticide, while Workers #3, and #6 reveal low
levels.   Worker   #1 is anomalous,   in that his   personal
samples   are   relatively high,   whereas the   rig   samples
point toward a moderate exposure.

Table VI.   Exposure Levels based on Personal Samples
(all values in micrograms/sq cm)

work #	outer chest		inner chest		outer back		inner back	
	D*	T*	D	T	D	T	D	T
1	12.45	6.83	1.10	.21	.99	.68	.04	--
2	11.94	7.20	--	.24	3.40	.62	.04	--
3	1.36	.19	--	--	.88	.13	--	--
4	11.39	1.70	.01	.28	6.30	.54	.12	--
5	4.23	.49	--	--	1.93	.17	--	05
6	.53	.07	--	--	.54	.08	--	--

Note: missing values were less than 2 times field blank
values
*   D = diazinon, T = tracer

In accord with many previous field observations, the
patches   placed   on the chest of five of the six   workers
are   markedly higher than those on the back.   Such   differential   exposure can be tentatively attributed to   two
factors: contamination of the samples during mixing and
loading,   and   the   forward motion of the   worker   during
spray operations causing greater deposition on the   front
of the body.
The   levels   beneath   the coveralls were too   low   to
quantify in most cases.   Four workers appear to have had
penetration   of low levels of pesticide or tracer.   Only
Worker #1,   whose outer chest patch is also high, appears
to have been significantly exposed beneath the   coveralls
based on these data   (i.e.,   pesticide exposure > 1 ug/sq
cm).
The personal samples on the chest and back allow   an
estimate   of   pesticide   exposure based on   the   standard
technique   of extrapolating from patch to total body   region.   The   standard method only   considers   unprotected
regions   of the body to be exposed.   In this case,   only
the head and neck of the workers are unprotected,   and in
four of six cases face shields were worn.   Thus, beyond a
comparison   of head and neck exposure for workers #1   and
#2,   it   is   not clear how the patch technique   could   be
applied   in this study.   Later in this paper   the   patch
data   will   be employed to make this   comparison.   These

exposure values will then be compared with those derived
from the video imaging analysis.

Results and Discussion: Video Imaging Analysis

The Before and After video images for each worker were
analyzed by the VITAE system to determine the extent of
exposure. Results are presented in Table VII. Workers
#3,#4,#5,and #6 exhibit only minor exposure. It should
be recalled that all of these workers wore face shields
throughout the study period, and two sprayed for relatively short periods.

Table VII. Diazinon Exposure*
(all values in micrograms)

Body Parts**	Worker No.					
	1	2	3	4	5	6
Hands	551.6	118.1	212.3	99.8	0	0
LF Arm	1014.3	61.2	0	0	0	55.8
RF Arm	1536.6	0	0	127.0	0	0
LU Arm	329.8	11.6	0	0	0	0
RU Arm	400.2	56.2	0	0	130.6	0
Torso	631.3	94.5	0	0	0	0
Head	995.7	146.2	0	35.9	115.0	0
TOTAL	5459.2	487.8	212.3	262.7	245.6	55.8

* Fluorescent tracer exposure values have been adjusted
    by ratio of diazinon to tracer from Table V.
** Regions protected by coveralls have also been adjusted
    by a clothing penetration factor of 3.4.
    For Workers #1 and #2 the penetration factor has been
    applied to the chest but not to the neck which re-
    mained unprotected.

The hand exposure of Worker #3 is undoubtedly due to
his unique practice of mixing and loading with gloves on,
but spraying with no gloves. His cautious practice of
spraying in only one direction to avoid drift appears to
have eliminated exposure to the aerosol itself. The
detection of exposure to the forearms of workers #4 and
#6 corroborates visual observations. It was noted during
examination that a ring of diffuse fluorescence extended
completely around the forearms, approximately 10 cm above
the wrists. Discussion with these workers revealed that
the exposure ocurred just at the top of the rubber gloves
which they all employed. Since the coverall sleeves are
not secured in any way, it appears that this exposure may
be due to movement of the gloves and coveralls at this
junction, rather than the result of clothing penetration.
The cause of the upper arm exposure of worker #5 is not
evident, but may have resulted from contact with contaminated equipment.

Exposure at the base of the neck of Worker #4 was apparent during the examination. It appeared as a high light intensity spot of circular shape. The worker suggested during discussion that the plastic helmet he wore during application may have collected the aerosol and allowed it to drip onto his back. While workers #4 and #5 received exposure to the head, only deposition to the sides of the face occurred. In fact, the point just in front of the ear at which the face shields ended was clearly demarcated. Thus, the face shields appear to have been very effective in reducing and in some cases eliminating facial exposure.

Quantifiable levels of tracer were detected on all body parts of Worker #1, and in 25 of 30 views. Based on data in Table VII, the highest levels occurred on the forearms. It is likely, however, that exposure to the head was greater than these figures reflect. As noted previously, a fixed f/1.4 aperture was employed throughout the study. Later analysis of the images revealed that a significant number of pixels from the head images were assigned the maximum grey level of 15, indicating detector saturation. Considering the extremely high exposure which this worker received to the face, it is likely that quenching also came into play, contributing to an artificially low value. These factors did not appear to obtain for any of the other images examined.

Worker #2 exhibits the pattern of exposure which might have been predicted for all workers. The exposed region of the head (no face shield) was highest. The hands were also high, despite the use of gloves. However, elevated levels were also detected beneath protective clothing. Since this worker wore a flannel shirt and T-shirt in addition to the T-shirt and coveralls issued, it was most surprising to detect exposure to the chest. The value for torso exposure in the table includes both a protected region (chest) and an exposed region (front of neck). Chest exposure alone accounted for 78 ug of the 94 ug exposure.

The calculation of exposure based on the patch technique traditionally employs the simplifying assumption that clothing penetration does not occur, or does not contribute significantly to total exposure. Based on the fluorescent tracer data it seems reasonable to argue that this assumption may be inappropriate. Table VIII presents the per cent of exposure occurring on both exposed and protected regions. Not surprisingly, the patterns are highly variable as they are affected by both protective clothing and work practices. For the two workers with exposure to nearly all body regions, protected areas accounted for 42% (#2) and 71% (#1) of total exposure. In some cases hands may account for all exposure (#3), while in others they may represent a relatively small contribution.

The calculation of exposure by the patch technique also assumes that deposition of pesticide is uniform over

Table VIII. Per Cent of Exposure to Body Regions

Region	Worker No.					
	1	2	3	4	5	6
Hands	10	24	100	38	0	0
Head	19	33	0	14	47	0
Coverall Protected	71	42	0	48	53	100

each body part represented by a patch. It is evident from qualitative examination of the workers and recorded images that the distribution of exposure over a given body region (e.g., head, hands, forearm) is not uniform. Such an exposure pattern would clearly be an exception. The more common pattern is the appearance of a "hot spot" adjacent to areas with little or no exposure. Thus, the extrapolation step in standard exposure calculations may underestimate exposure if the patch does not represent a high exposure spot, but would overestimate exposure if such a spot hit the patch. Since the patterns of exposure are highly variable and have not been well characterized, there does not appear to be any means of determining a priori where to place a patch to serve as a representative sample of a body region.

As methods of exposure estimation, neither the fluorescent tracer technique nor the patch technique have been validated. Nevertheless, it would be encouraging if a comparison of estimates by the two methods yielded roughly equivalent results. The only body region which can be reasonably compared is the head, as the patch method assumes no clothing penetration, and no hand wash was conducted in this study. Furthermore, four of the six workers must be excluded, as they wore face shields. Thus, the only comparison available is the head and neck exposure of workers #1 and #2. These data are presented in Table IX. Following the protocol outlined by Durham and Wolfe (4) and Davis (9), the amount of diazinon recovered from the dermal monitor on the chests of the two workers is employed to calculate exposure to the face and front of neck. A similar patch on the back allows calculation of exposure to the back of the neck.

Exposure for the head and neck of worker #1 appears to be 1026 ug by the tracer method. The estimation of exposure for these same areas derived from the patch technique is 10,069 ug, or 10 times greater. The patch estimate of 9926 ug for worker #2 is quite similar to that of #1, while here the tracer estimate is a much lower 163 ug. The current lack of any means of obtaining a "true" value for exposure independent of these methods allows only informed speculation as to which of these approaches is more correct.

Table IX. Dermal Exposure Estimation by
Patch and Tracer Techniques

Work No.	Body Part	Surface Area sq cm	Patch Exposure ug/sq cm	Calculated Exposure ug/part	Tracer Exposure ug/part
1	Face	650	12.45	8092	996*
	Back Neck	110	0.99	109	
	Front Neck	150	12.45	1868	30
			Total	10069	1026
2	Face	650	11.94	7761	146
	Back Neck	110	3.40	374	
	Front Neck	150	11.94	1791	17
			Total	9926	163

* Head region for tracer technique includes sides and
back of neck.

Although the accuracy of the methods remains in
question, one would expect each technique to provide
reasonable comparative exposure estimates within a study.
Based on visual observations of the tracer there is a
clear difference between facial exposure to tracer for
Workers #1 and #2. Such a difference is corroborated by
personal air sampling data, where these workers differed
by nearly an order of magnitude. A similar difference is
reflected in the tracer exposure values, while the patch
technique makes no distinction in the exposure of these
two subjects. Such comparisons are at this stage only
suggestive, and will require further investigation.

Directions for Future Research

The fluorescent tracer technique appears to hold a potential for providing far more detailed information concerning the magnitude and distribution of pesticide
exposure than existing techniques. This initial field
trial also illustrates many of the complexities of the
method. The quantitative relationship of the pesticide
and tracer as they are deposited on the skin surface
needs to be determined with a higher degree of accuracy.
A more careful determination of the ratio of the two
compounds in an aerosol, and of the chemicals' ability to
penetrate various types of fabric is clearly required.
Further comparative studies employing the tracer and
patch techniques would clarify the strengths and weak-
nesses of these two approaches.
    Quantification of exposure by means of the VITAE
system also requires refinement, particularly in regard
to the characterization of variable background levels in
pre-exposure images. A solution to this problem may lie

in an improved lighting/detector/filtration system. In addition, the problems of detector saturation and quenching currently limit the accuracy of the method. In general, such overloading of the skin surface with fluorescent material can be avoided by controlling the amount of tracer introduced into the spraying system. It appears that relatively high levels of tracer are necessary to detect protective clothing penetration, while much lower levels would be adequate to monitor deposition on exposed skin surfaces. A series of range-finding studies under controlled conditions could lead to an appropriate resolution of this problem.

Leaving such refinements aside for a moment, it is clear that the tracer technique as now practiced provides an investigator with a powerful qualitative tool for characterizing dermal exposure, and for developing recommendations concerning protective clothing use and changes in work practices. Further, the worker education potential of this approach cannot be overstated. The visualization of exposure allows workers to participate in their own evaluation. In many instances they come to recognize for the first time the nature of the hazard which they face in their day to day work, and we have seen marked changes in behavior literally overnight. As a simple and inexpensive means of evaluation, it is hoped that this approach will be adopted in the agricultural workplace despite the refinements required for quantitative analysis.

Nontechnical Summary

The use of fluorescent compounds as tracers of dermal exposure among pesticide applicators has been tested under normal working conditions. Six applicators introduced a Fluorescent Whitening Agent into their spray tanks with the organophosphate pesticide, diazinon. They were examined under long wave ultra-violet light (black light) after spraying to visualize the pattern of exposure on the skin surface. The fluorescence was quantified by means of the Video Imaging Technique for Assessing Exposure, or VITAE system. This system employs a television camera as a detector, and digitizes the video signal by means of a microcomputer. Quantifiable levels of tracer were detected beneath the cotton coveralls of five workers. The distribution of exposure over the body surface varied widely due to differences in protective clothing use, work practices and environmental conditions. Quantification of exposure with this technique is subject to further refinements. Qualitative assessment has proven very successful in regard to worker education and the evaluation of protective clothing performance.

Acknowledgments

This work was initially funded by the California State Department of Industrial Relations (Contract No. 4-6141), and was subsequently supported by the National Institute for Occupational Safety and Health (Grant No. 1 RO1 OH 01234-01A1) and the Environmental Protection Agency (Cooperative Agreement CR-810691-01-0). The work could not have been completed without the excellent technical support provided by Sharon Wong and William Gibb.

Literature Cited

1. Batchelor, G.S.; Walker, K.C. Arch. Ind. Hyg. 1954, 10, 522-529.
2. Franklin, C.A.; Fenske, R.A.; Greenhalgh, R.; Mathieu, L.; Denley, B.V.; Leffingwell, J.T.; Spear, R.C. J. Toxicol. Environ. Health 1981, 7, 715-31.
3. Fenske, R.A. Ph.D. Thesis University of California, Berkeley, 1984.
4. Durham, W.F.; Wolfe, H.R. Bull. World Health Organization 1962, 26, 75-91.
5. Gloxhuber, C.; Bloching, H. Toxicology Annual 1979, 3, 171-203.
6. Davies, J.E.; Freed, V.H.; Enos, H.F.; Duncan, R.C.; Barquet, A.; Morgade, C.; Peters, L.J.; Danauskas, J.X. J. Occup. Med. 1982, 24, 464-68.
7. Wolfe, H.R.; Durham, W.F.; Armstrong, J.F. Arch. Environ. Health 1967, 14, 622-33.
8. Wolfe, H.R.; Armstrong, J.F.; Staiff, D.C.; Comer, S.W. Arch. Environ. Health 1972, 25, 29-31.
9. Davis, J.E. Residue Reviews 1980, 75, 33-50.

RECEIVED September 24, 1984

Protective Clothing and Its Significance to the Pesticide User

RICHARD V. MORASKI[1] and ALAN P. NIELSEN[2]

[1]Office of Health and Environment Assessment, Office of Research and Development, Exposure Assessment Group, RD–689, Environmental Protection Agency, Washington, DC 20460
[2]Office of Pesticide Programs, Hazard Evaluation Division, TS–769C, Exposure Assessment Branch, Environmental Protection Agency, Washington, DC 20460

Until recent years, research devoted to the pesticide exposure of agricultural workers was essentially nonexistent. It has been established that a major source of exposure to toxic chemicals is the use of such chemicals in agricultural production. In general, applicators and mixer/ loaders have the highest exposure risk. Many studies have shown the exposure to applicators' skin to be well over 90% of their total exposure. The only significant type of barrier available to applicators to reduce dermal contact and hence exposure is protective clothing. Current chemical protective clothing technology clearly demonstrates the lack of knowledge and sound data to permit accurate and appropriate regulatory decisions in regard to specific personal protective devices for various exposure scenarios. Significant work on the effectiveness of personal protective devices in reducing pesticide exposure has recently been initiated. This paper reviews the current state-of-the-art knowledge of protective clothing technology and reviews the research being conducted in an effort to develop protective clothing recommendations with regard to pesticide users.

Pesticides are chemicals that are intentionally introduced into the environment for the control or destruction of pests. In agriculture, pest control is deemed important not only to produce more food but to produce a food product of higher quality. With at least 1400 chemicals serving as active ingredients, more than a billion pounds of pesticide products in various formulations are used yearly in the United States (1). Applicators, mixer/loaders, and workers who enter treated areas to perform tasks such as hand harvesting, cultivation and irrigation chores, scouting, thinning, maintenance, and many other operations, may be exposed to pesticidal residues. The intent of this paper is to present an overview of the current protective clothing technology as it applies to pesticide applicators and related workers.

By law the EPA is mandated to control exposure to chemical
substances including pesticides. The Federal Insecticide, Fungicide,
and Rodenticide Act as amended [FIFRA: §3(d)(1)(c)(i)] and the Code
of Federal Regulations - Title 40 (CFR-40: §162.10, 162.11, 170.2,
171.2, 171.4, and 171.5) state that EPA must establish the conditions
under which pesticidal chemicals are permitted to be used. Each use
of a pesticide requires its own risk assessment which is an expression of the acceptable levels of pesticide exposure. Since the
primary hazard associated with the use of pesticides is the chemical
itself, the potential for illness varies with the length of exposure
and the toxicity level of the pesticide (2, 3). In general, experience and research have shown that applicators and mixer/loaders have
the highest exposure risk. This is especially true of individuals
who perform both tasks. They must deal with exposure to the concentrated formulations while mixing/loading as well as the diluted
chemical during spraying operations.

Exposure Reduction

Pesticides may enter the body through the mouth, lungs, and
skin. The route of entry of greatest significance to the pesticide
user is entry through the skin. It is well documented that
percutaneous absorption of pesticides does occur (4, 5, 6). Dermal
exposure to pesticides, especially to the hands, usually accounts
for more than 90% of the total exposure received (7, 8, 9). Exposure
through inhalation rarely accounts for more than 10% of the exposure
received (7, 8, 9). The one major exception to these figures is
fumigants which are volatile and acutely toxic through inhalation.
Even though the National Institute of Occupational Safety and Health
and the Mine and Health Safety Administration have contributed a
considerable effort in the development of respiratory protection,
it should be noted that very little work has been done to determine
the effectiveness of respirators against pesticides. The least
significant mode of entry during spray operations is through the
mouth (10). Oral exposure usually occurs as the result of ingestion
caused by accidental splashing of liquid into the mouth or by wiping
the face with contaminated clothes, gloves, or hands. Any barrier,
then, that can be placed between the worker and the chemical to
reduce contact with it, should reduce the exposure level and increase
the margin of safety associated with its use.

Our assessment of available types of protective equipment
indicates that there are only two significant means for reducing
worker exposure to pesticides. One is through the use of passive
protective devices such as closed systems. Closed systems have the
potential for eliminating exposure during mixing/loading. Closed
systems, however, do not provide the applicator with any protection
and, because of some unresolved technical problems (11), they are
not universally available or acceptable. The other is through the
use of personal protective devices such as protective clothing whose
purpose is to shield the body from dermal contamination by pesticide
products.

Protective clothing offers the most important means for
minimizing exposure to pesticides during almost any operation
involving these chemicals. However, the protective clothing may

itself become a hazard by its functional and practical limitations,
such as poor design, lack of durability, and inability to be
decontaminated. These and other factors including thermal discomfort,
cost, or loss of dexterity may provide the rationale for workers not
wearing or removing portions of their protective outfits. Carelessness while using pesticides, improper use and inadequate care of
protective equipment may also contribute to reduced levels of protection. In recent years, the development of new types of protective
clothing, which are claimed by the manufacturer to be lightweight,
chemical resistant, strong, and disposable, has provided the needed
stimulation toward technological advances in this area.

Protective Clothing Assessment

Assessing protective clothing technology has become a major
initiative of the Agency. In 1981, a Protective Clothing Working
Group (PCWG) was established within the Office of Pesticide Programs
(OPP) to evaluate the complex problems associated with developing
protective clothing performance standards. The effectiveness or
availability of barriers to reduce or eliminate respiratory or oral
exposure are not within the scope of this effort.

Initial efforts focused on assembling information on the
availability of protective clothing. The "Catalog of Protective
Clothing/Safety Equipment for the Pesticide Applicator" (12)
provides for each entry such as protective clothing, respiratory
protection, and safety equipment, information which includes:
a basic description of the protective measure in terms of functional
and physical characteristics; recommended uses; work practices or
precautions related to use; practical evaluations; costs; advantages
and disadvantages; manufacturers and distributors; and references.
The information assembled suggested that protective clothing and its
effectiveness against pesticides had not received much attention by
clothing manufacturers.

To determine the extent of protective clothing research being
conducted, an exhaustive literature search as well as personal
communication with those in the forefront of protective clothing
research resulted in a second document called "Summary of Research
on Protective Materials for Agricultural Pesticide Uses" (13).
This document provides summaries of past and current (through 1982)
research in protective clothing and related areas. A listing of
all the individuals contacted is included. Based on the information
gathered, suggested research topics are identified for consideration.
Some of those are addressed later in this paper.

A third document was recently completed within the EPA. The
"Guidelines for the Selection of Chemical Protective Clothing,"
(14) for EPA's Office of Occupational Health and Safety is divided
into two volumes. Volume I is intended to be used as a field
manual which presents clothing recommendations for about 300
chemicals using fourteen garment and glove materials. Volume II
discusses permeation theory and test methodology and is more
technical in content. The protective clothing recommendations for
pesticidal compounds found in the Guidelines once again highlight
the fact that little research work has been done in the area of
pesticides and protective clothing.

In addition to these efforts, the PCWG has been working very closely with representatives of the agricultural industry through its trade association, the National Agricultural Chemicals Association, with representatives of the US Department of Agriculture, and with academia in writing a document entitled the "Safe Use of Pesticides During Mixing/Loading and Application." This document will be available to pesticide users as a pamphlet in the near future. It is intended to increase their awareness of the potential hazards of pesticides and the kinds of protective clothing and equipment that should be worn to minimize exposure. In addition, the pamphlet discusses properties of chemicals, types of formulations, cleaning, storage, maintenance of personal protective equipment, and closes with a section on personal hygiene.

Research Needs

Our assessment also indicates that, to date, total elimination of exposure can not be accomplished by the wearing of protective equipment (15, 16, 17). If the Agency is to satisfactorily develop performance standards on protective clothing materials, extensive research is needed in several areas:

1) Laboratory evaluation of the permeability and penetrability of various fabrics by different classes of pesticides and formulation types. Since exposure to the hands seems to be the location of greatest potential dermal exposure, especially during mixing/loading (15, 17, 18), the tesing of various glove materials should receive rather extensive initial attention. In addition, these evaluations could include "normal" clothing materials such as cotton whether treated with repellent finishes or untreated along with other commercially available non-woven clothing materials such as Tyvek or Gore-tex.

2) Field testing on the efficacy of different types of clothing materials in reducing pesticide exposure to applicators and mixer/loaders. Apparel such as coveralls, hats, suits, aprons, hand and foot coverings could be tested under actual agricultural use conditions.

3) The development and standardization of practical test methods to evaluate protective apparel. Two methods recently developed offer promise in the evaluation of the performance of protective clothing:

   a) ASTM Permeation Cell Test Method (19). This method developed by the American Society for Testing and Materials (ASTM) utilizes a test cell which is a dual chambered glass cell approximately 57 mm in width. A piece of the material to be tested is attached between the two chambers. The chemical is admitted into the challenge chamber where it undergoes diffusion/desorption in the material and, through a collection medium, is drawn out of the other side. It is then passed through a sample analyzer such as a gas chromatograph which measures the breakthrough time of the chemical. The test cell is now used for liquid materials and will be modified for use with vapors. This standard ASTM method for permeation testing can be used to determine breakthrough times for pesticides through various clothing or glove materials. It represents, however, a worst case scenario since it is a continuous liquid/fabric interphase, possibly analogous to spills or splashes on clothing. It probably would provide a very good benchmark system for testing protective clothing materials. ASTM also has subcommittees on developing a penetration test method for solids and on the classification of protective clothing.

b) DeJonge Permeation Test Method (20). When first developed, this test method used an enclosed hood over a variable speed conveyor belt where fabric and gauze were layered and attached to wooden frames. The fabric was then passed under a nozzle which sprays the material and the gauze was later analyzed for chemical residues. This method is closer to simulating exposure under actual use conditions, and is currently being modified.

4) The effects of decontamination procedures, such as laundering, on pesticide retention and the protective capability of various fabrics need to be determined.

5) The effects of clothing design, for example, seam leakage, on protective capability need to be determined.

6) The effects of material durability and degradation/wear on the efficacy of protective clothing need to be investigated.

7) A system for maintaining, updating, and disseminating state-of-the-art information for pesticide users needs to be developed so that an increased hazard awareness by more knowledgeable workers results in greater voluntary acceptability of protective clothing.

Currently, the Agency has directed its efforts in the following areas of research on chemical protective clothing:

1) The evaluation of dermal exposure to applicators by using fluorescent tracers in the spray tank to monitor the type and extent of worker exposure. This work is being conducted at the University of California-Berkeley under Richard Fenske and Thomas Leffingwell. A sophisticated computervideo processing system is being tested to quantify pesticide exposure to garments as well as the determination of the extent of pesticide residues penetrating the clothing to the skin.

2) At the University of Florida, Institute of Food and Agricultural Sciences, Agricultural Research and Education Center in Lake Alfred, Florida, Herbert N. Nigg is conducting research on the the efficacy of protective clothing while spraying dicofol (Kelthane) in citrus groves. In addition Dr. Nigg will be investigating thermal comfort of the protective clothing by directly measuring

temperatures both on the outside of the garment worn and on
the workers' skin using small thermistor probes.
3) The penetrability of garment materials by different classes
   of pesticides and formulation types is being investigated
   in the laboratory by Jacquelyn Orlando DeJonge, Head of
   the Department of Textiles, Merchandising and Design,
   College of Home Economics at the University of Tennessee in
   Knoxville.
   Dr. DeJonge will be screening different garment materials
   for Dr. Nigg's field studies in a contained spray apparatus
   to simulate some nozzle types and spray pressures used in
   the field.
4) Using the ASTM permeation cell, the Oil and Hazardous
   Materials Spills Branch of the Office of Environmental
   Engineering and Technology, Office of Research and
   Development, US EPA will initially test various glove
   materials including viton, natural rubber, butyl rubber,
   and nitrile rubber against organophosphorous pesticides
   currently in use.

Development of Protective Clothing Recommendations

Our goal is to develop recommendations that are consistent
with the toxicity of the chemicals being used. While there has
been an increased recognition of the limitations of protective
clothing, there has also been an increased awareness of the hazards
of exposure to potentially toxic pesticides without adequate or
appropriate protection. Our aims are to identify protective
clothing that the pesticide user, the pesticide registrant, and the
pesticide regulator would find effective and acceptable and to
recommend protective clothing and equipment on the pesticide label
where appropriate to protect against any unreasonable risk to man.

Protective clothing labeling recommendations are made not only
to protect the pesticide user against acutely toxic materials but
also to protect against potential chronic hazards. The toxicological
or precautionary statement matrix, consisting of prepared label
statements based on the four categories of toxicity levels as
determined by acute laboratory animal studies (CFR-40, §162.10),
provides guidance for protective clothing labeling recommendations.
The categories in the matrix to which the Working Group is paying
particular attention are Categories I and II for Acute Dermal
Toxicity (dermal LD_{50} Category I: $\leq$ 200 mg/kg and Category II:
200 − 2000 mg/kg). The only difference between Category I and II
label statements are the words, "Fatal if absorbed through skin..."
rather than "May be fatal if absorbed through skin..." The following
appears as a precautionary statement for chemicals in both
categories: "Wear protective clothing and rubber gloves...Remove
contaminated clothing and wash before reuse."

Day to day evaluation of potential pesticide hazards through
the various Agency registration review processes clearly indicates
the need for developing information on personal protective
equipment. When dealing with Category I and II pesticides, long
sleeved shirts and long legged pants may not provide adequate
protection from exposure. In addition, recommending the use of

impermeable clothing that has not been tested for its chemical
resistance in standardized laboratory and/or field trials may not
result in the level of protection sought. Making the proper
protective clothing recommendation depends not only on the toxicity
of the pesticide but on the physical-chemical interaction of the
protective clothing material and the pesticide formulation as well.
Testing protective clothing materials using the procedures described
in this paper will allow specific protective clothing recommendations to be made for specific pesticide use situations. EPA is
currently addressing protective clothing requirements as they relate
to farmworker safety under 40 CFR §170-Worker Protection Standards
for Agricultural Pesticides.

Protective clothing requirements, as a regulatory option, will
become more and more important not only when dealing with acutely
toxic pesticides but also for dealing with pesticides identified as
potentially causing chronic toxic effects. There is a need not
only to develop appropriate performance standards and to reflect
these standards on labels, but also to effectively communicate
these developments to those who use or are exposed to pesticides.
Educational programs that stress the relationship between toxicity
category of the pesticide and the protective clothing recommendation
are suggested. With this renewed emphasis in working more safely
with pesticides, it is hoped that the use of protective
clothing will become a reality.

Our overall opinion is that a well coordinated effort is
needed to eventually resolve the pertinent issues. We urge
scientists or organizations that have laboratory or field performance
data on pesticides and personal protective equipment to share that
information with us.

Nontechnical Summary

Protective clothing provides the most important means for
minimizing exposure to pesticides during mixing/loading,
application, and other pesticide operations. However, functional
limitations, thermal discomfort and cost are among the reasons
pesticide users may not wear their protective outfits. The US EPA
is evaluating current protective clothing technology for the
purpose of developing performance standards.   These standards will
be reflected in the precautionary statements found on pesticide
container labels which are made to protect the pesticide user
against not only acutely toxic materials but also against chronic
hazards. Current and future research needs are discussed.

Literature Cited

1. "Your Guide to the Environmental Protection Agency," U.S.
   Environmental Protection Agency. OPA 138/0, 1980.
2. Durham, W. F.; Wolfe, J. H.; Elliot, J. W. Arch. Environ. Health
   1972, 24, 381-387.
3. Maddy, K. T.; Smith, C. R.; Kilgore, S. L. "Occupational Illnesses and Injuries of Mixers and Loaders of Pesticides in
   California as Reported by Physicians in 1980," California Department of Food and Agriculture, Report No. HS955, 1981.

4. Maibach, H. I.; Feldman, R. J.; Milby T. H.; Serat, W. F. Arch. Environ. Health 1971, 23, 208-211.
5. Serat, W. F.; Feldman R. J.; Maibach, H. I. Natn. Pest Control Operator NEWS 1973, October.
6. Feldman, R. J.; Maibach, H. I.; Toxic. Appl. Pharmacol. 1974, 28, 126-132.
7. Wolfe, H. R. Weeds, Trees and Turf 1973, 12(4), 12.
8. Wolfe, H. R.; Durham, W. F.; Armstrong, J. F. Arch. Environ. Health 1967, 14, 622-633.
9. Wolfe, H. R.; Armstrong, J. F.; Staiff, D. C.; Comer, S. W. Arch. Environ. Health 1967, 25, 29-31.
10. Bohmont, B. L. "The New Pesticide User's Guide," Reston Publishing Company, Inc.: Reston, VA, 1983; Chap. 8.
11. Jacobs, W. W. "Closed Systems for Mixing and Loading," at the Determination and Assessment of Pesticide Exposure Workshop, USDA, NJAES, US EPA; Hershey, PA, 1980.
12. Russell, L. S. "Catalog of Protective Clothing/Safety Equipment for the Pesticide Applicator," U.S. Environmental Protection Agency, 1981.
13. Bodden, M.; Cioffi, J.; Fong, V.; McLaughlin, M.; Russell, S. "Summary of Research on Protective Materials for Agricultural Pesticide Uses," U.S. Environmental Protection Agency, 1983.
14. Schwope, A. D.; Costas, P. P.; Jackson, J. O.; Weitzman, D. J.; "Guidelines for the Selection of Chemical Protective Clothing," Volumes I and II, U.S. Environmental Protection Agency, 1983.
15. Dubelman, S.; Lauer, R.; Arras, D. D.; Adams, S. A. J. Agric. Food Chem., 1982, 30, 528-532.
16. Sheets, T. J. "Exposure of Hand Harvesters to MH in the Field, Final Report," 1980, Agricultural Research Service, North Carolina State University, Raleigh, NC.
17. "Applicator and Mixer/Loader Exposure to Pesticides During Ground Boom Spraying Operations," Draft Report, 1981, U.S. Environmental Protection Agency.
18. Maddy, K. T.; Winter, C.; Cepello, S.; Fredrickson, A. S. "Monitoring of Potential Occupational Exposure of Mixer/Loaders, Pilots, and Flaggers During Application of Phosdrin (Mevinphos) in Imperial County in 1981," California Department of Food and Agriculture, Report No. HS-899 Rev., 1982.
19. "Standard Test Method for Resistance of Protective Clothing Materials to Permeation by Hazardous Liquid Chemicals: Designation F 739-81," American Society for Testing and Materials, Annual Book of ASTM Standards, 1981.
20. Orlando, J.; Branson, D.; Ayers, G.; Leavitt, R. J. Environ. Sci. Health, 1981, B 16(5), 617-628.

RECEIVED September 24, 1984

Protective Apparel Research

JACQUELYN O. DeJONGE, ELIZABETH P. EASTER[1], KAREN K. LEONAS, and
RUTH M. KING[2]

Department of Textiles, Merchandising and Design, University of Tennessee, Knoxville,
TN 37996-1900

Recent studies on decontamination, penetration and
protective apparel selections by agricultural workers
have resulted in the following conclusions:
(1) pesticide decontamination is similar to other soil
removal studies, with oil based pesticides being more
difficult to remove from synthetic fabrics; (2) functional finishes have a significant effect on the
penetration of pesticides through fabrics; (3) cost has
greater influence over user preferences for protective
apparel than protection or thermal characteristics.
Captan removal was better on synthetic fabrics than
cotton where particles were entrapped in the weave.
Guthion (oil based) was more difficult to remove from
oleophilic synthetic fabrics. Both pesticides had
increased removal with increased wash temperatures.
Preliminary studies show fluorocarbon finishes may
impede penetration of pesticides. Successful
protective apparel must incorporate cost restraints
while providing both protection and comfort.

The University of Tennessee has an ongoing research program in
protective apparel for pesticide applicators. This research began at
Michigan State University in 1978 and was continued at The University
of Tennessee in 1980 where, up to this point, 4 Ph.D. dissertations
have been completed on this subject, and one is in progress.
Research topics which have been reported in the past include the
thermal comfort of protective apparel (1), the deposition on the
pesticide applicator during air blast spraying (2), users'
preferences for protective apparel (3), the decontamination of
pesticide contaminated fabric (4), and the penetration of pesticides
through fabric (5). This paper reports on 3 recent studies:
decontamination, penetration, and user preference for protective
apparel.

[1]Current address: Box 464, Irvine, KY 40336
[2]Current address: Kentucky State University, Frankfort, KY 40601

0097-6156/85/0273-0403$06.00/0
© 1985 American Chemical Society

Decontamination Study

The first project on the removal of pesticide residues from fabrics
by laundering or "pesticide decontamination" was a part of a doctoral
dissertation by Elizabeth Easter and is published in the March 1983
AATCC journal (4). This project was undertaken to determine if a
relationship does in fact exist between the removal of pesticide
residues and the removal of common soil. In textiles, "soiling"
denotes the undesirable accumulation of oily and/or particulate
materials on fabrics (6). As significant levels of pesticide
residues in workers' clothing have been reported by researchers,
these socalled "contaminated" fabrics may also be defined as "soiled"
fabrics (5, 7, 8).
        Previous research aimed at removing pesticide residues from
contaminated fabrics has been directed at removal of a particular
pesticide chemical and/or formulation of pesticide, with no effect
toward comparing the pesticide residue's composition to that of
common soil. Fabric selection for this study allowed a comparison of
both hydrophilic and hydrophobic fibers and the effect of fabric type
on soil removal. Two fabrics were identified for the study. Denim
was 100% cotton fabric of twill weave dyed with indigo dyes. This
fabric was 14 ounce, comparable to the heavy weight denim found in
jeans. The second fabric was Gore Tex, a three layer structure
consisting of an outer layer of rip-stop nylon and an inner layer of
nylon tricot laminated to a film. The film was a micro-porous,
polymeric film or polytetrafluoroethylene (PTFE). Previous studies
on pesticide penetration found Gore Tex to be impermeable to
pesticides. Thermal comfort studies found it to be relatively
comfortable, similar in comfort to the commonly worn denim jeans and
a chambray shirt.
        All fabrics were initially stripped of sizing by washing them
one complete cycle, using an adaptation of the procedure outlined in
AATCC Test Method 135-78: " Dimensional changes in Automatic Home
Laundering of Woven and Knit Fabrics." The fabrics were then cut into
a sample size of 6 x 6 inches. The denim fabric was clean finished
with a zigzig stitch.
        Two pesticides were used in this study: Captan, a fungicide,
and Guthion, an insecticide. The Captan formulation was an aqueous
suspension of pesticide particles in the 10 micron range. The actual
composition of the inert ingredients of this fomulation is proprietary information; however, it is sufficient to know that the
ingredients were clay-like materials. Based on the composition of
the formulation, Captan residues on the fabrics were considered to be
particulate soils. Guthion was used in the emulsifiable concentrate
formulation and was a homogenous dispersion of active ingredients in
an organic solvent, with an addition of an emulsifier. Based on the
composition of the emulsifiable concentrate formulation, Guthion
residues on the fabrics were considered to be oily soils.
        The study was designed as a factorial experiment with three
factors: fabrics (two); soil as pesticide residues (two); and wash
temperatures (three). Two replications were analyzed for each
combination of factors. For this study a chamber was designed to
simulate a field spraying application and was used to expose fabric
samples to a uniformly dispersed pesticide spray. A .12% pesticide

solution was delivered by a full-cone impingement nozzle, at a height of 10 inches above the fabric surface. The fabric samples were mounted on a tenter-frame type holder designed to fit into the chamber at a 90° angle to the nozzle. The contamination was accomplished by exposing the sample at 10 second intervals of the pesticide spray. The contaminated fabric was allowed to dry on the holder at room temperature.

The actual soil content (level of pesticide contamination) of the fabrics was determined by quantitative analysis procedures. In this approach, the amount of soil actually present in the fabrics before and after laundering is measured. The analysis procedure in this study involved the separation of the soil (pesticide residues) from the fabrics by solvent extraction and analysis of the extracts by gas chromotography.

Prior to contamination of the fabric sample, a 3 x 3 inch specimen was marked in the center of the sample. After contamination and/or laundering, the specimen was cut from the sample and transferred to a flask. A 50 milliliter portion of solvent was added, and the flask was shaken for 30 minutes using a Burrell Wrist-Action shaker. Preliminary testing of the extraction procedures showed that the acetone gave the highest percent recovery for the pesticide Guthion, and hexane was the most efficient solvent for the extraction of Captan.

The extracts were analyzed on a Varian 3700 gas chromatograph. A nitrogen-phosphorus specific thermionic detector (TSD) was used in the analysis of the Guthion and an electron capture detector (ECD) was used to analyze Captan. Conditions for analysis of Guthion were as follows: .318 cm x 1.8 m glass column (3% SE-30); gas carrier, helium; column oven 240C; detector 300C. Conditions for analysis of Captan were as follows: .318 cm x 1.8 m glass column (4% SE-30/6%OV-210); gas carrier, nitrogen; column oven 220C; detector 300C. The sample size was 2 microliters injected using a Hamilton 710-10 microliter syringe. Two replications per sample were injected and an average of the two reported in micrograms/square centimeter.

AATCC Test Method 61-75: "Colorfastness to Washing, Domestic; and Laundering, Commercial: Accelerated," and International Standard Method C06 were modified to establish the laundry procedure to simulate one home laundering cycle. An Atlas Launder-Ometer equipped with stainless steel canisters was used. Teflon liners were used in the lids to prevent retention of pesticides by the rubber gaskets. Abrasive action was provided by the placement of 25 steel balls in each canister.

Liquid-All, a heavy duty concentrate containing both anionic and nonionic surfactants, was used. The wash liquor was made up of .25% detergent concentration, based on the manufacturers' recommendation. The pH of the wash liquor was measured and found to be 9.20 ± .2. Variations in the water temperature were used to enable the evaluation of the effect of temperature on pesticide removal. The wash water temperatures were 38, 49 and 60°C. The corresponding rinse water temperatures were 28, 39 and 49°C. Following the completion of the wash and rinse cycles, the fabric samples were removed from the canisters and hung on a wire rack and allowed to hang at room temperature (25 ± 3C) until dry. The fabric samples were then extracted and the extracts analyzed.

An analysis of variance procedure was used to test for main effects (temperature, pesticide composition and fabric) and interaction of the main effects. Further examination of all possible pairwise comparisons of treatment means for the dependent variables which produced a significant $\underline{F}$ test was carried out with a Duncan's Multiple Range post hoc procedure. Overall, the laundry process removed a relatively high percentage of the initial pesticde contamination, as pesticide residues in the range of 72.7% to 99.8% were removed. Differences in removing pesticide residues by laundering were dependent on soil composition (pesticide residues), substrate (fabrics) and water temperature.

For the pesticide Captan, an analysis of variance showed that significant differences (.05 level) were attributable to fabrics during the removal of Guthion residues; post hoc analysis revealed that fabric means were significantly different for both denim and Gore Tex (Table I). The mean percentages removed from 100% cotton denim were lower in cumulative percent removal compared to Gore Tex. Denim retained the largest percentage of Captan residues, regardless of wash water temperatures. However, differences at 60°C were small. This finding may be attributed to fabric weave, fiber morphology and the formulation of the pesticide in combination with the denim fabric. The greater irregularities of the staple cotton yarn and the more open weave of denim strongly suggest more extensive physical opportunities for particulate soils to accumulate on them than on the smooth, round fibers such as nylon. The Captan residues performed similarly to a particulate soil. One possible explanation of this finding may be attributed to the clay-like materials of the inert ingredients of the Captan formulation. The possibility exists that these clay-like particles may be bound to the active ingredient of the pesticide. Geometric bonding was considered the principal mechnanism affecting the affinity of cotton toward particulate soils in the absence of oils; that is, particles are trapped in fiber surface crevices or trapped in fiber interstices.

Table I. Captan and Guthion Residues Retained by Fabrics and Removal by Laundering as a Function of Temperature

		Captan		Guthion	
		Denim	Gore Tex	Denim	Gore Tex
T_1					
	residue μg/cm	2.86	0.24	0.46	1.09
	removal %	72.70	97.80	94.30	86.40
T_2					
	residue μg/cm	0.24	0.03	0.30	0.76
	removal %	97.80	99.70	96.30	90.60
T_3					
	residue μg/cm	0.04	0.03	0.17	0.69
	removal	99.60	99.80	97.90	91.50
	T_1 = 38°C; T_2 = 49°C; T_3 = 60°C				

For the pesticide Guthion, residues retained by fabrics after laundering ranged from 86.4%-97.9%. An analysis of variance showed that significant differences (.05 level) were attributable to fabrics during the removal of Guthion residues; post hoc analysis revealed that fabric means were significantly different for denim and Gore Tex.

The lowest percentage removal of Guthion residues was shown by Gore Tex. An interpretaion of the finding must include a look at the chemical composition of the pesticide formulation as well as the fiber content of the fabric. Guthion 2S formulation was an oil based concentrate containing 43% petroleum distillates. The chemical composition of Gore Tex includes the nylon fiber as well as the PTFE film, both of which were expected to exhibit hydrophobic properties, and the oleophilic tendencies of the nylon fiber have been widely reported. This may explain both the increased removal of Captan residues exhibited by Gore Tex over 100% cotton denim, and the lower percent removal of Guthion residues. Suspended nonoily particulate soil should be more easily removed from the Gore Tex, since the soil should be concentrated mainly on the smooth surfaces and possess little affinity for nylon and the PTFE film. In addition, the lower surface energies of nylon and PTFE compared to cotton would facilitate removal of nonattractive soils. However, Guthion, with its oil based formulation, should possess greater affinity for nylon than cotton and so be less responsive to removal by laundering, as was found in this study.

The difficulty of removing oily soils involves not only the possibility of geometric entrapment of soils on the surface of the textile but also fiber/soil interaction. The components of oily soils have been shown to diffuse below the fiber surface and become molecularly entangled in the body of the filaments, or they may permeate the polymer itself. When this diffusion does occur, the soiled fabrics are more difficult to clean.

In looking specifically at the effects of temperature, an analysis of variance showed that the temperature effect was significant (.05 level) for both Captan and Guthion residue removal. Overall, an increase in temperature resulted in an increase in pesticide removal. This may be partially attributed to the theory that higher temperatures favor increased soil removal by increasing the kinetic energy of the particles. Other effects due to an increase in temperature may be due to a reduction in the viscosity of the wash liquor and/or the soil itself, which should intensify the Brownian motion of the particles. In addition, an increase in temperature may influence the solubility of the surfactant, and the surfactant may become less hydrated at higher temperatures and hence more surface active, thereby enhancing its cleaning power.

In conclusion, soil composition (pesticide residue) played an important role in controlling fabric/soil interactions. Captan, an aqueous suspension of particles, was more difficult to remove in 100% cotton denim. This was attributed to particle size and the clay-like nature of the materials comprising the pesticide formulation. Guthion, an oil based formulation, was more difficult to remove from Gore Tex. This fabric, predominantly nylon, has oleophilic tendencies. The difficulty of removing oily soils from oleophilic fibers has been reported by researchers as a serious problem in all soil removal studies. Based on the findings of this study, the removal of pesticide residues from fabrics contaminated with pesticides is similar to the removal of common soil.

Finishes and Pesticide Penetration

The second study is on the functional finish effectiveness in providing a barrier to pesticide exposure. This study is currently in progress at The University of Tennessee Karen Leonas, a Ph.D. candidate. The purpose of this study is to determine if fabrics treated with functional finishes are more effective in the prevention of pesticide penetration than the same fabrics that have not been treated. The study is being conducted with the Agriculture Experiment Station S-163 Regional Project.

The fabrics used in this study were prepared by the Southern Regional Lab especially for the 13 states involved in the S-163 Project. They include: 100% cotton, 100% polyester, and a 50/50 cotton/polyester blend. Fabrics are print cloth, woven construction, with a thread count of 70W x 78F, 3.5 ounce per square yard. All fabrics were wet finished and heat set. A durable press finish (DMDHEU) was applied to cotton and cotton/polyester fabrics. A water repellent fluorocarbon finish (Corpel) and an acrylic acid soil-release finish were applied to all three types of fabrics. Our preliminary findings for the AATCC spray test are reported here.

The AATCC Water Repellency Spray Test measures the resistance of fabrics to wetting by water. It does not measure penetration of liquid through fabric, but is a good preliminary scouting technique for penetration. The test specimen is fastened securely in the 6 in metal hoop. The hoop is then placed on the stand of the tester so that the fabric is uppermost in such a position that coincides with the center of the hoop. Two hundred fifty ml of distilled water at $27 \pm 1C$ is poured into the funnel of the tester and allowed to spray onto the test specimen. The hoop is then taken by one edge and the opposite edge tapped smartly once against a solid object, with the fabric facing the object, then rotated 180° and tapped once more on the point previously held. Then the wet or spotted pattern is compared with the rating chart. The test specimen is assigned a rating corresponding to the nearest standard in the rating chart. Intermediate ratings are not given. A mean score is then calculated from the replications for each sample.

This standard test was performed on each fabric, with and without the finishes. Each sample was tested without laundering and after 10, 30 and 50 launderings. The results for all of the samples except those with a fluorocarbon finish was 0, that is, a complete wetting of the whole upper and lower surfaces. All of the fluoro-carbon finished fabrics showed an increase in wetting with increased launderings (Table II). Overall, polyester performed the best followed by the cotton/polyester blend and then cotton. Based upon these findings, we are currently testing the cotton, cotton/polyester and 100% polyester fabrics with a fluorocarbon finish in our pesticide spray chamber with two pesticides: Galecron and methyl parathion.

Table II. Spray Test Ratings for Fluorocarbon Finished Fabrics
As a Function of Launderings

Fabrics	Times Laundered			
	0	10	30	50
cotton	80	70	63	50
cotton/poly	80	70	70	70
poly	100	77	80	80

User Garment Preference

The final study reported here was just completed by Ruth King, a
Doctoral student at The University of Tennessee. The intent of the
study was to evaluate the effects of perceived product attributes of
functionally designed protective apparel and of risk related factors
influencing the adoption/purchase decision (9). This discussion will
focus on the first objective, which was to determine if significant
differences existed between garment selection when information was
withheld relative to the product attributes of cost, comfort and
penetration.

A two part mailed questionnaire was used to ascertain subject
responses. Part I was limited to the illustration of protective
apparel products, with descriptions and fabric samples for each.
Part II consisted of five response categories: garment selection,
product attributes, risk perception, risk handling tactics and
demographic data. Four different questionnaire types were used for
Part I. One contained all of the information, whereas either
penetration, cost or comfort information was withheld from the
remaining three. A scaled response, 1 through 5 range, was employed
for each variable. Commercial catalogs were used in the final
selection of the 6 garments used in Part I of the questionnaire.
These 6 garments were randomly ordered for their presentation in the
questionnaire. They consisted of:

Garment #1. Gore Tex coveralls, style A, prototype, not available on
the consumer market – highly recommended for safety and comfort,
cost–$150;
Garment # 2. Tyvek coverall – minimum protection from pesticide
penetration, uncomfortable in hot weather, cost–$8.50;
Garment #3. Neoprene overalls, jacket and hat – highly recommended
for safety but not for comfort, cost–$60.75;
Garment #4. Tyvek treated with Sarenex coveralls – highly
recommended for protection from pesticide penetration, uncomfortable
in hot weather, cost–$26.50;
Garment #5. Denim jeans and chambray shirt – not recommended for
safety, comfortable in hot weather, cost–$19.48;
Garment #6. Gore Tex coveralls, style B – highly recommended for
safety and comfort, cost–$150.

In Part II of the questionnaire the subjects were instructed to
check the location on the scale that best described their likelihood
to purchase or not to purchase the garment. The scale ranged from
1 to 5, from "likely not to purchase" to "likely to purchase".

A higher rating would indicate a greater potential of adoption/
purchase intention.

Participants in this sample were selected from the 5 Agricultural Extension Service districts which include 95 counties in the
State of Tennessee. The sample population consisted of 906
agricultural workers likely to be involved in the application of
pesticides. The final data base was comprised of 421 respondents, a
47% response rate. Sixty-three percent of the subjects were actively
engaged in fruit growing, with a total acreage of 5 or less. Sixty
percent of the respondents were involved in tobacco growing , with an
acreage of 5 or less also. Field crops and livestock/dairy were the
major type of farm operations, either in combination or as separate
units. Over 80% of the respondents were the principal person
involved in pesticide application. Less than 10% was attributed to
commercial applicators. The greatest number of the sample was in the
25-34 years age group. Ninety-five percent of the total population
had at least attained high school or above education. Thirty five
percent had attained at least a high school education; forty four
percent an associate or 4 year degree; and 11 percent attended
graduate school.

The complete randomized, block design was used to profile the
four sample groups representing the four subsets of information
withheld in 6 garment choices. Group #1 consisted of all information
regarding garment characteristics. For group #2, penetration
information was withheld. Cost information was not provided subjects
in group #3. Information pertaining to comfort was denied subjects
in group #4. An analysis of variance was used to determine the
significance of information on respondents' choices of garment
selection. Garment selection was found to be significant for all
groups.

Once the garment selection was found to be significant, means
were partitioned via Duncan's Multiple Range Test to determine how
garment choices differentiated when information was withheld on
penetration, cost and comfort. The impact of withholding information
on subjects' garment choice varied across groups. Jeans and chambray
shirts were the first preference for three of the four groups, the
exception being group #3. When cost information was absent to group
#3, the mean of Gore Tex garment (A) was not significantly different
from the other groups. Jeans and chambray shirt were clearly the
first preference for all groups, with the exception of the group not
receiving cost information.

Contrast statements were then formulated to investigate the
change occurring in garment preferences when certain information was
absent. Data indicates there was a decisive shift in garment
selections in the presence of all information versus the absence of
information. Greater effects were observed when the cost variable
was not present for the two higher Gore Tex garments, (F value 31.61
and 28.7). The next significant difference was attributed to the
penetration variable when associated with jeans and chambray shirt,
and Gore Tex, style A, garment, an initial conclusion being: cost is
likely to have the greatest impact on subjects' choices. Also,
subjects are more likely to assume the risk associated with penetration, even when adequate information is available, if the cost factor
is apparent. Moderate variations were evident in the absence of

comfort information for the two Tyvek and Neoprene garments. No
significant changes were shown for the two Tyvek, Neoprene, nor Gore
Tex, style B, garments when penetration information was withheld.
The fact that jeans and chambray shirt were a first choice in the
presence of penetration information implies a greater value is placed
on cost versus safety or comfort. Subjects are willing to accept the
risk in lieu of paying the price.

Summary

Current research at The University of Tennessee in protective apparel
for pesticide applicators has investigated decontamination,
penetration and user preference for protective apparel. The
decontamination studies found pesticides behaved similarly to soil
removal, with oily based soils being more difficult to remove from
synthetic fabrics and particulate soil being more difficult to remove
from woven natural fabrics. Initial studies on the effect of fabric
finishes on pesticide penetration found a fluorocarbon finish was
most effective. There was, however, an increase in penetration with
increased launderings of the finished fabric. In a survey of user
preference of available garments, cost was the predominant factor
affecting choice, ranking above either safety or comfort.

Although additional studies are needed in the areas of
penetration of pesticides through fabric and in thermal comfort, the
acceptability of the final product to the consumer must not be
overlooked. This last study indicates the effect that cost has on
product acceptance. The cost factor is likely to be the more
influential criteria in purchase/adoption decisions and should not be
overlooked when the ideal garment is being designed for maximum
protection and comfort.

Literature Cited

1. Branson, D. H. Ph.D. Thesis, Michigan State University, 1982.
2. DeJonge, J. O.; Ayres, G.; Branson, D. Home Economics Research
    J. Submitted June, 1984.
3. DeJonge, J. O.; Vredevoogd, J.; Henry, M. S. Clothing and
    Textiles Research J. 1983-84, 2, 9-14.
4. Easter, E. P. Textile Chemist and Colorist 1983, 15, 47-51.
5. Orlando, J.; Branson, D.; Ayres, G.; Leavitt, R. J. Environ-
    mental Science and Health 1981, B16, 615-628.
6. Kissa, E. Textile Research J. 1971, 41, 750.
7. Finley, E. L.; Rogillio, J. R. B. Bulletin of Environmental
    Contamination and Toxicology 1969, 4, 343.
8. Finley, E. L.; Metcalfe, G. I.; McDermott, F. G. Bulletin of
    Environmental Contamination and Toxicology 1974, 12, 268.
9. King, R. M. Ph.D. Thesis, The University of Tennessee, 1984.

RECEIVED August 28, 1984

Minimizing Pesticide Exposure Risk
for the Mixer-Loader, Applicator, and Field Worker

ACIE C. WALDRON

North Central Region Pesticide Impact Assessment Program, Department of Entomology, Ohio
State University, Columbus, OH 43210

Final control in minimizing hazards from pesticides
rests with individual agricultural workers. Research
shows that use of proper protective clothing and equipment and observing re-entry intervals can provide adequate protection to workers. Approximately 97.5% of the
herbicides applied to major crops in Ohio in 1982 was
of the slightly toxic categories, but almost 60% of the
insecticides were highly or moderately toxic. Herbicides accounted for 90.5% of the 30 million pounds of
pesticide a.i. applied and insecticides for 9.0%. Over
99% of the corn and soybean acreages were treated for
weed control and 43% of the corn and alfalfa acreages
for insects. More than 80% of the farmers wore gloves,
head covering and long-sleeved, long-legged work
clothes in mixing/loading pesticides regardless of
toxicity but the percentages were far less for application and use of eye, face and respiratory protection.

Pesticides are evaluated based upon their toxicity, exposure, hazard,
efficacy and economics. But a distinction must be made between toxicity, exposure and hazard. The formulation and use pattern, to some
extent determine the potential hazard. The intrinsic toxicity of a
substance, per se, although of importance, is less significant in
determining hazard. Gathering information on the numbers and types
of people exposed to various concentrations of a pesticide may be
just as important in evaluating the hazard involved as is determining
the potential for toxicity. Some of the more toxic active ingredients are used at relatively low dosage rates by a limited number of
trained technical persons and may result in exposure hazards that may
be lower than that from less toxic active ingredients used at higher
dosage rates and perhaps by less adequately trained personnel.
 Pesticide related health hazards are more generally directed
towards the pesticide handler and applicator than any other segment
of the population. However, it is possible that the field worker,
who enters the pesticide treated field for various reasons, sometimes
soon after a pesticide application, may be a greater potential victim
because of less knowledge of and protection from pesticide residues.

0097-6156/85/0273-0413$06.00/0
© 1985 American Chemical Society

Thus, it is extremely important that all workers who come in contact with pesticide chemicals and/or residues be thoroughly familiar with and practice proper methods of protection. Research, extension teaching, pesticide regulations and legislation, and applicator certification programs have been directed to reduce the pesticide risks.

The bottom line in the determination of pesticide hazard to field workers, mixer/loaders and applicators of pesticides involves the evaluation of levels of exposure to the individual that result from given use patterns. Accurate assessment of the potential health impacts requires evaluation of the pesticide toxicity, the type and amount used, the procedures of handling and application, and the techniques of personal protection. The program of conducting pesticide use surveys, including also questions on user safety, has been a part of the Pesticide Impact Assessment Program (PIAP) in the states of the North Central Region (NCR), as well as in some other states in the nation, since 1978. Initially it started as a regional funded program, but it is now conducted in interested states from state PIAP funds. Agencies in the federal government have also, in the past few years, recognized the importance of obtaining factual pesticide use information, in contrast to earlier estimates, as vital to making the best decisions. The Interagency Pesticide Data Planning Group, chaired by the Office of Pesticide Programs (OPP) of the Environmental Protection Agency (EPA) and consisting of representatives from EPA, the United States Department of Agriculture (USDA), Food and Drug Administration (FDA), Animal and Plant Health Inspection Service (APHIS), Association of Agricultural Pest Control Officials (AAPCO), the Agricultural Census Bureau, and the State PIAP conduct an ongoing program of coordinated pesticide use surveys of importance to the decision making process.

Much NCRPIAP research has been directed toward the determination of the risk factors related to applicator and field worker exposure to pesticides. Several such research papers have been presented in this symposium and others have already appeared in print. This presentation may reiterate some data that have already been reported and attempt to correlate such with pesticide use and personal protection data obtained through surveys. Pesticide usage data reported herein are that obtained in the 1982 survey of major field crops in Ohio (10) but are applicable to most states, particularly in the North Central Region, involved in corn, soybean, grain and alfalfa production as noted in the regional survey of 1978 (11).

Pesticide Use in Ohio

The Ohio Crop Reporting Service (OCRS) reported that there were 93,000 farms in Ohio in 1982 with a total of approximately 16,200,000 acres. Approximately 69.5% of the acreage was planted to major field crops and 15% in pasture. Almost 16% of the major field crop acreage was in Integrated Pest Management (IPM) programs. Conventional land tillage practices prevailed for 67.4% of the acreage followed by 27.2% for minimum tillage and 5.4% for no-tillage. The largest percentage of no-tillage acreage was 9.8% for corn. Ninety-six percent of the farmers used chemical pest control practices, but 87.6, 78.2, 68.2, 8.2, 4.9 and 0.9% also used crop rotation, resistant varieties, cultivation, biological control, organic farming, or no control, respectively.

In 1982, farmers producing major field crops in Ohio used 29,334,000 lbs of pesticide active ingredient (a.i.) with 90.5% of that being herbicides (10), 9.0% insecticides, and 0.5% fungicides and other materials. Over 99% of the corn and soybean acreages was treated for weed control with considerably lower percents for other crops. Approximately 43% of the corn and alfalfa acreages was treated for insect control.

Farmers applied 81% of the herbicides, 93% of the insecticides and 92% of the fungicides to 82, 94 and 92%, respectively, of the pesticide treated acreage. Of those farmers involved in handling pesticides, 97.3% performed the complete process of mixing, loading and applying the pesticides and 72% were certified applicators.

Approximately 91.4% of the pesticides applied to Ohio major field crops was of toxicity category III or IV (Table I). Only 2.5%

Table I. Quantities of Pesticides Applied to Major Field Crops in Ohio in 1982 Relative to Dermal Toxicity

Class of Pesticide	Pesticide Active Ingredient Applied 1000 lbs. a.i. & (percent of class)			
	Category I	Category II	Category III	Category IV
Herbicides	126.1 (0.5)	533.9 (2.0)	25051.6 (94.3)	855.4 (3.2)
Insecticides	809.8 (30.1)	1044.5 (28.8)	819.5 (30.5)	16.4 (0.6)
Fungicides	0	0	14.3 (31.4)	31.2 (68.6)
Other[a]	0	6.2 (19.8)	25.1 (80.2)	0
Total	935.9 (3.2)	1584.6 (5.4)	25910.5 (88.3)	903.0 (3.1)

[a]Includes paraquat in Category II as a defoliant for soybeans and Maleic hydrazide in Category III for sucker control in tobacco.

of the herbicides, none of the fungicides and 19.8% of the chemicals used for "other" control (paraquat as a defoliant for soybeans) were more toxic than category III. However, over 30% of the insecticides applied were of category I and almost 29% of category II. Greater than 93% of the acre-treatments with herbicides consisted of chemical products in the slightly toxic or lower categories (Table II). The major exceptions are listed in Tables IV and V. On the other hand 78.3% of the acre-treatments with insecticides consisted of those products classified as highly or moderately toxic, including "restricted use" (Table III).

Five pesticides in the slightly toxic category constituted 91.4% of all herbicides used on corn and 80.5% of the acre-treatments. These were atrazine, alachlor, metolachlor, cyanazine and butylate (Table VI). Alachlor and metolachlor constituted 62.1% of the quantity of herbicide use on soybeans but only on 38.9% of the acre-treatments. Metribuzin, linuron and chloramben of category III and trifluralin from category IV were used for 52.7% of the soybean acre-treatments. EPTC was the prevalent herbicide used for alfalfa and MCPA for small grains. In addition to the herbicide data listed in Table VI, 9,500 lbs of propachlor were used on corn; 90,500 lbs of acifluorfen, 18,300 lbs of naptalam, 7,300 lbs of oryzalin, 19,300 lbs of profluralin and 9,700 lbs of vernolate were used on soybeans;

Table II. Acreages of Major Field Crops in Ohio Treated With
           Herbicides of Various Toxicities in 1982

| Crops | Acres | | Percent of Acre-Treatments with Toxicity | | | | |
| | Treated (1000) | Percent of Planted | Restricted Use | I | II | III | IV |
					(percent)		
Corn	4,320.0	99.3	2.5	0	5.4	90.1	1.9
Soybeans	3,716.0	99.1	0.8	1.1	0	92.3	5.9
Wheat	108.0	7.2	0	0	58.1	41.9	0
Oats	116.0	30.5	0	0	62.1	37.9	0
Alfalfa	53.0	11.7	20.6	0	0	49.7	29.7
Other Hay	11.0	1.3	0	0	46.8	53.2	0
Pasture	144.0	6.0	65.4	0	24.1	10.6	0
Tobacco	10.6	73.5	0	0	0	75.8	24.2
Total	8,478.6	62.1	2.4	0.5	4.0	89.4	3.7

Table III. Acreages of Major Field Crops in Ohio Treated With
            Insecticides of Various Toxicities in 1982

| Crops | Acres | | Percent of Acre-Treatments with Toxicity | | | | |
| | Treated (1000) | Percent of Planted | Restricted Use | I | II | III | IV |
					(percent)		
Corn	1,879.0	43.2	2.1	36.1	41.4	29.2	----
Soybeans	124.0	3.3	0.7	0.6	16.0	83.7	----
Wheat	6.0	0.4	----	----	----	36.7	----
Oats	2.0	0.6	----	----	----	50.0	----
Alfalfa	189.0	42.0	11.5	2.0	80.6	38.6	11.9
Other Hay	14.0	1.7	13.6	----	27.9	71.4	----
Pasture	5.0	0.2	100.0	----	----	----	----
Tobacco	7.3	50.8	----	2.2	----	84.9	----
Total	2,226.3	16.3	3.1	32.3	42.9	33.5	1.0

and 6,000 lbs of profluralin were used on alfalfa. Herbicides from
the slightly toxic category used for tobacco included 6,700 lbs of
pendimethalin, 5,800 lbs of pebulate and 5,700 lbs of diphenamid.
For pasture 7,800 lbs of dicamba and 6,000 lbs of glyphosate were
used mostly for spot treatment.

     Four insecticides constituted the majority of use of slightly
toxic products on major field crops (Table VI). Additions to the
data presented in the Table are 800 lbs of phosmet applied to alfalfa
and 1,800 lbs of diazinon and 600 lbs of malathion applied to
tobacco. The major fungicide or other chemicals in the slightly
toxic category were 25,100 lbs of maleic hydrazide and 8,400 lbs of
metalaxyl applied to tobacco and 800 and 5,100 lbs of carboxin
applied to soybeans and small grains, respectively.

     The use of Category IV pesticides on major field crops is shown
in Table VII. The only additional data not shown in this table is
3,700 lbs of benefin applied to tobacco acreage and 700 lbs of
captan and 500 lbs of maneb used in seed treatment for small grains.

Table IV.   Use of Highly Toxic Pesticides on Major Field Crops
in Ohio in 1982 [b]

Pesticide	Quantity Used on Crop				
	Corn	Soybeans	Alfalfa	Tobacco	Pasture
Herbicides:		(1000 lbs a.i.)			
Dinoseb	–	7.5	–	–	–
Naptalam + Dinoseb	–	118.5	–	–	–
Insecticides:					
Carbofuran	–	–	3.0	3.1	–
Disulfoton	1.7	–	–	1.9	–
Fonofos[a]	675.7	–	–	–	–
Isofenphos[a]	69.4	–	–	–	–
Oxydemeton methyl	1.9	–	–	–	–
Parathion[a]	–	1.4	6.0	–	0.3
Phorate	50.4	1.1	–	–	–

[a]Restricted Use pesticide.
[b]Based on dermal LD_{50} of commonly used formulations.

Table V.   Use of Moderately Toxic Pesticides on Major Field Crops
in Ohio in 1982[a]

Pesticide	Quantity Used on Crop				
			Small	Alfalfa	
	Corn	Soybeans	Grains	& Hay	Pasture
Herbicides:		(1000 lbs a.i.)			
2,4-D	261.3	–	81.2	2.5	65.6
Paraquat[b]	104.5	22.6	–	–	2.4
Picloram[b]	–	–	–	–	250.6
Insecticides:					
Azinphosmethyl[b]	–	–	–	0.7	–
Chlorpyrifos	151.9	–	–	–	–
Dimethoate	2.8	1.9	–	53.9	–
Lindane	50.7	2.3	c	–	–
Methidathion[b]	–	–	–	13.7	–
Methomyl[b]	1.7	–	–	a	–
Methyl Parathion[b]	–	–	–	2.6	–
Profos	11.9	–	–	–	–
Terbufos	672.2	–	–	–	–
Toxaphene[b]	78.2	–	c	–	–

[a]Based on dermal LD_{50} of commonly used formulations.
[b]Restricted Use pesticide.
[c]Quantity not published when less than 500 acres treated.

Precautions in Pesticide Use

Evaluation of the data presented in relation to the toxicity of the
pesticides used, the general cropping practices and the assumption
that the farmer follows the proper precautions in handling and applying pesticides, indicates that the potential for excessive personal
contamination is probably well within the limits of safe use.   The

Table VI. Use of Slightly Toxic Pesticides on Major Field Crops
in Ohio in 1982[a]

Pesticide	Quantity Used on Crop			
	Corn	Soybeans	Small Grains	Alfalfa & Hay
Herbicides:	(1000 lb a.i.)			
Alachlor	3299.6	3608.4	–	–
Atrazine	5316.4	–	–	–
Bentazon	8.1	342.3	–	–
Butylate	1861.1	–	–	–
Chloramben	–	983.6	–	–
Cyanazine	1995.4	–	–	–
2,4-DB	–	8.9	2.2	13.2
Dicamba	228.0	–	8.9	2.4
Diclofop-Methyl[b]	–	11.9	–	–
EPTC	415.2	–	–	25.8
Fluchloralin	–	46.6	–	–
Glyphosate	44.1	44.3	5.8	–
Linuron	18.0	786.9	–	–
MCPA	–	–	21.0	–
Metolachlor	2476.0	1966.5	–	–
Metribuzin	–	975.5	–	1.3
Pendimethalin	13.4	76.2	–	–
Pronamide[b]	–	–	–	11.2
Insecticides:				
Carbaryl	26.4	93.5	2.5	47.9
Carbofuran	547.8	–	–	–
Diazinon	31.8	17.6	–	2.5
Malathion	–	9.0	0.8	18.9

[a]Based on dermal LD_{50} of commonly used formulation.
[b]Restricted Use pesticide.

history of pesticide use on major crops in Ohio in relation to reported cases of poisoning, etc., seems to substantiate that observation. However, it is not wise to make such an assumption and
dismiss the problem as inconsequential. The safe use of pesticides
and the reduction in exposure to the farmer is of vital importance.
Earlier surveys showed that farm workers, for the most part, wear
ordinary work clothing (long-sleeved cotton shirt, long-legged work
pants, duck-billed cap, leather work shoes or boots and cotton or
leather gloves) for most farm work operations. Education in pesticide
use, as required in certification training, hopefully has caused a
greater awareness for use of certain protective apparel to reduce the
potential for dermal exposure. The ideal for protection from dermal
exposure is total body covering with moisture and dust impenetrable
materials, but the availability, costs and complete wearer comfort of
such body coverings precludes widespread acceptance by the farmer.

The Role of Protective Clothing

A proper evaluation of the farm worker exposure potential to

Table VII. Use of Relatively Non-Toxic Pesticides on Major Field
Crops in Ohio in 1982[a]

Pesticide	Quantity Used on Crop		
	Corn	Soybeans	Alfalfa & Other Hay
Herbicides:		(1000 lbs a.i.)	
Benefin	----	----	2.2
Bifenox	----	36.8	----
Simazine	297.4	----	12.5
Trifluralin	----	502.8	----
Insecticides:			
Methoxychlor	----	----	20.9
Fungicides:			
Captan	16.9	3.8	----
Mancozeb	9.3	----	----
Maneb	----	----	----

[a]Based on dermal LD_{50} of commonly used formulation.

pesticides must take into consideration the prevention of skin and
respiratory contact provided by different types of protective clothing and equipment. Farm worker safety regulation and applicator
training needs to approach the problem from a factual viewpoint.
Considerable research has been done through PIAP funding in the North
Central Region as well as other regions relative to the protection
from pesticide exposure provided by different fabrics and different
use practices. Included in the NCRPIAP research have been studies to
determine the areas of the body profile or clothing that are most apt
to receive the highest deposition of pesticide residue during different types of application and thus the most vulnerable areas for
dermal exposure. The maximum pesticide deposits from air blast
orchard spraying of Guthion occurred on the lower and upper arm in
both front and back, the hood area, and the front upper and lower
leg (6). For applicators to turf areas, although the diazinon residue levels were considerably lower than expected, the highest levels
of contamination were the thigh scrotal area (29.4 to 592 ng/100
cm^2) associated generally with the proximity to the spray solution
and the hand-wrist area (3.9 to 130.2 ng/100 cm^2) nearest the spray
nozzle (2). Mixer/loaders in all pesticide use operations are much
more apt to become contaminated in the hand-forearm area than any
other.
    Almost all the data evolving from fabric penetration studies (7)
show the dermal contact with pesticides to be reduced to very minute
concentration levels when the appropriate protective gear is worn.
For instance, protective clothing made from Gore-Tex, Tyvek and
Crowntex materials reduce the exposure to Guthion approximately 200
fold from residue levels of 3.2-3.4 ug/cm^2 on exterior selected
clothing sites to .014-.023 ug/cm^2 on corresponding interior skin
adjacent surfaces (7). Treated chambray-cotton clothing reduced
exposure 6 fold (2.95 to 0.46 ug/cm^2) and untreated chambray-cotton 5
fold (2.83 to 0.564 ug/cm^2) on corresponding surfaces. Different types
of protective gear worn by choice by carbaryl applicators in Nebraska

reduced exposure from 14 to 53 fold as measured from pads placed outside and inside the clothing or device. The external exposure to clothing was reduced from 3.85 ug/cm^2/hr to 0.26 for internal, for gloves from 4.77 to 0.09, for boots from 2.97 to 0.08 and for respirator from 3.02 to 0.06 ug/cm^2/hr (4).

Evaluation of the data from the NAPIAP interregional project on EBDC exposure of applicators and mixer/loaders (1) showed high levels of protection to the mixer/loader provided by protective clothing with the major concentration of potential exposure in the forearm area. It also appeared that those involved in ground application operations might have a greater potential for exposure than those in aerial application operations. The differences in exposure potential for pilot and tractor driver applicators was not significant. In most cases the protection provided by the airplane cockpit or the location of the tractor driver in relation to the spraying equipment was sufficient to prevent residue deposit on the exterior surfaces of the clothing, etc. Likewise, the use of a partially enclosed tractor cab for orchard application of captan (3) greatly reduced the dermal and inhalation exposure. Research shows that the covering of body surfaces by the normal everyday clothing of the backyard gardener provides satisfactory protection from dermal exposure to pesticides (1). The body areas of greatest potential exposure to such persons were the ankles and thighs followed by the forearm.

Another excellent example of the contrast between protected and unprotected exposure to pesticides and the influences of different handling systems and formulations is found in the research of Putnam, et al, in 1981 with nitrofen (8). Exposure to the exterior surface of the clothing or equipment on the various parts of the applicator's body in contrast to the residues determined on the interior surface of the clothing showed a reduction in exposure with an emulsifiable concentrate (EC) formulation, open handling system of from 17,100 to 39.2 ng/cm^2 in the hand area, 838 to 13.7 ng/cm^2 on the head and 17.7 to 3.1 ng/l for the air filter. By contrast the exterior exposure from a closed system for those same body areas was 780, 59 and 112.6, respectively, and the interior surface exposure was essentially the same as for the closed system. Wettable powder (WP) handling systems showed much greater potential exposure with exterior concentrations of 14,960, 2202, 136 ng/cm^2 for the hands, legs and head and 3307 ng/l for the air filter. The corresponding protected interior surfaces ranged from 16 to 52 ng. Consequently, the daily total potential exposure for applicators in contrast to the reduction in exposure afforded by protective clothing and devices was 17,720 to 248 ug for the EC open system, 3916 to 226 ug for the EC closed system and 40,040 to 535 ug for the WP system. Additional research by Putnam (8) showed that the potential exposure to mixer/loaders was far greater than for the applicator, particularly for those body areas in closest proximity to the pesticide formulation. The protection provided by protective clothing and equipment was about the same for both mixer/loaders and applicators.

The Use of Protective Clothing and Equipment in Ohio

The final criteria in ascertaining farmer protection in handling and applying pesticides is his adherence to the principles of safe use.

The 1982 survey of Pesticide Use on Major Crops in Ohio provided
some data on farmer personal protection (10). Although the data presented is on a composite sampling and report, it is possible to
correlate the data to individual farmer responses by referring to the
individual survey returns. Most farmers wear gloves, a long-sleeved
shirt, long-legged work pants, and a head covering when mixing/
loading pesticides regardless of the toxicity of the material (Table
VIII).However,the percent of farmers who use other items of protective equipment including a respirator, eye or face shield and rubber
boots is much lower. With the exception perhaps of a respirator, the
selection of protective clothing did not show much difference between
pesticide toxicity classes. This may be a reflection on the type of
formulation used that required less sophisticated protection; i.e.
granular vs emulsifiable concentrates or wettable powders. Protective measures taken during mixing/loading, however, were more pro-
nounced than when applying the pesticide, which could also be a
reflection on the equipment used in application and the proximity to
that equipment. It should be noted that approximately 1/4 of all
applicators have enclosed tractor cabs regardless of the toxicity of
the pesticide. This is probably a reflection more of the type and
convenience of current day equipment rather than concern for protection against pesticide contamination.

Table VIII.   Protective Clothing and Equipment Used by Farmers in
Ohio for Mixing/Loading and Applying Selected Pesticides

| Protective Gear | Percent of Farmers Using Gear for Pesticide Category | | | | | |
| | Mixing/Loading | | | Applying | | |
	Highly Toxic	Moder- ately Toxic	Slightly Toxic	Highly Toxic	Moder- ately Toxic	Slight- ly Toxic
Gloves	81	78	77	38	34	37
Long Sleeved Shirt	81	79	79	67	66	67
Head Covering	88	85	85	75	74	75
Spray Suit (Coveralls)	20	17	18	19	16	17
Rubber Boots	20	15	16	17	12	12
Dust Mask	16	14	14	11	9	10
Eye or Face Shield	32	31	30	14	13	15
Respirator	13	8	9	10	7	8
Closed Delivery	4	3	4	--	--	--
Enclosed Cab	--	--	--	26	22	22
None	2	3	3	11	14	12

[a]Includes "Restricted Use" pesticides.

The Ohio farmer does exhibit respect for pesticides of different
toxicity levels. An example can be seen in Table IX relative to the
use of organophosphates of different toxicities on alfalfa. Notice-
able contrasts can be seen in the wearing of rubber gloves, spray
suits, eye or face protection and respirators in the handling and
applying of parathion, dimethoate, and malathion which are represent-

ative of the three toxicity categories. The data in Table X show some difference in use of protective gear between the carbamate categories, carbofuran (I) and carbaryl (III), but essentially none between the organophosphates, fonofos (I) and chlorpyrifos (II), applied to corn. The formulation may be a deciding factor in these cases. Although the differences are not outstanding relative to the application of herbicides of different toxicity categories, the trend is still evident (Table II) with the higher percentage of protective gear use associated with the increase in toxicity or restricted nature of the product.

Table IX.   Comparison of Farmer Use of Protective Gear Relative to Toxicity of Organophosphate Pesticides Applied to Alfalfa in Ohio in 1982

| Protective Gear | Percent of Farmers Using Gear With Pesticide Use[a] | | | | | |
| | Mixing/Loading | | | Applying | | |
	Para-thion	Dime-thoate	Mala-thion	Para-thion	Dime-thoate	Mala-thion
Gloves	83	73	63	83	45	27
Long-Sleeved Shirt	74	82	82	74	61	73
Head Covering	87	86	91	87	77	91
Spray Suit (Coveralls)	30	16	9	39	16	27
Rubber Boots	26	34	18	26	32	9
Dust Mask	22	18	18	22	16	27
Eye or Face Shield	35	30	18	22	20	9
Respirator	35	11	0	35	16	9
Closed Delivery	0	5	0	--	--	--
Enclosed Cab	--	--	--	17	14	27
None	4	5	0	4	9	0

[a]Toxic Category: Parathion (Highly); Dimethoate (Moderately); Malathion (Slightly).

The comparison between the reported use of protective clothing and equipment in the 1982 survey and that of the 1978 survey (9) shows some improvement and trend towards better understanding and compliance by the farmer. However, the increase in the percent of farmers using more personal protective measures, except for the enclosed cab, is relatively small. With the exception of wearing gloves (which may or may not be rubber gloves), long-sleeved shirts, long-legged work pants, and head coverings, the Ohio farmers who use other pesticide protective gear are far in the minority. There is still much to do in educating the farmer and instilling compliance with personal safety practices to further minimize the worker exposure risks from pesticides.

Summary

Research on the parameters and kinetics of pesticide absorption from human dermal contact, on the measurement of absorbed residue

Table X. Comparison of Farmer Use of Protective Gear Relative to
Toxicity of Carbamate and Organophosphate Pesticides
Applied to Corn in Ohio - 1982

Protective Gear	Percent of Farmers Using Gear With Pesticide Use[a]							
	Mixing/Loading				Applying			
	Carbo-furan	Carb-aryl	Fono-fos	Chlor-pyrifos	Carbo-furan	Carb-aryl	Fono-fos	Chlor-pyrifos
Gloves	79	71	75	79	45	27	22	32
Long-Sleeved Shirt	79	71	78	79	70	59	58	59
Head Covering	88	86	84	85	77	73	66	68
Spray Suit (Coveralls)	25	11	15	21	23	11	15	18
Rubber Boots	22	14	14	12	19	13	8	9
Dust Mask	15	13	16	24	15	7	8	15
Eye or Face Shield	26	38	33	47	13	9	12	12
Respirator	14	11	5	9	12	13	4	3
Closed Delivery	2	4	7	6	--	--	--	--
Enclosed Cab	--	--	--	--	23	27	36	38
None	3	2	1	3	14	9	11	21

[a]Toxic Category: Carbofuran and Fonofos (Highly); Chlorpyrifos
(Moderately); Carbaryl (Slightly).

concentrations in body tissue and fluid in relation to dermal contact, on health aspects of exposure, and on the preventive measures
to reduce or eliminate the risks involved are vital to a proper
benefit/risk evaluation for the use of pesticides. Likewise, studies
on human behavior under field conditions and the development of
functional protective clothing and equipment are vital toward minimizing the risks of dermal exposure to workers using agricultural
pesticides. Exposure potential must take into consideration a knowledge of what pesticide chemicals are being used by the farmer-
producer including the formulations used, the relative toxicities of
such products, how and where they are used, the equipment used in
handling and applying, and the user/worker utilization of personal
protective measures. But in spite of all the research done, the
knowledge accumulated and subsequently published and taught, the
bottom line in the safe use of pesticides and the control of the
risk potential is the individual mixer/loader, applicator, and field
worker. Even after an effective program in safety training and the
availability of the best in protective gear and equipment, a momen-
tary lapse in memory accompanied with an unintentional or habitual
act of carelessness can cause an unwarranted pesticide exposure.
Sometimes such exposure may be inconsequential, but at other times it
may produce dire results.

     Factors for consideration in minimizing the pesticide exposure
potential to the agricultural worker include the following: (a) knowledge of what pesticide is being used including the formulation,
where and by whom it is used, what equipment systems are used for

delivery and application, etc., (b) manufacturing processes to reduce
the toxicity of pesticides, (c) changes in formulations and methods
of handling to reduce worker contact, (d) improvements in application
equipment, (e) the development of satisfactory, low-cost, comfortable

Table XI. Comparison of Farmer Use of Protective Gear Relative to
           Toxicity of Herbicides Applied to Corn in Ohio in 1982

| Protective Gear | Percent of Farmers Using Gear with Pesticide Use[a] | | | | | |
| | Mixing/Loading | | | Applying | | |
	Para-quat	Metol-achlor	Alachlor	Para-quat	Metol-achlor	Alachlor
Gloves	85	78	77	45	34	39
Long-Sleeved Shirt	82	78	79	71	63	68
Head Covering	90	83	85	80	69	76
Spray Suit (Coveralls)	23	17	19	24	15	20
Rubber Boots	27	17	16	24	14	12
Dust Mask	19	12	14	13	7	10
Eye or Face Shield	36	28	33	18	11	16
Respirator	16	9	8	13	6	8
Closed Delivery	4	3	3	--	--	--
Enclosed Cab	--	--	--	22	25	19
None	3	3	3	9	13	12

[a]Toxic Categories: Paraquat (Restricted Use); Metolachlor
              (Moderately) and Alachlor (Slightly).

protective clothing and then the acceptance and wearing of such
clothing, (f) continued education of pesticide handlers and applicators through effective applicator training and certification
schools and then effective programs to monitor the compliance of
personnel with the education received and the information on pesticide labels, (g) restrictions or closer controls on the registration
of pesticides particularly those with a history of problem use, (h)
cancellation of the registration of certain pesticide products if
other action cannot promote the safe use. It must be remembered
that all activities addressed in this symposium are geared toward
protecting the agricultural field worker from the potential hazards
of pesticide use, but in the final analysis that individual is the
determinate factor in whether or not such activities are of any
consequence.

Literature Cited

1. Brandes, Gordon A. "Applicator, Mixer/Loader Exposure Studies,
    Mancozeb (Dithane M-45)." Unpublished preliminary report for
    NCRPIAP Project Nos. 129 (132-NC-MN-F), 130 (133-NC-MI-F), 131
    (134-NC-OH-F) and 132 (135-NC-OH-F) by H. L. Bissonette; F.
    Tschirley and H.S. Potter; J. Farley; and C.C. Powell, respect-
    ively, and WRPIAP-Oregon Project by J.M. Witt and F.N. Dost.
    1981.

2. Daniels, W.H., R.P. Freeborg and V.J. Konopinski. "Evaluation of the Utilization of RPAR'd Pesticides Applied to Residential and Public Turf Sites and the Potential Exposure to Applicators." NCRPIAP Project No. 74 (25-NC-IN-O) Unpublished Final Research Report. 1980.

3. Deer, H.R. "Dermal and Inhalation Exposure of Commercial Applicators to Captan." NCRPIAP Project No. 108 (41-NC-MN-F) Unpublished Final Research Report. 1981.

4. Gold, R.E., J.R.C. Leavitt, T. Holsclaw and D. Tupy. "Exposure of Urban Applicators to Carbaryl." Arch Environ Contam Toxicol 11: 63-67. 1982.

5. Laughlin, J., R.E. Gold, C.B. Easley and R.M. Hill. "Fabric Parameters and Pesticide Characteristics that Impact on Dermal Exposure of Applicators." NCRPIAP Project No. 170 (166-NC-NE-I). Unpublished progress reports and private communication 1982-1984.

6. Orlando, J., D. Branson, G. Ayers, and M. Henry. "Development of Functional Apparel for the Reduction of Dermal Exposure to Pesticide Applicators." NCRPIAP Project Nos. 119/133/169 (34/136/165-NC-MI-I). Unpublished progress reports and private communication. 1980-1984.

7. Orlando, J., D. Branson, G. Ayers and R. Leavitt. "The Penetration of Formulated Guthion Spray through Selected Fabrics." J. Environ. Sci. Health, B 16 (5): 617-628. 1981.

8. Putnam, A.R., M.D. Willis, L.F. Binning and P.F. Boldt. "An Assessment of Exposure of Pesticide Applicators and Other Field Workers to Nitrofen (TOK) Herbicide." NCRPIAP Project No. 157 (160-NC-MI-H). Unpublished Final Research Report. 1982.

9. Waldron, A.C., H.L. Carter and M.A. Evans. "Pesticide Use on Major Crops in Ohio-1978." Research/Extension Bulletin 1117/666. The Ohio Agricultural Research and Development Center and the Ohio Cooperative Extension Service, The Ohio State University, April 1980.

10. Waldron, A.C., H.L. Carter and M.A. Evans. "Pesticide Use on Major Field Crops in Ohio-1982." OCES/OARDC Bulletin 715/1157, Agdex 100/600. The Ohio Cooperative Extension Service, The Ohio State University. February 1984.

11. Waldron, A.C. and E.L. Park (In cooperation with State Pesticide Impact Assessment Liaison Representatives of the North Central Region). "Pesticide Use on Major Crops in the North Central Region-1978." Research Bulletin 1132, The Ohio Agricultural Research and Development Center. July 1981.

RECEIVED July 17, 1984

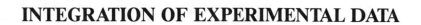

INTEGRATION OF EXPERIMENTAL DATA

Occupational Exposure to Pesticides and Its Role in Risk Assessment Procedures Used in Canada

CLAIRE A. FRANKLIN

Environmental Health Directorate, Department of National Health and Welfare, Ottawa, Ontario, Canada K1A 0L2

The process whereby pesticides are registered in Canada is not unlike that in many other countries. The manufacturer is required under Federal law to submit, at the time of application for registration, a package of data supporting the safety and efficacy of the product. If after review of these data, the product is judged to be acceptable, it is registered and food tolerances are established if required. Over the past 5 years there has been an increased awareness of the potential health hazards to those involved in the application of pesticides and those inadvertently exposed during application (bystanders). To properly analyze these risks, more accurate estimates of exposure are essential. The problems associated with current methods of exposure, the importance of analysis of urinary metabolites, the correlation of dermal exposure and urinary metabolites and the determination of percutaneous penetration are discussed.

In most developed nations, the sale and use of pesticides are regulated through legislation. In Canada, the primary legislation under which pesticides must be registered before they can be legally sold is the Pest Control Products Act. This Act is administered by the Department of Agriculture, and numerous other departments and agencies are requested to provide advice to Agriculture before a regulatory decision is made on any product. The Department of National Health and Welfare advises on all human health related matters and, under the provisions of the Food and Drugs Act and Regulations, maximum residue limits are set where appropriate.

The assessment of potential human health hazards resulting from the use of pesticides requires knowledge of both the amount of exposure to the person and the inherent toxicity of the product. Whereas there has been considerable effort in the past to monitor pesticide residues left on food after normal agricultural usage, it

0097–6156/85/0273–0429$06.00/0
© 1985 American Chemical Society

is only in recent years that regulatory agencies have emphasized the need to quantitatively assess the amount of pesticide to which the applicator is exposed. There are many other situations in which a potential human exposure exists occupationally in the manufacture, formulation and domestic or commercial application of pesticides and inadvertently for bystanders in or near sprayed areas.

Although the potential human exposure may be highest in the manufacture and formulation of the technical pesticide, it is also feasible that technological controls can be implemented to minimize exposure. However, once the pesticide is available in the open market, control of exposure becomes the responsibility of the individual user. Since there is a wide range of expertise in handling the products, it is essential that there be a wide enough margin of safety to encompass the anticipated excursions above normal in levels of exposure. Eight of the ten provinces in Canada have licencing procedures for commercial pesticide applicators. This situation is currently being re-evaluated and the feasibility of developing a core program and reciprocal licencing is being discussed. At the present time there are no provisions in any of the provinces to licence farmers. However, the implemention of some type of training and certification program for farmers is also being considered.

Steps in Risk Assessment

The process whereby the risks associated with the use of pesticides are assessed has become increasingly complex over the years, and even the definition of the term risk assessment is widely variable. However, most include the concepts of hazard and probability of occurrence and require information on toxicology and exposure. In the ideal situation (Table I) there should be accurate data on the actual amount of pesticide to which the worker was exposed (including the primary route of exposure), the absorption should be known (enabling correction of the exposure estimate) and there should be a well defined no effect level (NOEL), preferably derived from a study in which the route of exposure was similar to that in man. These data would enable a realistic calculation to be made of the margin of safety (MOS). In the case of non-threshold effects, there should be adequate data to allow a quantitative risk estimate to be calculated using suitable statistical models. The remaining step would be to determine the acceptability of the margin of safety. If the margin were unacceptable, steps would then have to be taken to determine the risk management strategy that would reduce or eliminate the risk.

Unfortunately, ideal conditions do not prevail, and the variance in each of these components can have a profound effect on the validity of the risk estimation as discussed below.

Exposure Estimate. Although considerable effort has been expended in the characterization of toxicity, there has not been an equivalent effort directed towards systematically estimating human exposure following use of these products. It has been shown that the dermal route of exposure is predominant in many types of

Table I. Proposed Steps in Risk Assessment

RISK ASSESSMENT

Exposure Estimate
Dermal/Inhalation Absorption Correction
Estimated Dosage
NOEL from Toxicity Data

Margin of Safety = $\dfrac{\text{NOEL}}{\text{Exposure}}$ or   Quantitative Risk Assessment

Acceptability of Margin

RISK MANAGEMENT STRATEGIES

Minimization of Exposure - closed systems
- personal protective clothing
- formulation
- equipment
- education, training, licensing
- restriction of uses
- cancellation/suspension

---

application (1) and historically, absorbent patches have been utilized to estimate the amount of pesticide which impinges on the skin. Durham and Wolfe (2) developed the technique of placing patches at points close to the body parts which would come in direct contact with the pesticide. This resulted in regional patch deposition densities being used to calculate deposition to the face, V of chest, back of neck, lower arms and hands. The problems associated with the assumptions of the patch technique have been discussed elsewhere (3). Regardless of these problems, the patch technique has gained acceptance as an indicator of dermal exposure, and this is reflected in the number of published studies using the technique (4,5,6). One of the obvious advantages of the patch technique is that it is non-invasive and is adaptable to any use situation. Unfortunately there is a wide range in the exposure values reported in the literature even in studies where similar application techniques were used (Table II).

More recent studies, and especially those submitted in support of new registrations, exhibit a wide variation in the location and number of patches used to measure impingement on different body parts and in the method for determining exposure. Closer analysis of these studies must be carried out before a "standardized" protocol is adopted. It remains to be determined whether the variations seen are due to true variations in exposure (due to personal handling differences, formulation type or wind) or whether they simply reflect differences in the method of calculation of the data.

Table II. Summary of Published Studies on Potential
Exposure of Workers Using Air Blast Equipment from
Patch Data and Hand Swabs or Hand Washes (6)

References	Pesticide	Dermal Exposure mg·hr^{-1}
Jegier (1964)	parathion	2.4
Jegier (1964)	malathion	2.5
Simpson (1965)	azinphosmethyl	9.9
Jegier (1964)	azinphosmethyl	12.9
Jegier (1964)	parathion	19.0
Simpson (1965)	carbaryl	24.9
Jegier (1964)	carbaryl	25.3
Wolfe (1967)	azinphosmethyl	27.2
Wolfe (1967)	malathion	30.0
Wojeck (1982)	arsenic	68.0
Batchelor (1954)	parathion	77.7
Wojeck (1981)	ethion	288.0
Wassermann (1963)	azinphosmethyl	541.0
Wassermann (1963)	azinphosmethyl	755.0

It has been suggested that correlation of exposure with the amount of pesticide applied rather than with the time taken to complete the application would reduce the variability, particularly in operations which might take some applicators considerably longer to complete than others. There is also considerable variation between studies in the placement of patches and whether or not hand washes are included in the estimate. The reliability of patch data to estimate actual exposure is questionable. Body areas such as hands and face are extremely difficult to patch yet are probably the most highly contaminated areas. Some studies do not include any patches under the clothing, yet it has been shown on many occasions that pesticides may permeate clothing or enter through garment openings. Early studies done with fluorescent markers clearly showed this was true and also that the hands and face were highly exposed (7).

Only recently has the problem of the loss of pesticide from patches used in the field been addressed (8). Many studies do not report laboratory or field recovery data for sampling substrates or comment on correction for recovery of the data (9). Serat (8) found that cotton gauze retained only 30% of extractable parathion and 70% of extractable dicofol under field conditions. He concluded that in the absence of adequate controls to determine the quantity of chemical lost from the fabric collectors there is no assurance that the extracted depositions represent anywhere near the actual values. This factor seriously limits the usefulness of many older exposure studies. New techniques using fluorescent markers (10) are promising and will undoubtedly lead to more quantitative estimates of contact exposure.

Another practice which may result in a large difference in the exposure estimate is the extrapolation of data collected for a portion of the spray operation to that of a full day. This needs to be more fully investigated because of the trend to conduct studies for one hour and then to extrapolate to 8 hours.

Measurement of hand exposure. This measurement alone can have a tremendous effect on the exposure estimate. Three techniques are used to estimate hand exposure: wrist patches, cotton gloves and hand washes.

The use of cotton gloves has been criticized as unduly overestimating hand exposure due to absorption of liquids. It is also apparent that extrapolation from a wrist patch to hand exposure would underestimate exposure. Swabbing or washing have been suggested as alternatives (11).

Davis (11) compared hand exposures of apple thinners using gloves and hand washes. He found that hand exposures obtained by rinsing were significantly lower than those obtained by using either cotton or nylon gloves. The mean exposures for cotton or nylon gloves were approximately 4-5 times larger than those obtained by using hand rinses. Davis concluded that the use of gloves to monitor hand exposure grossly exaggerates estimates of total potential exposure. However, hand washes measure that pesticide which has not been absorbed or is not irreversibly bound in the layers of the skin. It has been found that regardless of solvent rinsings, pesticides can remain on the skin for long periods of time (12). The true value for hand exposure probably lies somewhere between the two measurements.

Studies showing the portion of dermal exposure that has been attributed to the hands are summarized in Table III. Regardless of the method used to measure hand exposure these studies show that the hands contribute from 27% to 99% of the total dermal exposure. In mixer/loader situations where the worker is more likely to contact the concentrate, the majority of dermal exposure is to the hands regardless of whether extra protective gloves were worn over the cotton gloves or a closed mixing system was used.

Wojeck (13) used eight outside patches and the palms and back of cotton gloves to estimate total dermal exposure to mixer/loaders or airblast applicators of ethion. Mixer/loaders received 76% of the total dermal exposure to the hands and applicators received 42% of the total dermal exposure to the hands. If the original patch method of Durham and Wolfe (2), which did not include a hand exposure estimate is used to recalculate the data, the total dermal estimate, was 10 times lower than the total body method used by Wojeck. This emphasizes the importance of using hand exposures to more accurately estimate total exposure.

In another study using the same method, Wojeck (14) measured exposure of mixer/loaders and airblast applicators using arsenic spray. Hand exposure accounted for 52% and 41% of total dermal exposure for mixer/loaders and applicators respectively.

In several studies carried out during aerial agricultural applications, a large portion of the total exposure was also seen on the hands, especially for mixer/loaders. Peoples (15) monitored the potential dermal and inhalation exposure of mixer/loaders, pilots

Table III. Hand Exposure Expressed as a Percentage of Total Dermal Exposure

	Pesticide	Method	Mixing System	Hand Exposure (% of total)				Respiratory Exposure (% of total)
				Mixer/Loader (%)	Applicator (%)	Pilot (%)	Flagger (%)	
Orchard								
Wojeck (1981)	ethion (E.C.)	cotton gloves	open	76	42	–	–	1
Wojeck (1982)	lead arsenate (liquid)	cotton gloves	open	52	41	–	–	0.01
Aerial								
Peoples (1979)	DEF (E.C.)	handwash*	closed	57	–	73	41	–
Maddy (1982)	mevinphos (E.C.)	handwash*	closed	74	–	27	42	–
Everhart (1981)	benomyl (W.P.)	cotton gloves*	open	96	–	–	–	–
Ground								
Dubelman (1982)	diallate (E.C.)	cotton gloves	open	99	64	–	–	1
		cotton gloves*	closed	n.d.	–	–	–	5

* workers wore protective gloves   – not sampled   n.d. not detected

and flaggers during the performance of duties associated with the aerial application of DEF. Multi-layered patches were attached to seven body areas in such a way that estimates of deposition exposure to exposed areas and clothed areas could be calculated. Hand exposure was measured using a hand wash and accounted for 57% of the total dermal exposure. It is likely that hand exposure was reduced in this study for mixers by the provision of a closed mixing system and the use of neoprene gloves. Surprisingly the pilot received 73% of his dermal exposure to the hands. The authors attributed this to the pilots adjusting nozzles of the aircraft without using the required protective gloves. It should be noted that good field observations are valuable in some cases to explain unusual values. Also, if hand exposure had been based on extrapolation from lower wrist patches such unexpected but important exposures might have been missed. The flagger received only 42% of the dermal exposure on the hands. As flaggers are exposed to the airborne spray cloud, other areas such as the head and shoulders become more important areas for pesticide deposition.

Maddy (16) monitored dermal and inhalation exposures for mixer/loaders, flaggers and pilots associated with the aerial application of mevinphos, using the methods described in Peoples (15). In this study the mixer/loaders operating closed transfer systems wore gloves but others associated with the spray operation did not. The mixer/loaders received 74% of their total dermal exposure on the hands, flaggers received 42% and pilots received 27%. Pilots received a considerably lower proportion of the total exposure to the hands than in the study by Peoples (15).

The use of closed systems did not appear to modify the proportion of the total exposure that occurred on the hands in either aerial studies or in the orchard studies. However it is premature to draw conclusions relative to the suitability of closed systems. This is an important area to be considered for reduction of exposure and more studies on the magnitude of reduction would be very useful.

Everhart (17) monitored 8 mixer/loaders who each prepared one tankful of benomyl for aerial application. Five gauze pads and cotton gloves were used to measure exposure. Most workers wore additional protective gloves over the cotton gloves. Regardless of this additional precaution 96% of the total dermal exposure was found on the cotton gloves. In almost all other cases the forearm patches had the highest levels of contamination.

In a different use situation Dubelman (18) measured dermal and inhalation exposure to mixer/loaders and applicators associated with the boom application of the herbicide diallate. The body was patched at 5 locations for the 6 open mixing trials and 12 locations for the 9 closed mixing trials. Hand exposure was measured using cotton gloves. For the closed mixing trials neoprene gloves were worn over the cotton gloves but no additional gloves were worn during the open system mixing trials. In the open mixing trials hand exposure for the mixer/loaders accounted for 99% of the total exposure. In the closed mixing trials no hand exposure was detected and in fact total dermal exposure was reduced to less than 1% of that found during open mixing. It cannot be ascertained whether this exposure reduction was due to the closed system or to the use of the neoprene gloves. The applicators were observed to have 64% of the total dermal exposure on their hands.

Although various patch techniques were used as well as different methods of estimating hand exposure in these studies, they all emphasize the importance of including an estimate of hand exposure in calculating the total dermal exposure. The available data do not clearly indicate which procedure for estimation of hand exposure is the most accurate. Since it has been suggested that cotton gloves overestimate hand exposure it would be prudent from the point of view of health protection to use this method until better methods are designed.

Metabolite Analyses. The current difficulties surrounding the use of patch data to quantitatively estimate exposure have led to the development of alternative methods such as the measurement of urinary metabolite levels. Studies in which both urinary metabolites have been measured and patches analyzed have emphasized the unreliability of patches (3,7,9). Unfortunately there are also difficulties in using metabolite excretion as a quantitative indicator of exposure, and it is essential that consecutive 24 hour urine samples be taken (7). Failure to do so results in a lack of correlation between metabolite excretion and patch data (13). The collection of accurate 24 hour samples over several days requires the cooperators to be highly motivated, and this is a major problem with this method.

The detection of pesticide metabolites in the urine of workers indicates prior exposure. However, it is difficult to relate this level of urinary metabolite to the actual worker exposure, and it is equally difficult to interpret the toxicological significance of the level. A preliminary study conducted in rats exposed dermally to 100, 200 and 400 ug of azinphos-methyl showed a significant linear correlation between the dermal dosage and the urinary alkyl phosphate metabolite levels (19). Further studies are being conducted in other species to determine whether a similar type of relationship occurs and to develop a standard curve in which urinary metabolite levels could be utilized to estimate the amount of dermal exposure.

Exposure Studies. Although submission of applicator exposure studies (or suitable exposure estimates) are currently a registration requirement in Canada, it is our intention to ascertain whether exposure scenarios can be developed to provide a "worst case" or maximum expected exposure level. Considerable effort has gone into the development of a forestry scenario (20,21) in which the estimated exposure levels appear to be comparable to those observed in actual field studies (22). Whether other scenarios can be developed and validated is currently being evaluated in a collaborative venture between industry and government.

Dermal/Inhalation Absorption Correction. Since it is generally presumed that 100% of the inhaled pesticide dose is absorbed, little work is being done to refine this. It has also been shown that in most agricultural applicators the dermal route is the predominant route of exposure. However, the patch methods which are used only estimate the amount of pesticide which impinges on the skin and do not give any indication of the actual amount absorbed (the potentially toxic dosage). This in itself would not pose as large a a problem if the predictive toxicity data were generated using the dermal route of exposure, but this is not generally the case. Therefore, due to the wide variations in the absorption of various pesticides (23), the contact dosage should be corrected by the actual absorption of the pesticide in question.

The use of percutaneous penetration data to correct dermal exposure estimates is in its infancy, and there are numerous aspects which must be investigated before this becomes an accepted regulatory procedure.

It has been shown that there is species variability in percutaneous penetration and that the skin of miniature pigs and rhesus monkeys most closely estimate absorption in man (23). The site of application (24), single versus multiple exposure (25,26) and environmental factors such as temperature, humidity, light and air flow also affect penetration. Work in my laboratory using ^{14}C labelled Guthion (azinphos-methyl) according to the method of Maibach, in which a correction factor for incomplete urinary excretion of the pesticide is applied to the dermally administered dosage, confirms these earlier findings (Table IV). Technical Guthion was totally absorbed in both rats and rabbits and less than

Table IV. Percutaneous Penetration of ^{14}C-Guthion (azinphos-methyl) Expressed as % of Applied Dose

Compound	Rat	Rabbit	Rhesus Monkey	Man
Guthion in propylene glycol	50.0+14(IM)	31.7+5(IM)	70.4+2(IM)	
Guthion in acetone	107.0+11(D)* (36 h)**	116.0+38(D)* (7 h)	47.4+10(F)* (23 h)	36.1+11(F)* (31 h)
			32.0+9(A) (23 h)	
Guthion W.P. in H$_2$O			82.8+27(F) (27 h)	
			39.9+4(A) (26 h)	

IM intramuscular
 D intrascapular dermal
 F forehead dermal
 A forearm dermal
 *corrected for incomplete urinary excretion
 **t$\frac{1}{2}$ - excretion half-life

50% absorbed in monkeys and man (Table IV). There was greater
penetration from the forehead (47%) than the forearm (32%) in
monkeys although the difference was not as large as seen with other
products which are currently being tested. These data suggest that
the best predictor for man is the monkey and that for this
particular product either the forearm or forehead would give a
reasonable estimate of absorption. Derivatization of the Guthion to
the wettable powder increased penetration from the forehead but was
without effect on the forearm. The wettable powder was applied as a
suspension in water which may account for the differences or simply
emphasize the real differences between application sites. The
wettable powder is currently being tested in man to see if a similar
effect occurs. Another parameter which varied amongst species was
the excretion half-life with a much more rapid excretion in rabbits
(7 h) than in monkeys (23 h), man (31 h) or rats (36 h).

   There has been increased emphasis on the development of in
vitro models to estimate absorption. These models have the
advantages of being faster and less expensive than in vivo models
but will require parallel in vivo studies to validate their
suitability for estimating human absorption of pesticides. At the
present time we assume that all of the pesticide which impinges on
the skin as estimated in the exposure study is absorbed unless there
are acceptable data which allow a specific correction to be made.
Although in many instances the correction of the exposure data does
not significantly alter the risk estimate, it can become an
important factor in the cases of high exposure and/or high toxicity.
It is therefore important that we have reliable and accurate
estimates of the amount of pesticide absorbed. One additional
sequela of the dermal penetration studies on formulations is that
information may be gained which would prove useful in designing
products which are not well absorbed by humans.

No Observed Effect Level (NOEL) from Toxicity Data. The types of
toxicity studies that are submitted in support of registration are
similar throughout the world. In Canada there are no specific
protocols delineated for the conduct of toxicity tests but most
comply with those set under FIFRA, WHO, or OECD guidelines. The
data requirements include the tests outlined on Tables V, VI, and
VII. These are guidelines, not rigid requirements, and the
manufacturers are encouraged to discuss their data packages before
completion.

   One of the primary shortcomings of the standard data package
with regard to worker/bystander risk assessment as it exists today
is the emphasis on the oral route of exposure. Others are the
limited data on kinetics of the chemical, lack of attention to
determining the effect of the route of exposure on toxicity and the
inability to test combinations of pesticides in a manner which would
approximate the type of mixed exposure that applicators receive.
These issues complicate the risk assessments for applicators, for
whom the primary route of exposure is dermal and generally is
intermittent.

Risk Estimation. For pesticides which exert toxicological effects
that demonstrate a no observed effect level (NOEL), the standard

Table V. Acute Toxicity Tests Required for Registration
(Technical and Formulations)

LD_{50} - oral, dermal, inhalation

Irritation - dermal, eye

Sensitization

Delayed neurotoxicity

Table VI. Subacute Toxicity Tests Required for Registration
(Technical and Formulations)

---

90 day oral (rat and dog)

12 month oral (dog)

90 day dermal

90 day inhalation

Delayed neurotoxicity (if acute test positive)

Table VII. Long Term and Special Tests Required for
Registration (Technical)

Chronic feeding (rat)

Oncogenicity (rat and mouse)

Pharmacokinetic (appropriate routes)

Mutagenicity

Teratology

Multi-generation reproduction

Exposure

---

procedure for risk estimation is to use "safety" factors. This
approach has been developed over a number of years, and one chapter
in an early Food and Drug Administration (FDA) publication addressed
the issue of safety evaluation (27). The recommendations on the use
of safety factors by the Food Protection Committee of the National
Research Council (28) were adopted by the Joint Food and
Agricultural Organization and World Health Organization Expert
Committees on Food Additives (29) and Pesticide Residues (30). In
addition to the one hundred fold safety factor suggested by Lehman
(31), safety factors ranging to 5000 are used dependent upon a
number of factors, including the severity of the toxicological
lesion, quality of the data base and sample size.

For pesticides which have been shown to be animal carcinogens,
the risk estimation becomes more complicated, relying heavily upon
statistical models which express the probability of occurrence as a
function of dose. All of the statistical models need an exposure
estimate expressed as a daily dosage to enable comparison with the
exposure estimate from the chronic study.

If exposure to the population under study occurs on a daily
lifetime basis, the procedure is relatively straight forward.
However, in many agricultural use situations the exposure to the
applicator or bystander is intermittent.

In most cases there may be only a few days of exposure a year
but in some there may be more frequent exposure over the entire
year. One approach that has been taken to obtain a lifetime daily
exposure under these circumstances has been to conduct a worker
field study and measure the exposure received for one day. This is
multiplied by the number of days worked in a year and then by the
number of working years. This is an Amortized Daily Exposure.

AMORTIZED EXPOSURE (ug/kg BW/day)

$$= \frac{\text{dosage* x application rate x acres treated x duration}}{\text{working lifespan (days)}}$$

This approach results in a very small estimated daily exposure and
ignores the toxicological significance of high pulses of exposure.
There are generally no toxicology data to support this approach.

In the absence of these supporting data it would be more
prudent to assume the worst case; that is the dosage as determined
from the exposure study would be received every day for the working
lifetime of the applicator. This is a Peak Exposure.

PEAK EXPOSURE (ug/kg BW/day)

$$= \text{dosage* x application rate x acres treated}$$

*dosage (ug/kg BW/lb ai)
$$= \frac{\text{corrected dermal exposure + corrected inhalation exposure}}{\text{body weight (kg) x ai applied (lb)}}$$

It is obvious that this peak exposure approach is also not the true
case, and if quantitative risk assessment is to be feasible this
very serious impediment will have to be rectified through experi-

ments designed to elucidate both the mechanism of action and the effect of intermittent exposure.

The decision to use an amortized exposure value or a peak exposure value has a profound impact on the outcome of the quantitative risk assessment. To illustrate this point, data from an actual field exposure study were used. The average daily dermal exposure level as measured by the patch technique was used to calculate the amortized exposure level and the peak exposure level (Table VIII). Estimates of risk at low doses were obtained using linear extrapolation from the 1% excess risk point based on a fitted Weibull model (32) and the Armitage–Doll multi-stage model (33). While both models gave similar results, the effect of the exposure estimates had a dramatic effect on the risk estimates. The amortized exposure estimates lowered the estimates of risk substantially.

The shortcomings pertaining to the estimation of exposure which have been described are very serious, and these issues will have to be resolved before statistical risk assessment models can be utilized as the basis for regulatory decisions on the registration of pesticides.

Table VIII.   Effect of Exposure Level on Quantitative Risk Assessment

Model	95% Upper Confidence Limit on Excess Risk			
	Amortized Exposure (mg/kg/da)		Peak Exposure (mg/kg/da)	
	3×10^{-6}*	8×10^{-5}	0.2*	2.75
Linear Extrapolation based on a fitted Weibull Model	1.0×10^{-8}	2.7×10^{-7}	7.3×10^{-4}	9.3×10^{-3}
Multi-stage Model	1.3×10^{-8}	3.6×10^{-7}	9.5×10^{-4}	1.2×10^{-2}

*Workers wore protective rubber gloves

Conclusion

The estimate of exposure to workers involved in the application of pesticides and to bystanders is a critical component of risk assessment. The deficiencies of existing methods need to be rectified to ensure reliable and accurate estimates of actual exposure. Emphasis should be placed on development of novel methods as well to assist in assessing exposure. One of the more serious impediments to the use of quantitative risk assessment models is the resolution of the problem of exposure estimation following intermittent exposure.

Nontechnical Summary

The process whereby the risks associated with the use of pesticides are assessed has become increasingly complex over the years, and even the definition of the term risk assessment is widely variable. However, most include the concepts of hazard and probability of occurrence and require information on toxicology and exposure. In the ideal situation there should be accurate data on the actual amount of pesticide to which the worker was exposed, including the primary route of exposure, the absorption should be known, enabling correction of the exposure estimate, and the amount of pesticide necessary to cause toxic effects in test animals should be known. From these data, it could be determined whether the product could be used safely.

Given that the margin between exposure to humans and the level which was toxic in animals was unacceptable, steps would then have to be taken to determine the risk management strategy that would reduce or eliminate the risk.

Unfortunately the ideal situation does not exist and there are many difficulties which must be overcome before accurate risk assessments can be conducted. For pesticide applicators, the dermal route has been shown to be the most important one. However, the methods used to measure the amount of pesticide landing on the skin are not very reliable and many studies conducted in the past did not try to estimate hand exposure. This omission is a serious one because it has been shown that a very large percentage of the total dermal exposure is to the hands. New methods using fluorescent tracer techniques are promising and will undoubtedly lead to more quantitative estimates of contact exposure.

A definite shortcoming of all of these existing techniques for measuring exposure is that they measure the amount of pesticide that lands on the skin (contact exposure) and give no estimation of the actual amount of pesticide that is absorbed through the skin. It is this absorbed dosage which is potentially toxic to a target tissue. There are many factors which must be considered when conducting absorption studies, including site of application such as forehead or forearm, solvent or formulation and the actual pesticide itself. The effects of these parameters must be more fully understood before correction of contact dosage can be done with certainty.

Another way to estimate exposure is to measure urinary metabolite levels. However, it is difficult to relate this level to the actual amount which contacted the skin and work is currently underway to elucidate this relationship.

Another factor which complicates the risk assessment is the intermittent nature of pesticide exposure to applicators who may only use a specific product for a few days a year.

Resolution of these issues is essential if we are to be able to scientifically support quantitative risk assessment.

Acknowledgments

The author wishes to thank Nancy Muir for her invaluable assistance in preparing the manuscript and Linda Bradley who typed it.

Literature Cited

1. Durham, W.F.; Wolfe, H.R.; Elliot, J.W. Arch. Environ. Health. 1972, 24, 381–387.
2. Durham, W.F.; Wolfe, H.R. Bull. WHO 1962, 26, 75–92.
3. Franklin, C.A.; Muir, N.I.; Greenhalgh, R. in Pesticide Residues and Exposure, ACS Symposium Series 182, 1982, p. 157–168.
4. Nigg, H.N.; Stamper, J.H. Arch. Environ. Contam. Toxicol. 1983, 12, 477–482.
5. Atallah, Y.H.; Cahill, W.P., Whitacre; D.M. Arch. Environ. Contam. Toxicol. 1982, 11, 219–225.
6. Wolfe, H.R.; Durham, W.F.; Armstrong, J.F. Arch. Environ. Health. 1967, 14, 622–633.
7. Franklin, C.A.; Fenske, R.A.; Greenhalgh, R.; Mathieu, L.; Denley, H.V.; Leffingwell, J.T.; Spear, R.C. J. Toxicol. Environ. Health. 1981, 7, 715–731.
8. Serat, W.F.; VanLoon, A.J.; Serat, W.H. Arch. Environ. Contam. Toxicol. 1982, 11, 227–234.
9. Lavy, T.L.,; Shepard, J.S.; Mattice, J.D. J. Agric. Food Chem. 1980, 28, 626–630.
10. Fenske, R.A.; Leffingwell, J.T.; Spear, R.C. Presented at 184th ACS National Meeting, Kansas City, Mo, Sept. 1982.
11. Davis, J.E.; Stevens, E.R.; Staiff, D.C. Bull. Environ. Contam. Toxicol. 1983, 31, 625–630.
12. Kazen, C.; Bloomer, A.; Welch, R.; Qudbier, A.; Price, H. Arch. Environ. Health, 1974, 29, 315–318.
13. Wojeck, G.A.; Nigg, H.N.; Stamper, J.H.; Bradway, D.E. Arch. Environ. Contam. Toxicol. 1981, 10, 725–735.
14. Wojeck, G.A.; Nigg, H.N.; Braman, R.S.; Stamper, J.H.; Rouseff, R.L. Arch. Environ. Contam. Toxicol. 1982, 11, 661–667.
15. Peoples, S.A.; Maddy, K.T.; Datta, P.R.; Johnston, L.; Smith, C.; Conrad, D.; Cooper, C. Calif. Dept. Food and Agr. Report HS–676, Nov. 1976, p. 34.
16. Maddy, K.T.; Winter, C.; Cepello, S.; Fredrickson, A.S. Calif. Dept. of Food and Agr. Report HS–889, Jan. 1982, p. 34.
17. Everhart, L.P.; Holt, R.F. J. Agric. Food Chem. 1982, 30, 222–227.
18. Dubelman, S.; Lauer, R.; Arras, D.D.; Adams, S.A. J. Agric. Food Chem., 1982, 30, 528–532.
19. Franklin, C.A.; Greenhalgh, R.; Maibach, H.I. in: IUPAC Pesticide Chemistry: "Human Welfare and the Environment," Pergamon Press, 1983; p. 221–225.
20. Houghton, E.R. Standardized scenarios of pest control situations as a means of assessing human exposure to pesticides. Agriculture Canada, Ottawa, 1978.
21. Crabbe, R.; Krzymien, M.; Elias, L.; Davie, S. National Research Council of Canada. Report No. LTR–UA–62, Part I, 1982.
22. Franklin, C.A.; Muir, N.I. National Research Council of Canada, 1984, in press.
23. Feldman, R.J.; Maibach, H.I. Toxicol. Appl. Pharmacol. 1974, 28, 126–132.

24. Maibach, H.I.; Feldman, R.J.; Milby, T.H.; Serat, W.F.; <u>Arch.</u>
     <u>Environ. Health.</u> 1971, 23, 208–211.
25. Wester, R.C.; Noonan, P.K.; Maibach, H.I. <u>Arch. Dermatol. Res.</u>
     1980, 267, 229–235.
26. Wester, R.C.; Noonan, P.K. Int. J. Pharm. 1980, 7, 99–110.
27. Appraisal of the Safety of Chemicals in Foods, Drugs and
     Cosmetics. Association Food and Drug Officials of the United
     States (AFDOUS) 1959.
28. NRC/NAS (National Research Council/National Academy of
     Sciences) Food Protection Committee, Food and Nutrition Board.
     Evaluating the Safety of Food Chemicals Washington DC.   NAS
     1970.
29. Joint FAO/WHO Expert Committee on Food Additives, 1972.   WHO
     Tech. Report Series 505.
30. Joint FAO/WHO Expert Committee on Pest. Residues, 1965.   FAO
     Meet Rep. No. PL/1965/10, WHO/Food Add/26–65.
31. Lehman, A.J.; Fitzhugh, O.G.   <u>Assoc. Food Drug Officials Q.</u>
     <u>Bull.</u> 1954, 18:33–35.
32. Krewski, D.; Van Ryzin, J. <u>in</u> Statistics and Related Topics,
     North–Holland Publishing Co. 1981, p. 201–231.
33. Howe, R.B.; Crump, K.S. Global 82: Report for Office of
     Carcinogen Standards, Dept. of Labour Contract YIUSC252C3.
     1982.

RECEIVED August 28, 1984

Risk Assessment of Excess Pesticide Exposure to Workers in California

K. T. MADDY, R. G. WANG, JAMES B. KNAAK, C. L. LIAO, S. C. EDMISTON, and C. K. WINTER

Worker Health and Safety Unit, California Department of Food and Agriculture, Sacramento, CA 95814

Pesticides are selected because they have specific adverse biological effects on certain organisms. Unfortunately, many pesticides are also toxic to humans and beneficial organisms. The pesticide safety program of the California Department of Food and Agriculture involves evaluation of measurements of: (1) amounts of pesticide vapors, mists, or dusts in the breathing zone of persons who may be exposed; (2) amounts of pesticide dusts, powders, or liquids that reach the skin of persons applying pesticides; (3) levels of pesticide residues, including the more toxic breakdown products on foliage and soil of fields and other places where work is to take place subsequent to application; (4) urine excretion rates; and/or, (5) any biologic adverse effects in exposed persons. In order to better evaluate human exposure risk, the following data may be required of registrants either before or after registration: (1) indoor exposure data; (2) mixer, loader, and applicator exposure data; (3) dislodgeble leaf residue and soil residue data; and, (4) dermal absorption rate data. In the past, little of this type of information was available nor was it supplied by pesticide registrants. Separate studies to monitor exposure levels of pesticides in the workplace are being conducted by CDFA for certain pesticides currently registered. These measurements are of value in designing methods to keep user exposures at low levels and to determine if adequate safety margins exist to protect against identified or suspected adverse health effects.

The Environmental Protection Agency (EPA), when first created in 1970, continued the approach of its predecessor, the United States Department of Agriculture (USDA), in evaluating the overall toxicity of a particular chemical. In assigning signal words, which suggest the potential hazard, the USDA and then the EPA emphasized acute toxicity, often focusing on the hazard of accidental ingestion. They did not place a high priority on evaluating workplace exposure.

0097–6156/85/0273–0445$06.00/0

In 1971, new California laws began to emphasize requirements for assessing total workplace hazards for pesticide users (including long-term exposure hazards) and ways of mitigating these hazards. This has resulted in specific California requirements for data which may be used to estimate such hazards.

During the EPA's Rebuttable Presumption Against Registration (RPAR) process (now called Special Review), it became apparent that if uses of certain pesticides with identified potentials for causing adverse effects were to be continued, user exposure data would be needed that demonstrated minimal exposure hazards when certain use procedures were followed. Scientists of both the EPA and the Scientific Advisory Panel (SAP) to EPA then realized that they could not make satisfactory risk assessments and evaluate the impact of continued use without actual workplace exposure data.

California Program

The pesticide worker safety program of the California Department of Food and Agriculture (CDFA) includes the consideration of: 1) amounts of pesticide vapors, mists, or dusts in the breathing zone of exposed persons; 2) amounts of pesticide dusts, powders or liquids on the skin of persons mixing, loading, and/or applying pesticides; 3) levels of pesticide residues, including the more toxic breakdown products, on foliage and soil of fields where work is to take place subsequent to application which may later contact skin; 4) residues in the air, on floors, counters, etc., following application of pesticides indoors that may be inhaled or be contacted by skin. In the past, little of this type of information was available; nor was it supplied by pesticide registrants. Studies of worker exposure levels in the workplace are conducted by the CDFA for certain pesticides currently registered. Also in California, these kinds of data are currently required of the registrants prior to registration of certain pesticides, particularly those with high acute or subacute toxicity or a potential to produce certain chronic effects.

These measurements are of value in designing methods to reduce exposure of all persons, including persons who use pesticides in apartments, houses, and yards. CDFA evaluates basic toxicology data, exposure measurements and the manner in which the pesticide product is to be used. By modifying the way the pesticide is to be used, establishing reentry intervals, or suggesting changes to EPA of precautionary statements on pesticide labels, the risk of exposure to a potentially hazardous pesticide may be greatly reduced. The CDFA gathers and analyzes detailed information on more than 2,000 illness reports per year from physicians who describe possible occupational exposures to specific pesticides, as well as more than 12,000 inquiries handled each year by poison information centers in California on non-occupational exposures. This information is used to assist in developing training programs, developing worker safety regulations, and in evaluating proposed registrations, in an effort to minimize exposures. In order to complete the risk assessment process, the CDFA also examines exposure data generated by registrants.

A major difficulty in making hazard assessments for any persons who might be exposed before, during, and after a pesticide application is the lack of information on the amount of pesticide that may be inhaled or may reach the skin, the extent of dermal absorption, the rate and pathway of biotransformation, and the route of elimination from the body.

The following are some of the data that may be required by CDFA to assist in making exposure estimates of persons involved in various activities involving the use of pesticides: indoor exposure; field reentry; mixer, loader, and applicator exposure, dermal absorption, and dermal dose response data.

Indoor Exposure.   Products to be used indoors (houses, institutions, greenhouses, etc.), may have potential exposure (inhalation, dermal, and ingestion) hazards both during the application and upon reentry. An appropriate ventilation period may be needed to protect residents, inhabitants, or workers in the treated area from inhalation of hazardous chemicals as well as from contacting residues on carpets, countertops, etc. A study outline has been developed and used by the CDFA for studies it conducts to acquire needed data; this is available upon request for others to use to plan their studies.

Field Reentry.   Certain pesticides pose a potential hazard to field workers if they enter a treated area and have significant contact with treated plants or soil (1). Currently, CDFA places major emphasis on exposure to the foliage of citrus, grapes, peaches, nectarines, and apples. EPA now also has guidelines for developing field worker reentry data. The following is a guide suggested and used by CDFA in deciding if reentry data is needed.

Such data may be needed if the product is to be applied to a commercially grown crop, particularly to its foliage or the soil, and cultural practices (such as pruning or harvesting) of that particular crop involving substantial body contact with the foliage, bark, or soil, or exposure to pesticide residues shaken from the foliage or bark, and the product contains: (a) a cholinesterase inhibitor; or (b) a significantly toxic principle that can cause a detrimental acute systemic toxic reaction or is suspected of causing a chronic effect, and may be readily absorbed through the skin or inhaled following exposure to pesticide residues contacted while conducting usual cultural practices; or (c) a chemical which causes a significant primary skin irritant reaction in appropriate test animals or man; or (d) a chemical which is a significant skin sensitizer in appropriate test animals or man.

Reentry intervals are now established on the basis of: (1) data on dermal absorption or dermal dose response; (2) inhalation, dermal, and oral acute toxicity studies in animal models; (3) foliar and soil residue dissipation data; and, (4) available human exposure data. CDFA recommends several sources as useful guides for determining residues of pesticides on soil and leaf surfaces (dislodgeable residue) and conducting field reentry studies involving human volunteers (1-5). Human exposure studies may not be required if adequate animal data from (1) through (3) above are available.

Mixer, Loader, Applicator Exposure. In order to make an appropriate
hazard assessment, information is needed on the amount of pesticide
that may be inhaled, and/or reach the skin and more importantly the
amount being absorbed during a "typical" application. A study outline is available from CDFA. It places emphasis as follows:

Testing should be performed using the formulated product to be
marketed, and used in accordance with the proposed label. It is
preferable for the applications being studied to be at the maximum
rate specified and the least dilution permitted in the use instructions. The period of exposure studied should be on at least three
different workdays in which sufficient work is accomplished during
each day to allow the investigators to collect meaningful and representative samples; a minimum of four hours of work per day is desirable. Sufficient numbers of workers should be monitored during the
study to gather meaningful and representative data. Reported values
should include data from at least four different workers if
possible. The workers should be employees who are routinely engaged
in the mixing/loading or application of pesticides. Informed consent and appropriate human subjects review may be required for
studies done in California if the pesticide or the use of the pesticide being studied does not have Federal Experimental, Federal or
California Conditional, or full California registration. Exposure
should be as realistic as possible. Only the protective items
proposed or already required on existing or proposed labeling--for
example, protective clothing such as long-sleeved cotton coveralls,
and protective equipment such as impervious gloves and impervious
foot covering--are to be worn. If additional protection is specified on the label or proposed label, it should be carefully complied
with in the study. Toxicity Category I liquid pesticides should be
transferred from their original containers to mixing or application
tanks through closed transfer systems. Exposures of persons should
not be conducted with excessively dusty toxicity Category I pesticides until dustiness is reduced to a level acceptable for use in
California. (A summary of a number of studies conducted in
California by CDFA is included in Appendix One.)

Dermal Absorption and Dermal Dose-Response. These data are needed in
the risk assessment of field workers, mixers/loaders, applicators,
and flaggers; they may also be used in the development of reentry
intervals. The data gathered informs CDFA of how much of the chemical actually enters the body once it comes into contact with the
skin. Guides for these types of studies in test animals are available through, and were conducted by, the CDFA. At times, data from
human volunteer studies are available; when available, this type of
information usually takes precedence over animal test data.

Hazard Evaluation (Risk Assessment)

The CDFA, in its hazard evaluation process, determines whether an
adequate hazard assessment can be made immediately, or if additional
data are needed, based on the consideration of the following
factors:

1.   Review of the basic toxicology data submitted by the registrant;

2. Review of other toxicology data available to the Unit (journal articles, unit studies, computerized national data banks, texts, etc.);
3. Human illness information developed by the unit or others involving the pesticide under consideration or similar pesticides;
4. Available exposure data on this pesticide or this class of pesticides developed by this unit or any other group; and,
5. Work practices known about or expected in California for the proposed use.

The CDFA develops and continues to update data on pesticide-related illnesses for specific pesticides as to when, why, and how they occur. The Unit also measures how much exposure occurs in the wide variety of use situations.

The basic toxicology review informs the Department of the extent and adequacy of the data base upon which the evaluation of a potential use hazard is to be made.

A hazard evaluation differs considerably from a basic toxicology review. For example, a specific pesticide can be found in the toxicology review to be extremely toxic. However, in the hazard evaluation process, it may be determined that the product is to be used in such small quantities with specialized equipment that a person could only be overexposed in the unusual case of equipment failure. On the other hand, a product could be found to be of low toxicity; but, the most common use might involve long hours of exposure to many workers in orchards while using hand-held spray wands (spraying the pesticide above their heads) with no protective clothing due to lack of specification in the precautionary label statements. In another example, the basic toxicology data for a product may only indicate a moderate toxicity; however, in assessing the proposed use of the product mid-summer in a citrus grove in the San Joaquin Valley, there could be substantial conversion of the active ingredient to a highly toxic degradative product under actual field conditions which would be hazardous to field workers.

Often the data submitted by the registrant to meet EPA requirements is also adequate for the CDFA to complete a hazard evaluation, especially for many of the low toxicity and low hazard products. The CDFA may require additional data, as discussed above, to complete the hazard evaluation.

The CDFA review may include:
1. Determining the use pattern of the proposed product;
2. Determining significant human exposure hazards;
3. Evaluating the adequacy of use instructions and/or regulations that are in place to inform users of the possible use hazards and how to avoid excess exposure.
4. Evaluating the adequacy of information provided to recognize illness due to exposure if it occurs;
5. Determining the adequacy of first aid information; and,
6. Examining the availability of data to support medical management.

Data from the toxicology base, plus those from the additional Health and Safety studies that are sometimes required, allow for the

estimation and calculation of potential exposure hazards. For some
products, experience already gained allows for a quick determination
that adherence to the use instructions should result in a low hazard
situation. On the other hand, a small percentage of the pesticides
considered for registration have significant hazards from either a
short-term or long-term exposure standpoint. These hazards are
estimated and/or calculated to determine if a favorable recommendation on the proposed registration can be given and, if not, whether
additional restrictions would be expected to acceptably reduce the
hazards of use.

For example, a particular product might be a highly dusty wettable powder with only moderate acute toxicity but with demonstrated
potential for producing chronic effects. The calculations for the
hazard evaluation are based upon the total workday measurement of
the skin and inhalation exposure to this pesticide when it is used
in accord with the label instructions. This potential daily dose is
then adjusted by the estimated 24-hour dermal absorption rate. This
final figure is compared to animal test data for the dose expected
to produce a specific adverse effect. The safety factor for this
specific effect will then be calculated to determine if it is adequate to protect the workers. In some cases, results of calculations might not give an acceptable safety factor for a mixer/loader;
but, if this product were packaged in water-soluble packets or if it
were to be used as a liquid product and required to be transferred
through a closed system, the hazard might be acceptably reduced.

Of particular concern are potential adverse effects such as
carcinogenicity, fetotoxicity, and teratogenicity. The following is
given to illustrate the assessment process by CDFA of these types of
adverse health effects.

Cancer Risk Assessment. Based on chronic animal bioassay and mutagenicity testing results, an in-depth review is conducted to determine whether the product is an animal carcinogen. If positive
results have been confirmed, the chemical undergoes further evaluation. The possible mode of action is then determined to be: (1) a
genotoxin (exhibited positive results in a chronic animal bioassay
in at least one animal species tested, in conjunction with a battery
of positive mutagenicity tests); or, (2) an epigenetic toxin (minimal or weakly positive results in a chronic animal bioassay and a
battery of negative mutagenicity tests). A ranking system (modified
Squire) (6, 7) is then used which takes into consideration a variety
of vital parameters; such as number, species and sex of animals
affected, tumor type, organs involved, malignancy and rarity of
tumor, tumor incidence in comparison to the incidence of spontaneous
tumors, dose range and dose response, and the results of a battery
of mutagenicity tests.

Then, from the worker exposure data, an average and a maximum
exposure level for each type of work activity involved with pesticide use is taken into consideration. The number of workers in each
job category, the total yearly body dose (which may be derived from
number of hours/days/months exposure in performing the job), and the
total dermal absorption is all taken into consideration. Residue
levels (including degradation products) found in treated crops or a
particular product are used to assess consumer risk.

A cancer risk assessment is made using the currently available mathematical models, as suggested by the EPA.
(See Appendix Two for an example of a CDFA assessment of carcinogenic risk.)

Fetotoxicity and Teratogenicity Risk Assessment.   The CDFA has developed a guideline for evaluating fetotoxicity and teratogenicity (8).   A number of vital parameters are considered in this ranking of teratogens.   These include, but are not limited to, the nature of major and minor malformations, maternal toxicity and lethality, at which dosages morphological changes of the embryoes and fetuses are being observed, effective dose range, and maximum no observable effect level (NOEL), and the route of administration.

Since fetotoxic and teratogenic responses differ qualitatively, so does the "potency" of an embryotoxin or a teratogen.   CDFA differentiates   between   high   dose   and   low   dose   teratogens;   for instance, a chemical which exerts a fetotoxic/teratogenic effect with a dose as little as 0.1 mg/kg/day when given during organogenesis is notably more potent than another product which does not exert a fetotoxic/teratogenic response until a dose of 300 mg/kg/day is given.   The ranking that a fetotoxin/teratogen receives determines the acceptable safety factor needed to mitigate the health hazard during exposure.   The total body dose (mg/kg/day) actually absorbed by the worker during a typical workday divided by animal NOEL (mg/kg/day) represents the safety factor that is obtained for that particular work activity.   This is then compared to the acceptable safety factor.   From this, it is determined whether adequate safety is reasonably achievable.   In such cases when there is an inadequate safety factor, additional mitigation measures are taken to ensure adequate worker protection if registration is to be granted or maintained.

Safety Factors.   The following is CDFA's current guideline for safety factors required to mitigate various toxicological effects. If the desired safety factor cannot be achieved, use of that product is in question, unless additional practices to increase safety can be applied such as use of closed system transfer, water-soluble packaging, specifying less hazardous work practices, or requiring special protective clothing.

For each of the following effects, a minimum safety factor is applied to the No Observable Effect Level (NOEL) in test animals. In acute animal exposure studies, the maximum dose level which produces no detectable clinical illnesses, no biochemical changes, no histopathological changes and no deaths is considered to be the NOEL.

Adverse Effects	Safety Factors
1. Acute Effects	
a. Cholinesterase inhibition	10-fold
b. Other acute effects	20-fold
2. Effects on Reproduction	

    a. General reproduction (including reductions
       in (1) number of off-spring, (2) fertility,
       (3) sperm counts, and (4) size of testes, etc.)   50 fold
    b. Embryotoxic/fetotoxic effects   50 fold
    c. Teratogenic effects   50 to 300 fold
3. Delayed-Onset Neurotoxic Effects   50 fold
4. Oncogenicity (including mutagenicity) Risk
    Assessments   *

*The lifetime risk of cancer is usually calculated by using one of
three models: (1) the one-hit model (9, 10); (2) the multi-stage
model (11, 12); and, (3) a choice of a third model usually the
Weibel model or the improved Mantel-Bryan model (13, 14). The risk
calculations are made by comparing the dose response curve obtained
from animal exposures to the human exposure data.

a. For consumers of   Not more than one additional esti-
    treated crops   mated case of cancer in the
                       lifetime of 1,000,000 persons.

b. For field workers   Not more than one additional esti-
                       mated case of cancer in the
                       lifetime of 300,000 persons.

c. For mixers, loaders,   Not more than one additional esti-
    applicators   mated case of cancer in the
                       lifetime of 100,000 persons. For
                       a few years, a risk as high as 1
                       in 10,000 may be tolerated in the
                       case of extreme need.

Adequacy of Mitigation Measures After all relevant data are
evaluated, an assessment is made as to the adequacy of the possible
mitigation measures to protect workers from hazards of use. The
product label may be accepted and the product may be registered
without further concern. On the other hand, one or more of the
following conditions may be required before the product is considered for registration by the CDFA: (1) the EPA may be advised of
the desirability of requiring a label change, or the registrant may
recognize the need to ask EPA for a label change; (2) a California
regulation on the use may be enacted (which will have the same
effect as a label change, but this can take a number of months to
accomplish); (3) the product may be made a California restricted
material which will allow imposition of specific permit requirements
(this process can also take a number of months); (4) closed system
transfer of liquid pesticides may be required, (this is currently
required for all toxicity Category I liquids, when specified on
labels regardless of the toxicity category and when specifically
required by regulations); (5) change in the product's formulation
may be required to reduce excess hazards (e.g., reduce dustiness);
(6) water-soluble packaging of the more toxic powders may be
required; (7) minimum field reentry intervals may be set by regulation (a several-month process unless they are adequately specified
on the label); (8) medical supervision may be required by regulation; and/or (9) detailed safety training may be required for specific pesticides.

If hazards of use cannot be mitigated by means that can be reasonably employed, the product will not be registered.

CONCLUSIONS

Excessive unnecessary warnings on every use of every product could lead to workers taking a casual attitude in their use of all products. On the other hand, there has been so much scrutiny and concern about the use of pesticides in recent years that it is important to warn of real hazards and to base information on how to reduce exposure to pesticides on the best possible technical information. This information clearly stated on the product is of benefit to: (1) the manufacturer who has spent millions of dollars in developing a product and who wishes to sell and/or continue to sell it; (2) the users who may collectively receive financial benefits or a more comfortable pest-free situation from the proper use of the product; (3) the person who handles the pesticide, since he is told exactly what the use hazards are and how to avoid them; as well as, (4) the many members of the general public who have concerns that pesticides are not being used carefully enough.

Literature Cited

1. Knaak, J.B.; Schlocker, P.; Ackerman, C.R.; and, Seiber, J.N. Bull. Environ. Contam. Toxicol. 1980, 24.
2. Iwata, Y.; Knaak, J.B.; Spear, R.C.; and, Foster, R.J. Bull. Environ. Contam. Toxicol. 1977, 18, 649.
3. Spencer, W. F.; Iwata, Y.; Kilgore, W.N.; and, Knaak, J.B. Bull. Environ. Contam. Toxicol. 1977, 18, 656.
4. Iwata, Y.; Knaak, J.B.; Carman, G.E.; Dusch, M.E.; and, Gunther, F.A. Journal of Agricultural and Food Chemistry 1982, 30, 215.
5. Kahn, E. Residue Reviews 1979, 70, 27.
6. Squire, R.A. Science 1981, 214, 877.
7. Wang, R.G. 1984, In-House Document, Worker Health and Safety Unit. State of California.
8. Wang, R.G. 1984, In-House Document, Worker Health and Safety Unit.   State of California.
9. Armitage, P. J. Nat´l. Cancer Inst. 1959, 23, 1313.
10. Crump, K.S.; Guess, H.A.; and, Deal, K.L. Biometrics 1977, 33, 437.
11. Van Ryzin, J.; and, Rai, K. In H.R. Witschi (ed.), Elvesier/North Holland Biomedical Press 1980, 273-290.
12. Crump, K.S. Biometrics 1979, 35, 157.
13. Armitage, P. Biometrics (Supplement) 1982, 38, 119-129.
14. Mantel, N.; Bohidar, N.R.; Brown, C.C.; Ciminera, J.L.; and, Tukey, J.W. Canc. Res. 1975, 35, 865.

Appendix One: Dermal Exposure Monitoring of Mixers,
Loaders, and Applicators of Pesticides in California

Some pesticides possess the potential to cause adverse health
effects in workers who are exposed to these chemicals during the
application process (1-3). Concerns about these health hazards
have led to the development of exposure monitoring techniques
designed to help understand the factors influencing pesticide
exposure. Data generated from these techniques assist in the
development of preventive measures including the use of protective clothing and equipment, medical supervision of employees,
increased awareness of the need for proper personal hygiene
practices, improved label statements and government regulations.
     Early attempts at monitoring worker exposure to pesticides
during application were performed by Batchelor and Walker (4) and
Durham and Wolfe (5). They measured dermal exposure by placing
small filter pads on the skin of the workers in areas not protected
by clothing. Analysis of the collected residues and extrapolation
of the results to the entire unprotected surface area gave rise to
an estimated total dermal exposure. Potential inhalation exposure
was also monitored by analyzing respirator pads of face masks for
pesticide residue. Results indicated that dermal exposure to
pesticides being applied outdoors to foliage was by far, of greater
concern than inhalation exposure during application for its potential
to cause acute health effects. These results are consistent with
those obtained from other studies (6-8).
     Durham and Wolfe (5) assumed that workers involved in pesticide
applications usually wore shoes, socks, long trousers, a short-
sleeved open-necked shirt, but no hat, respirator, or gloves. They
reasoned that the majority of the dermal exposure of the workers
would occur on the unprotected skin areas of the face, hands,
forearms, back of neck, front of neck, and the "V" of the chest.
Exposure to other areas is protected by clothing, although some
penetration may still occur (9-11). The capacity to penetrate
clothing depends on the individual chemical, as well as its formulation, the amount used, and the specific fabric used in the clothing.
     California regulations require daily provision and use of clean
coveralls or other clean outer clothing to mixers, loaders, flaggers,
and applicators of any pesticide in toxicity Categories I and II
(12). These requirements serve to reduce the potential dermal
exposure of workers to pesticides by decreasing the area of bare
skin available for contact with the chemicals.
     The California Department of Food and Agriculture (CDFA) has
attempted to estimate pesticide exposure of body areas protected by
clothing. This report summarizes experimental studies which attempt
to estimate total dermal exposure and the different amounts of this
exposure which occur on various parts of the body.

Methods

CDFA conducted dermal exposure monitoring of workers involved in the application of parathion, mevinphos (Phosdrin), nitrofen (TOK), DEF/Folex, and chlorobenzilate (Acaraben) (13-18). Exposures of mixers/loaders, ground applicators, mixers/loaders/ground applicators (workers performing all three activities during a single application), aerial applicators, and flaggers were determined in a total of 102 individual exposure situations.

In all the exposure situations, workers wore cloth coveralls. Rubber or some other type of waterproof gloves were worn by all workers except the aerial applicators and flaggers. Respirators and other protective devices were used when required by pesticide labels.

Hand exposure was determined by rinsing the hands in a predetermined solvent containing either water, soap and water, ethanol, or a combination of the three. Hands were rinsed prior to and upon completion of the applications. Wettable and soluble powders are usually well removed with soap and water; for other formulations, solvents such as ethanol often were more efficient.

Exposures to the head, face, and neck were estimated by placing small cloth pads on the upper collar of the coveralls in the front and back, or, in some cases, placing smaller pads directly on the face. Amounts of chemicals in these pads were extrapolated to the entire surface areas of these body parts.

Potential exposure to skin protected by cotton coveralls was measured with pads measuring 49 cm^2 made of an outer layer of seven-ounce 65 percent dacron polyester, 35 percent cotton twill, and an inner layer of 100 percent cotton gauze backed by aluminum foil. The pesticide found on the gauze portion was assumed to simulate the amount which would penetrate the coverall material and reach the skin.

The composition of the outer pad was consistent with most commercially available coveralls. As in the case of the head, face, and neck exposures, values were extrapolated to estimate exposures of the total surface area.

Results

Tables I, II, and III summarize the average percentage of total dermal exposure found on various regions by individual chemical and job activity, respectively. The hands are not considered to be a protected area, as such, even though waterproof gloves were usually worn. Table IV summarizes the amounts of pesticide that were estimated to have reached the skin.

Discussion

The results presented in the Tables show that estimated exposure to protected body areas represented, on the average, 23.3 percent of the total dermal exposure. Statistical analysis utilizing one-way analysis of variance was performed to determine whether the average percentage of total dermal exposure found on the unprotected areas differed by chemical or job activity. Calculated F-values of 1.84 and 1.21, respectively, were below the value of 2.49 required for statistical significance at the p=0.05 level. It was concluded, that the average contribution of the unprotected areas to the total dermal exposure did not appear to strongly depend upon the chemical or job activity involved in the situations monitored by CDFA.

The fact that hand exposure exceeded exposure to all other areas was not surprising; other studies have shown similar results (10, 11, 19) even when gloves were worn. Workers who wore water-proof gloves still experienced hand exposures, representing 40.9 percent of their total dermal exposure. Possible explanations for the relative ineffectiveness of the gloves include: (1) contamination of the inside material of the gloves; (2) removal of gloves during mechanical adjustments to the application equipment; and, (3) the handling of the outside of contaminated gloves while putting them on or taking them off. This does not imply that the wearing of gloves would be expected to increase exposure to pesticides; the data merely suggests that the potential for waterproof gloves to prevent exposure of the hands is not routinely maximized. Quantitative data for actual penetration of glove materials by specific chemicals is often not available to CDFA, but there is some evidence that this is only a minor factor in contamination of the hands.

Questions arise as to the necessity of monitoring protected areas if only 23.3 percent of the total dermal exposure occurs in these areas. A qualitative study of worker exposure using fluorescent tracers led to the conclusion that "results depend critically on knowing where to place the pads" (11). This study also demonstrated that the principal exposure was to the face, hands, and neck.

In some studies, particularly screening studies, more attention should be given to the monitoring of the hands, head, face, and neck, and less attention to monitoring protected areas. The ability of a chemical to penetrate protective clothing and, thus, present hazards to protected skin areas, could be quantitated in the laboratory prior to the commencement of a field study in order to determine whether sampling protected areas might be necessary. Current techniques in hand monitoring could be improved by performing additional hand-washes and calculating the extraction efficiencies of the various solvents used (19). Thin cloth gloves can be used as inserts in the usually-worn waterproof gloves to be extracted periodically to estimate the amount of chemical which reaches the skin. Direct methods for face and neck monitoring, such as swabbing (6) or skin washing (20), are possibilities for improving accuracy over the current pad exposure techniques. These techniques would place less emphasis on extrapolative methods, and would also enable identification of the protective capabilities of faceshields, goggles, and respirators in the reduction of dermal exposure.

The actual biological monitoring of workers to detect evidence of exposure such as a drop in blood cholinesterase levels or the presence of a urinary metabolite is superior to the indirect techniques employed in this study. Realizing the difficulties in accurately determining the dermal exposures of mixers, loaders, and applicators to pesticides, the employment of simpler monitoring techniques than the ones performed by CDFA in this report might

Table I. Pesticides Used in 102 Different Applications to Farm Fields in California During Which Exposure of Workers Involved in the Applications Were Monitored

Chemical	Application Type	Formulation Type	Pounds Per Acre of Active Ingredient	Acres Treated Per Hour
Parathion	Air Blast—Ground	WP 25%	2.5	4
Mevinphos	Airplane/Helicopter	EC 25%	0.5 to 1	50 to 75
TOK	Boom—Ground	EC 24%, WP 50%	3.5	12
DEF/Folex	Airplane	EC 70%	1.5	175
Chlorbenzilate	Oscillating Boom/Handwands	EC 45%	2.2 to 2.7	2

See specific studies as referenced for more details.

Table II. Relative Contributions to Total Dermal Exposure of Body Areas to Pesticides as Studied by the California Department of Food and Agriculture

Chemical	Number of Exposures Monitored	Average Percentage on Hands	Average Percentage on Head, Face, and Neck	Average Percentage on Hands and Head, Face, and Neck	Average Percentage on Protected Areas
Parathion	3	23.4	67.4	90.8	9.2
Mevinphos	22	48.0	34.6	82.6	17.4
TOK	24	49.2	22.7	71.9	28.1
DEF/Folex	32	46.8	23.7	70.5	29.5
Chlorobenzilate	21	27.1	59.4	86.5	13.5
Total	102	42.9	33.8	76.7	23.3

Table III. Relative Contributions to Total Dermal Exposure of Body Areas by Job Activity

Chemical	Number of Exposures Monitored	Average Percentage on Hands	Average Percentage on Head, Face, and Neck	Average Percentage on Hands and Head, Face, and Neck	Average Percentage on Protected Areas
Mixer/Loader, Ground Applicator	4	18.1	57.5	75.6	24.4
Mixer/Loader	36	50.7	22.0	72.7	27.3
Aerial Applicator	18	54.6	27.4	82.0	18.0
Ground Applicator	25	30.4	47.9	78.3	21.7
Flagger	19	38.7	38.6	77.3	22.7
Total	102	42.9	33.8	76.7	23.3

Table IV. Estimated Dermal Exposure of Workers to Pesticides Adjusted for a Seven-Hour Work Period as Studied by the California Department of Food and Agriculture[1]

Mg/Day Chemical Activity	Hands Median	Hands Range	Head, Face, & Neck Median	Head, Face, & Neck Range	Protected Areas Median	Protected Areas Range	Total Median	Total Range
Parathion	7.335	4.954– 19.106	7.332	5.003– 73.396	3.042	1.940– 6.736	15.380	14.226– 99.238
Phosdrin	0.081	0–3.383	0.028	0–1.691	0	0–6.951	0.254	0–8.856
TOK	0.943	0.148– 25.255	0.634	0.023– 4.9896	0.707	0–3.967	5.285	0.259– 29.883
Def/Folex	4.626	0.293– 17.270	1.811	0.053– 23.072	2.139	0.403– 24.516	10.240	4.087– 40.190
Chlorobenzilate	.96	0– 91.787	1.837	0.087– 20.650	0.262	0– 7688.000	12.775	0.175– 7523.425
Mixer/Loader, Ground Applicator	6.145	0.148– 19.106	6.168	1.713– 73.396	3.653	1.940– 6.736	14.803	6.63– 99.238
Mixer/Loader Only	1.400	0.097– 91.787	1.662	0– 12.950	0.425	0– 24.516	5.853	0.299– 94.500
Aerial Applicator	2.641	0– 15.960	0.200	0– 3.989	1.663	0– 2.629	6.027	0– 17.733
Ground Applicator Only	0.767	0– 8.400	0.850	0.030– 20.650	0.606	0– 7513.000	3.5	0.175– 7523.425
Flagger For Airplane	0.866	0– 78.910	1.030	0– 23.072	0.953	0– 10.241	5.111	0– 29.389

1/ Studies were based on 102 use situations. Amounts are expressed in milligrams of active ingredient that reached the skin. Absorption rates are not given.

yield useful results particularly for pilot studies or range-finding
studies. For example, since hand exposure was, on the average,
responsible for more than 42 percent of the total dermal exposure,
estimates of total dermal exposure could be derived by multiplying
the hand exposure by a factor of 2.5. This rough estimate should be
accurate within one order of magnitude and, as such, would generally
enable adequate determination of potential health risks for regulatory purposes.

Caution should be exercised in comparing the dermal exposure
values found in these studies with other studies. These dermal
exposure levels are as much as one-tenth of the amount found for
other similar applications of similar pesticides outside of California. All persons were working in accord with California Worker
Safety and Restricted Materials Regulations and all applications
were made by trained employees of California Pest Control Operators.
All of these formulations studied were California Restricted Pesticides and almost all were toxicity Category I liquids which are
required to be mixed and loaded through closed systems. All workers
put on clean outer clothes daily and all wore impervious gloves when
contact with the concentrate was a possibility. On the other hand,
caution was exercised to avoid special training, extra instructions
or excessive observation because the employers and employees had
been instructed to apply the pesticides in the usual manner.

References

1.   Kay, K. L.; Monkman, L.; Windish, J. P.; Doherty, T.; Pare', J.;
     and Racicot. C.A.M.A. Arch. Indust. Hyg. 1952, 6, 252.
2.   Sumerford, W. T.; Hayes, W. J.; Johnston, J. M.; Walker, K.;
     and Spillane, J. A.M.A. Arch. Indust. Hyg. 1953.
3.   Jegier, Z.: Health Hazards in Insecticide Spraying of Crops.
     Arch. Environ. Health 1964, 8, 670.
4.   Batchelor, G. S. and Walker, K. C. A.M.A. Arch. Indust. Hyg.,
     1954, 10, 522.
5.   Durham, W. F. and Wolfe, H. R. Bull WHO 1962, 26, 75.
6.   Durham, W. F. Arch. Environ. Health 1965, 10, 842.
7.   Hartwell, W. V.; Hayes, G. R.; and Funckes, A. J. Arch.
     Environ. Health 1964, 8, 820.
8.   Durham, W. F.; Wolfe, H. R.; and Elliott, J. W. Arch. Environ.
     Health 1972, 24, 381.
9.   Davies, J. E.; Freed, V. H.; Enos, H. F.; Duncan, R. C.;
     Barquet, A.; Morgade, C.; Peters, L. J.; and Danauskas, J. X.
     J. Occup. Med. 1982, 24, 464.
10. Leavitt, J. R.; Gold, R. E.; Holcslaw, T.; and Tupy, D. Arch.
     Environ. Contam. Toxicol. 1982, 11, 57.
11. Franklin, C. A.; Fenske, R. A.; Greenhalgh, R.; Mathieu, L.;
     Denley, H. V.; Leffingwell, J. T.; and Spear, R. C. J.
     Toxicol. Environ. Health 1981, 7, 715.
12. California Administrative Code, Title 3, Sect. 2477 (h),
     Sacramento, California.
13. Maddy, K. T.; Winter, C. K.; Saini, N.; and Quan, V. HS-888,
     Worker Health and Safety Unit 1982. State of California.
14. Maddy, K. T.; Winter, C.; Cepello, S.; and Fredrickson, A. S.
     HS-876, Worker Health and Safety Unit 1981. State of Cali-
     fornia.

15. Maddy, K. T.; Winter, C.; Cepello, S.; and Fredrickson, A. S. HS-889, Worker Health and Safety Unit 1982. State of California.
16. Maddy, K. T.; O'Connell, L. P.; Winter, C. K.; and Margetich, S. HS-903, Worker Health and Safety Unit 1982. State of California.
17. Maddy, K. T.; Johnston, L.; Smith, C.; Schneider, F.; and Jackson, T. HS-745 Worker Health and Safety Unit 1980. State of California.
18. Peoples, S. A.; Maddy, K. T.; Datta, P. R.; Johnston, L.; Smith, C.; Conrad, D.; and Cooper, C. HS-676, Worker Health and Safety Unit 1981. State of California.
19. Davis, J. E. Residue Reviews 1980, 75, 34.
20. Keenan, R. R. and Cole, S. B. Am. Ind. Hyg. Assoc. J. 1982, 43, 473.

Appendix Two: Cancer Risk Assessment for Persons
Involved in Application of Chlordimeform as a
Pesticide to Cotton Fields in California

Summary

Chlordimeform is used as a pesticide on cotton fields in two counties in California under a closely regulated worker exposure control
program. Animal test data indicates that this chemical is a carcinogen. Urinary metabolites (aniline derivatives) of this chemical
were measured in workers who were involved in this application.
These values were used in estimating cancer risk of exposed workers.
It was determined that with very close attention to mimimizing
inhalation and dermal exposure to this chemical, if exposure were
limited to five days a week, 10 weeks a year, for only 10 years,
cancer risk might be kept as low as one chance in 500,000 of an
extra case of cancer in the lifetime of such an exposed person. On
the other hand, if only average attention were given to minimizing
exposure for the same number of days and years, the risk of an
exposed worker acquiring cancer might rise to as high as one chance
in 24,000.

Analysis

According to the data submitted by the registrant to this Department, when mice were fed chlordimeform, a significant increase in
the incidence of malignant hemangioendotheliomas was observed as
compared to the control mice. This tumor incidence is presented in
Table I.

Table I. Malignant Hemangioendothelioma Incidence
Induced by Chlordimeform in Mice

Dose Level (ppm)	Male	Female	Combined
0	1/42	1/41	2/83
20	0/42	2/44	2/86
100	15/47	22/44	37/91
500	39/47	35/46	74/93

Dr. Bernard Hanes, our Consulting Biostatistician, assisted us
in carrying out a series of risk estimates based on this mouse bioassay data, using three recognized mathematical models (multi-hit,
multi-stage, and one-hit). Table II provides a print-out of "point-
estimate" doses at given response values (risk).

With the data presented in Table II, it is possible to make
risk estimations, by interpolation, for workers who are exposed to
certain levels of chlordimeform.

Table III shows cancer risk assessments for chlordimeform exposure based on urinary excretion of chlordimeform in man and malignant tumor incidence from the mouse bioassay study (male and female
mice data combined). Three commonly used mathematical models
(multi-hit, multi-stage, and one-hit) are used in the risk estimations.

Table II. Computer Output of Risk Assessment Data

I. From Male Mouse Data

Risk	Multi-Hit	Estimated Dose (ppm) Multi-Stage	One-Hit
10^{-2}	7.98	3.65	3.00
10^{-3}	1.44	3.64×10^{-1}	2.99×10^{-1}
10^{-4}	2.62×10^{-1}	3.64×10^{-2}	2.99×10^{-2}
10^{-5}	4.79×10^{-2}	3.64×10^{-3}	2.99×10^{-3}
10^{-6}	8.74×10^{-3}	3.64×10^{-4}	2.99×10^{-4}
10^{-7}	1.60×10^{-4}	3.64×10^{-5}	2.99×10^{-5}
10^{-8}	2.91×10^{-5}	3.64×10^{-6}	2.99×10^{-6}

II. From Both Sexes Combined Data

Risk	Multi-Hit	Estimated Dose (ppm) Multi-Stage	One-Hit
10^{-2}	2.79	2.89	2.89
10^{-3}	2.72×10^{-1}	2.88×10^{-1}	2.88×10^{-1}
10^{-4}	2.66×10^{-2}	2.88×10^{-2}	2.88×10^{-2}
10^{-5}	2.60×10^{-3}	2.88×10^{-3}	2.88×10^{-3}
10^{-6}	2.54×10^{-4}	2.88×10^{-4}	2.88×10^{-4}
10^{-7}	2.49×10^{-5}	2.88×10^{-5}	2.88×10^{-5}
10^{-8}	2.43×10^{-6}	2.88×10^{-6}	2.88×10^{-6}

Table III. Worker's Cancer Risk Due to Chlordimeform Exposure

Chlordimeform Levels in Urine	Multi-Hit	Multi-Stage	One-Hit
50 ppb (0.05 ppm)	2.2×10^{-6} (1 in 450 K)	2.1×10^{-6} (1 in 480 K)	2.1×10^{-6} (1 in 480 K)
100 ppb (0.1 ppm)	4.4×10^{-6} (1 in 230 K)	4.2×10^{-6} (1 in 240 K)*	4.2×10^{-6} (1 in 240 K)
250 ppb (0.25 ppm)	1.1×10^{-5} (1 in 91 K)	1.0×10^{-5} (1 in 100 K)	1.0×10^{-5} (1 in 100 K)
500 ppb (0.5 ppm)	2.2×10^{-5} (1 in 45 K)	2.1×10^{-5} (1 in 48 K)	2.1×10^{-5} (1 in 48 K)
1,000 ppm (1 ppm)	4.4×10^{-5} (1 in 23 K)	4.2×10^{-5} (1 in 24 K)	4.2×10^{-5} (1 in 24 K)

*For instance, this means a probability of 1 in 240,000 of inducing cancer in one worker due to chlordimeform exposures.

The following assumptions were made to calculate the above risk estimates:

1) Humans are as sensitive to the carcinogenic effects of chlordimeform as are the laboratory mice.
2) For the mouse, 1 ppm chlordimeform in the diet equals 0.1 mg chlordimeform per kilogram of body weight based on average food intake.
3) Average worker weight is 70 kg (154 pounds).
4) The average amount of urine excreted per day is 1.5 liters.
5) Exposure to chlordimeform will occur five days per week, 10 weeks in a year, and for 10 years of a 70-year life span.
6) Carcinogenic effect is determined by the total accumulated dose, i.e., (dose) x (time) = tumor yield.
7) Based on human and laboratory animal data, the amount of chlordimeform measured in urine represents 35% of the dermally absorbed dose.

During the summer of 1982, the California Department of Food and Agriculture's Worker Health and Safety Unit staff monitored worker's exposure associated with the use of chlordimeform as a pesticide on cotton in Imperial County, California, under a very tightly regulated exposure reduction program. Table IV gives a summary of chlordimeform (as aniline derivatives) measured in the urine of workers involved in applications of this pesticide.

Table IV. Summary of the Levels of Chlordimeform Measured
in the Urine of Workers Involved in Applications
of this Pesticide in Imperial County in 1982

Urine Sample	Total Number of Samples	Average Chlordimeform Levels ppm**
"A" samples only (urine collected at end of workshift)	537	0.12
"B" samples only (urine collected 8-12 hours after end of workshift)	556	0.10
"A" and "B" samples	1,093	0.11
"A" and "B" samples (higher of the two values only)	598	0.13

**All non-detected levels were given the value of 0.05 ppm, the limit of detection.

Table IV shows that the averge chlordimeform levels among the urinary samples taken are in the range of 100 to 130 ppb (0.10 to 0.13 ppm). The cancer risk for a worker having been exposed to this amount of chlordimeform can be estimated from the data presented in

Table III. For example, if a worker has a urine concentration of 100 ppb of chlordimeform, the extra risk of acquiring cancer due to chlordimeform exposure is approximately 1 in 240,000 according to the multi-stage model. For the majority of the monitored workers whose urinary chlordimeform levels were below 50 ppm, their increased risk might be as low as 1 in 500,000.

Due to the intrinsic uncertainty associated with the mathematical extrapolation, from a few animal data points to a low dose response, the risk shown in Table III from exposure to a specific level of chemical should be considered as a probability distribution or risk profile. For example, for a risk with a "best point-estimate" of 10^{-6}, there might be a five percent chance that the true level of risk might be one or two orders of magnitude greater or smaller than the point-estimate value. Thus, for the person excreting an average level of 1 ppm chlordimeform in urine, for the conditions that apply in Table III for the multi-stage model, the increased risk of acquiring cancer has a 95% probability of being in the range between 1 chance in 240 and 1 chance in 2,400,000.

Although these statistical methods are currently being used to estimate cancer risk, because of the small number of animals exposed and the small numbers of dose levels used, considerable caution should be exercised not to over-interpret these statistical estimates of what will happen in a biological system such as the exposed person.

An additional variable not dealt with completely in these risk analyses, is the expected type of tumor. The tumors produced in the mouse were hemangioendotheliomas in the abdominal organs and tissues. Aniline residues passing through the human bladder are suspect as having the potential of producing more serious tumors at this site. This variable adds to the uncertainty of cancer risk assessment for human exposure based on laboratory animal data.

RECEIVED November 14, 1984

The Use of Exposure Studies in Risk Assessment

JAMES T. STEVENS and DARRELL D. SUMNER

Agricultural Division, CIBA-GEIGY Corporation, Greensboro, NC 27419

The extrapolation of animal toxicology data and
combination with human exposure data may be used to
estimate risk for those situations where exposure is
likely. Methods for integrating these data as well
as the assumptions for extrapolation from the animal
studies are dependent upon the safety data. Risk
assessment includes consideration of; the type of
toxicity involved and its potency, species comparisons, time considerations, dose response, kinetics
of homeostatic mechanisms, and mechanisms of toxicity. When the essential components for extrapolations are well understood, more precise estimates
can be made. In the absence of such understanding,
more conservative approaches are appropriate.

Exposure and risk assessment procedures are often combined to
evaluate use practices for handling toxic materials. In order to
adequately consider the marriage of these two techniques, it is
important to examine both the virtues and frailities of the
approaches. Risk assessment involves several unprecise and sometimes unverifiable assumptions as well as a deceptive, comforting
assurance of specific number resolution; exposure assessment
helps to define quantitatively the situation but often with an
artificial air of exactitude. The following article attempts to
discuss some of the intimacies of these procedures in the final
safety assessment.

For purposes of this discussion, risk assessment is defined
as an estimate of the probability of an adverse effect. In virtually all cases, a quantitative value for the probability is
expressed. Exposure shall be defined as the amount of material
in immediate contact with an inanimate or a living system (including man). In man, exposure may result from inhalation into
the respiratory tract, ingestion into the gastrointestinal tract
or deposition and absorption through the skin. From a toxicological viewpoint, materials outside the body may not present a
particular hazard, with the possible exception of local effects.

0097-6156/85/0273-0467$06.00/0

For simplicity, materials inhaled or ingested are generally considered to be completely absorbed; whereas, materials deposited on the skin may or may not receive the same treatment since it is recognized that total penetration through the skin is unlikely. The ability to remove the materials from the skin by washing may reduce the time of exposure so that actual dermal absorption may be diminished. The amount present within the body is better defined as a body burden. It is this body burden that is regarded as of toxicological concern.

Risk is a function of the body burden and the inherent toxicity of the material (1). Clearly, Botulinum toxin, which is an extremely hazardous toxicant, constitutes no risk when body burdens are zero. Body burden may be best illustrated in kinetic terms, as shown graphically in Figure 1.

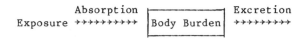

Figure 1. Body burden illustrated in kinetic terms.

It is clear that the body burden increases as absorption increases and excretion decreases. Since toxicology studies often involve ad libitum feeding or bolus administration into the GI tract, where complete absorption is assumed, they inherently evaluate the excretion rate; in dermal exposure, absorption is the prominent variable in the evaluation (2).

Hence it becomes important to define this variable as precisely as possible. It is generally recognized that the skin is a relatively poor protection barrier to most organic chemicals. But, in the absence of specifically designed studies, 100 percent absorption is often assumed. Data to estimate dermal penetration may be collected from a variety of sources: humans, rats, mice (hairless), rabbits, monkeys, pigs, or excised human skin (3). Human skin grafted to the trunks of immunologically compromised nude mice offer interesting possibilities for the future (4).

The skin of the domestic pig has been suggested to be the most similar to man. Like human skin, it is nearly hairless; but pigs are large and somewhat difficult to handle (3). However, despite these considerations, the rat skin appears to be nearly as good a model for human skin as the pig (5).

Although more predictive approaches may be possible in the future, with the ethical considerations of utilizing humans in studies with pesticides, currently the laboratory rat appears to be a suitable model. Dermal absorption studies with the rat allow the calculation of a penetration rate; and hence, assist in the estimation of a potential body burden in man. Indeed, the extrapolation of a dermal penetration rate in the rat to man may represent a worst case approximation. Studies with one pesticide, malathion, in the rat and man have revealed the absorption/penetration rate in the rat to be approximately 3-fold higher than man (6).

Work habits and personal hygiene may impact on exposure. In an informed work force, showering or washing is a common practice that can be routinely expected. These procedures may reduce the exposure burden. In an uninformed work force, showering may not occur, so longer exposure times may need to be incorporated.

That a laboratory animal may qualitatively and quantitatively be extrapolated to man is a basic premise of toxicology (Paracelsus, 1493-1541). Paracelsus stated that, "All things are poisons, for there is nothing without poisonous properties; it is only the dose which makes a thing poison" (1). Inherent in this interpretation is the concept that quantitatively there will be an exposure level below which no discernable adverse effects occur. In addition, logical extrapolation of the premise of Paracelsus includes the concept that responses due to chemicals will be qualitatively similar in animals and man.

Based on these principles, quantitative and qualitative toxicology data on pesticides are generated from animal studies and extrapolated to man. The extrapolation, however, is usually not direct and may include several assumptions. Species susceptibility, species metabolism differences, and extrapolations of dose response relationships below the experimental range should be considered (7). In a work situation, the human body burden is determined by the exposure, absorption, and excretion rates. The same is true in animal studies, although continuous exposure is usually incorporated in the study design. Absorption is usually considered relatively complete. Excretion rates are usually specific to the physico-chemical properties of the chemical and the species; however differences in excretion rates are not usually incorporated into extrapolations to man (8).

Administration of the test material in animal diets at 3 or 4 concentrations is most often the approach taken. The duration of feeding as well as the unrealistic levels of feeding often used constitute an exaggerated worst case situation. Since animal feeding levels are usually much higher than man is expected to encounter, extrapolation of the dose response relationship outside the range of administration is often required. Furthermore, animal studies usually involve continuous exposure without affording a time for healing or recovery. Clearly many considerations may be envisioned which may encumber the qualitative and quantitative response seen in animals relative to human exposure.

For adverse responses which demonstrate thresholds, the usual evaluation involves identification of a no observable effect level -- NOEL -- in the most sensitive animal species or, in some cases, the calculation of the threshold for the effect. The NOEL is divided by a suitable safety factor, to establish an acceptable daily intake (ADI) in man (9). Safety factors vary from 10 to 2,000 depending upon the toxic response observed as well as the duration of the animal studies. The ADI refers to the amount ingested and this amount is considered to be totally absorbed.

An example of such a calculation illustrated by a NOEL of 50 mg/kg/day in a lifetime rat feeding study. Applying a safety factor of 100, an ADI of 0.5 mg/kg/day may be calculated. A maximum permissible intake of 30 mg/day may then be calculated for a 60 kg worker. If the amount absorbed in a work day were 25%, the maximum permissible dermal exposure would be 120 mg/day.

This example illustrates the assumed equivalency of toxicity regardless of exposure route. This premise is consistent with the concept of body burden and is applicable in most cases.

Despite the simplicity and attractiveness of the no-effect level or threshold concept of biological systems to toxicants, concern has risen in respect to the possibility that carcinogenesis in general does not follow this pattern. Scientific information has accumulated which suggests that some agents which cause cancer produce their endpoint by irreversible combination with DNA. This hypothesis encompasses the idea that this response is produced by such a small amount of material that no threshold exists. Additionally, there are growing hypotheses, being built on an experimental foundation, which suggests chemical carcinogens can be separated into two classes: genotoxins and nongenotoxins (10). Although it is strongly believed by some that nongenotoxic agents should be grouped into the class of compounds which have a threshold, it is difficult to simply ascribe the classical approach of safety assessment to any carcinogen without further assurances in the area of biological evidence of such a threshold.

This uncertainty leads us into an integrated approach for the evaluation of hazard due to exposure to a tumorigenic agent in mammals (11, 12). The components of this approach include not only attempts to assess what the response means quantitatively to man by extrapolation mathematically, but also assessment of the response qualitatively to attempt to determine the mechanism.

In order to relate the probability of tumorigenic response at a given environmental exposure, it is necessary to first extrapolate from the high doses in animal studies producing the response to low doses, and second from animals to humans. The first extrapolation for an oncogenic response can be made using a model which reflects some form of a dose-response; varying from the nonthreshold linear reaction to more complex multi-stage or multicompartment processes.

The animal to human extrapolation involves an estimation of exposure equivalent to the body burden based on mg/food intake/day, mg/kg of body weight/day, or mg/day interpolated from surface area. Traditionally species comparisons are made on a mg/kg dose basis, but this technique does not allow for differences in metabolism rate. Alternatively basing species extrapolations on body surface area affords such a correction. The use of ppm in the diet also reflects differences in metabolism rates. Dietary ppm may be converted to mg/kg/day by incorporation of food consumed per day and animal body weight. If compounds are metabolized (as most are) the use of ppm in the diet is probably superior. Furthermore its use will usually result in the most conservative estimates (13).

As one attempts to assign risks that are acceptable to humans (1 in 10^5 or 10^6), it is clear that an enormous sample size is needed. Actual statistical sensitivity of the toxicology tests is dependent upon the number of animals used, the background incidence of the tumors seen and the doses administered.

As more precise biological data are obtained one can begin to select individual models for evaluation of a given oncogenic

response as qualitative understanding is obtained about how the
response is elicited.

Various mathematical models have evolved that attempt to
incorporate some of the biological concepts and hypotheses. Some
of the most commonly used models are the Probit, the Multi-Hit,
the One-Hit, the Multi-Stage, and the Weibull. All of these
models have the defined property that for zero dose, the risk is
zero. However, since the spontaneous background incidence is not
zero for most tumors, the models incorporate background, utilizing the concept of independence as ascribed by the correction
of Abbott (14); i.e.,

$$P(d) = Po + (1-Po) R(d)$$

where P(d) is the observed tumor incidence at dose d.

Po is the spontaneous tumor risk.

R(d) is the probability of tumor incidence due to dose d.

A comparison of background using Abbott's correction vs.
simple background subtraction may show substantial differences
when low probabilities are involved.

Grieves (14) has reviewed the theoretical mathematical properties of these five common models and indicated that there is
no single approach which allows one to choose which model is
most appropriate. All models have utility provided that properly
spaced feeding levels are used. However, as mechanisms of carcinogenesis become better understood, it may be possible to
select the models that appropriately fit the data on a biological
basis.

Despite the minimal biological basis or lack of proven
applicability in the probability ranges where applied, we continue to rely on mathematical models. The models most commonly
relate:

$$R(d) = f(d,\underline{n})$$

where R(d) is the carcinogenic risk for a dose d; f is some function; and $\underline{n}$ is a vector of the inherent parameters (13).

The One-Hit model

$$P(d) = 1-exp(-kd)$$

is based upon the one-hit theory of infectious titrations (15).
At low doses it is essentially linear and has been the basis of
the linear risk models. The dose response for dimethylnitrosamine heptatocarcinogenicity in rats (16) shows that, in fact,
the response is more complex than a one-hit process. (Figure 2)

The Probit model

$$P(d) = \Phi[\alpha + \beta \log_{10}(d)]$$

has its roots in the mathematical processes developed to describe
LD_{50} observations (17). It utilizes a log dose/probit transfor-
mation of the tumor incidence to describe the dose response rela-

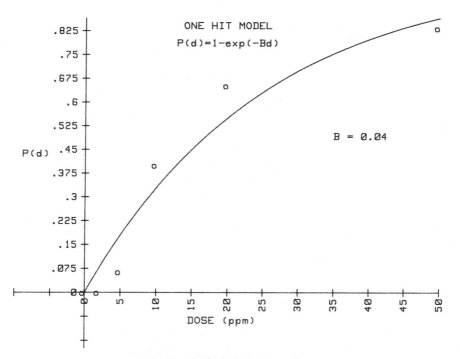

Figure 2.   Incidence of Hepatocellular Carcinoma in rats fed diets containing Dimethylnitrosamine.

tionship. The effectiveness of the model can be demonstrated in small populations where significant percentages of individuals are involved. However, when one extrapolates the relationship from 1 in 3 or 4 to 1 in a million or more, the practical basis of the statistically normal distribution is poorly supported. The Multi-Hit model

$$P(d) = \int_0^\Theta \frac{d e^{-u} u^{k-1}}{\Gamma(k)} \, du$$

where k = the number of hits
and Θ = a model parameter greater than 0.

is based upon a projected mechanism of carcinogenesis which involves several independent events, each of which has an independent probability of occurrence (18). The Multi-Hit model uses a projected Poisson distribution of population susceptibilities. The Multi-Stage model

$$P(d) = 1-exp^{-}(-Q_0+Q_1 d+Q_2 d^2 \ldots)$$

is based upon a sequential or multi-step process of carcinogenesis (k-steps), each with its own probability of occurrence (19). The model was originally developed as a time/dose model, but for the sake of practicality, time was considered constant (lifetime). The model utilizes a prescribed number of stages or it calculates the number of steps based upon the data. The solution of the equation limits the number of possible steps to one less than the number of doses tested. In the standard NCI Bioassay, two test doses and a control are utilized. Such data can only support a model involving two steps in the process of carcinogenesis.

An additional limitation of the Multi-Stage model, in fact of all the models discussed, is that generally the maximal incidence is assumed to be 100%. This, in practice, may not be possible since increasing administration may result in death rather than tumor formation. When the Multi-Stage model is used to evaluate the dose response for dimethylnitrosamine, hepatocarcinogenicity in the rat (16), it shows a better fit than the One-Hit, but the data does not fit the curve particularly well (Figure 3). The less than perfect fit is possibly because the model forces the maximum incidence to be 100% -- a condition not apparent in the data.

When used with the saccharin data (20), the Multi-Stage model appears to fit the dose response very well (Figure 4). Since 7 doses were used in the saccharin study, the number of doses is not a limiting factor and the full potency of the model can be utilized to calculate the theoretical 4-step process which fits the data nicely. The Weibull model

$$P(d) = 1-exp(-Ad^x)$$

can be viewed as a special case of the Multi-Stage model in which

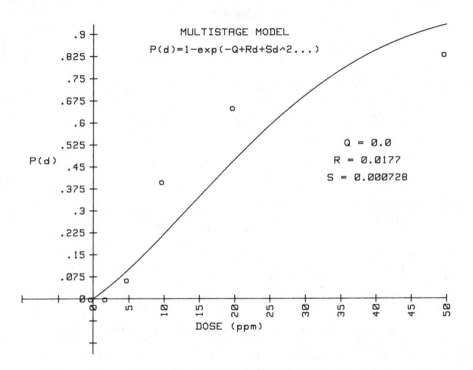

Figure 3.   Incidence of Hepatocellular Carcinoma in rats fed diets containing Dimethylnitrosamine.

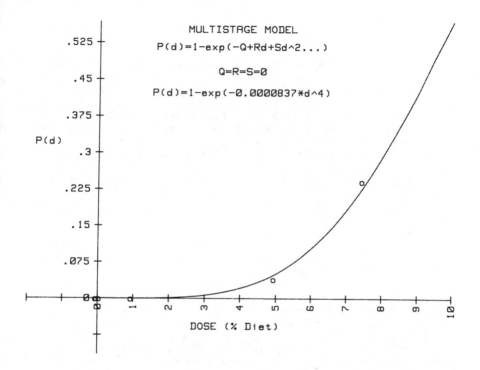

Figure 4.   Incidence of bladder tumors in rats fed diets containing sodium saccharin.

only one of the k-stages is rate limiting and, therefore, only
one step is dose dependent (21). Incorporating this limitation
is attractive because it allows identification of a larger multi-
step process (k>2) without the multiple dose levels required of
the Multi-Stage model.

Furthermore, it also allows reincorporation of the time
factor

$$P(d) = 1-\exp^{-}(Ad^x + Bt^y)$$

thus, it is one of the models providing a mechanism to evaluate
both dose and time in the animal data.

All the models are based upon standard statistical distributions. The Multi-Hit model is based upon a Poisson distribution. The Probit model is based upon a normal distribution, and
the One Hit, Multistage and Weibull models rely upon linear probabilities. Such distributions have proven applicability in
dealing with substantial percentages of the population (up to 1
in 20). However, the models lose precision when they are pushed
to extremes such as 1 in 10^6, such as encountered in risk assessment. Furthermore, homeostatic mechanisms such as DNA repair and
immunological surveillance may be poorly evaluated in risk assessment. Such high doses are administered to achieve the maximum
tolerated dose, that these mechanisms are surely overwhelmed in
the animal studies. Additionally it should be noted that a risk
of one in a million does not mean one tumor in the lifetime of a
million people, it means that each individual has one chance in a
million of developing a tumor in a lifetime.

In order to conduct a risk assessment, a suitable risk model
and toxicology data base must be selected. With these a dose
corresponding to an acceptable level of risk may be calculated.
This dose is usually referred to as the Virtually Safe Dose (VSD)
and corresponds to a risk of 10^{-5} to 10^{-8}, with 10^{-6} chosen most
commonly. Considering the statistical approximations, such a
risk probably constitutes no risk at all. It should be noted
that these values are based upon daily exposure for a lifetime,
since that is the manner in which the animal studies are conducted. Much human exposure is intermittent in nature; allowing
potential time for recovery or healing. Although the specific
consideration of continuous vs. intermittent exposure is still
open to question, it would appear that genotoxins and nongenotoxins should be handled separately.

Conversion of the VSD to a work situation commonly involves
averaging of the exposure over a lifetime. If one assumes a
person may handle the product up to 6 months per year for 40
years and that only 25% of the material is absorbed, a series of
correction factors are often included (VSD x 6/12 x 40/70 ÷ 4) to
determine a maximum safe exposure level.

Although mathematical treatments are appropriate when the
toxicological mechanisms are unknown, if the mechanism of car-
cinogensis for a material is sufficiently understood to demonstrate a threshold, there is no reason that this threshold cannot
be utilized. It may not be feasible to completely eliminate the

possibility of additional underlying carcinogenic activity, but such is equally true of all "non-carcinogens" since they, too, may have underlaying oncogenic activities which are so weak they elude the power of the statistical detection.

The use of linear correction factors is compatible with the basic assumptions of the One Hit model and depending upon the biological steps involved the Multistage and Wiebull models as well.   By analogy the risk is dependent upon a total cumulative lifetime dose and this accumulation constitutes an "averaging" of exposure.   A recent publication by Crump (22) addresses this issue in a more mathematically eloquent fashion.

In the case of melamine, such considerations on carcinogenic mechanisms are appropriate.   The material has been associated with an increased incidence of bladder carcinomas in male rats. No other tumors were observed.   High doses of melamine cause bladder calculi.   It is these calculi, through chronic bladder irritation, that result in the neoplasia.   The compound is not a mutagen in a large variety of mutagenicity tests (23).

Therefore, melamine appears to exert its effect via precipitation and chronic mechanical irritation.   Since chronic irritation is a known promoting function, this is a likely hypothesis of the mechanism of toxicity.   This hypothesis is further supported by the absence of carcinogenicity in doses below the dose which results in bladder calculi.   The conclusions reached from this mechanism indicate that a threshold exists at the dose resulting in calculi and safe limits on exposure for melamine should be based upon the acceptable daily intake even though the compound by some definitions is a carcinogen.

The acceptable daily intake should not be ignored in situations involving carcinogens.   It is conceivable that for a product used only a few days a year that the permissible exposure level calculated from the virtually safe dose could be greater than that calculated from the ADI.   Therefore, these values should be compared and the lower value adopted.

In summary, the use of risk assessment should include a review of the applicability and precision of the values based upon the theoretical and practical principles involved.   Although the combination of exposure, toxicokenetic, and risk assessment provide information to support safe work practices many assumptions and extrapolations are involved.

Literature Cited

1.   Casarett, L. J.; Bruce, M. C.   In "Casarett and Doull's Toxicology, The Basic Science of Poisons"; 2nd ed., Doull, J.; Klaassen, C. D.; Andur, M. O., ed.; MacMillan Publishing Co., Inc., New York, 1980; Chap. 1.
2.   Dugard, P. H.   In "Dermatotoxicology"; 2nd ed.; Marzulli, F. N.; Mailbach, H. I., Eds.; Hemisphere Publishing Corp.: Washington; New York; London, 1983; Chap. 3.
3.   Bronaugh, R. L.; Mailbach, H. I.   In "Dermatotoxicology"; 2nd ed.; Marzulli, F. N.; Maibach, H. I.; Eds.; Hemisphere Publishing Corp.:   Washington; New York; London, 1983; Chap. 4.

4. Krueger, G. G.; Chambers, D. A.; Shelby, J. J. Exp. Med.
    1980, 152, 1329-1339.
5. Bartek, M. J.; Labudde, J. A.; Maibach, H. I. J. Invest.
    Dermatol., 1972, 58, 114-123.
6. Wester, R. C.; Maibach, H. I.; Bucks, D. A. W.; Guy, R. H.
    Toxicol. Appl. Pharmacol., 1983, 68, 116-119.
7. "Drinking Water and Health," National Academy of Sciences,
    1977.
8. Klaassen, C. D. In "Casarett and Doull's Toxicology, The
    Basic Science of Poisons"; 2nd ed.; Doull, J.; Klaassen, C.
    D.; Andur, M. O., Eds.; MacMillan Publishing Co., Inc., New
    York, 1980; Chap. 2.
9. "Principles for Evaluating Chemicals in the Environment,"
    National Academy of Sciences 1975.
10. Weisburger, J. H.; Williams, G. M. In "Casarett and Doull's
    Toxicology, The Basic Science of Poisons"; 2nd ed.; Doull,
    J.; Klaassen, C. D.; Andur, M. O., Eds.; MacMillan Publish-
    ing Co., Inc., New York, 1980; Chap. 6.
11. Stevens, J. T.; Sumner, D. D. J. Toxicol. - Clin. Toxicol.,
    1983, 19, 781-805.
12. "Chemical Carcinogens; Notice of Review of the Science and
    its Associated Principles," Office of Science and Technology
    Policy, Fed. Reg., May 22, 1984, 21593-21661.
13. Hoel, D. G.; Gaylor, D. W.; Kirschstein, R. L.;
    Schneiderman, M. A. J. Toxicol. Environ. Hlth., 1:133,
    1975.
14. Grieve, A. P. Presented at Internationale Brometrische
    Gesellschaft Region Oesterreichs Schweiz; Basel, Schweiz,
    September 1983.
15. Armitage, P. J. Natl. Cancer Inst., 1959, 23, 1313-1326.
16. Terracini, B.; McGee, P. N., and Barnes, J. M. Brit. J.
    Cancer, 1967, 21, 559-565.
17. Mantel, N.; Bryan, W. R. J. Natl. Cancer Inst., 1961, 27,
    455-470.
18. Rai, K.; Van Ryzin, J. Biometrics, 1981, 37, 344-352.
19. Crump, K. S.; Guess, H. A.; Deal, K. L. Test of Hypothesis,
    1977, 33, 437-451.
20. Taylor, J. M. and Friedman. L. Tox. Appl. Pharmacol., 1974,
    29, 154.
21. Krewski, D.; Van Ryzin, J., In "Current Topics in Probabil-
    ity and Statistics"; Csorgo, M.; Dawson, D.; Rao, J. N. K.;
    Salek, E., Eds., North-Holland, New York, 1981.
22. Crump, K. S. and Howe, R. B., Risk Analysis 1984 in press.
23. "Carcinogenesis Bioassay of Melamine," National Toxicology
    Program Technical Report Series No. 245, March 1983.

RECEIVED November 15, 1984

Assessment of Farmworker Risk from Organophosphate-Induced Delayed Neuropathy

BARRY W. WILSON[1], MICHAEL HOOPER[1], EDWARD CHOW[1], JAMES N. SEIBER[2], and JAMES B. KNAAK[3]

[1]Department of Avian Sciences, University of California, Davis, CA 95616
[2]Department of Environmental Toxicology, University of California, Davis, CA 95616
[3]California Department of Food and Agriculture, Sacramento, CA 95814

Organophosphate Induced Delayed Neuropathy (OPIDN)
is an axonal neuropathy characterized by delayed
onset, species and toxicant specificities. This
paper discusses special features of OPIDN with
regard to the workplace and the environment, body
surfaces, metabolism, target cells and molecules,
gene regulation and toxicity identification. Among
the examples used is isofenphos, the active
ingredient in the registered pesticide Oftanol;
evidence regarding its neurotoxicity in hens at
single doses of 100 mg/kg is reviewed. Reasons for
the lack of recognition of its neuropathic potential
in the past are discussed with respect to EPA
regulations for screening for neuropathic
organophosphorus esters.

Organophosphate Induced Delayed Neuropathy (OPIDN) and other
long-term problems of organophosphorus ester (OP) agricultural
chemicals pose special problems for risk assessment. Procedures
have been developed over the years to evaluate the dangers from
acute exposures to OPs, but the insidious effects of repeated
exposures to toxic chemicals are more difficult to anticipate and
to detect.

The acute effects of OPs are usually due to their inhibition
of AChE at the motor end plates of the peripheral and the
synapses of the central nervous systems. Unfortunately, OPIDN is
not related in any simple way to these inhibitions.

OPIDN is an axonal neuropathy caused by some but not all
OPs (1). It is characterized by delayed onset, axonal destruction
followed by myelin degeneration and death of the nerve cell
bodies in the central nervous system (Table I). Sensitive
animals include man, cat, dog, sheep, water buffalo and the
chicken but not rodents. The chicken is usually the experimental
animal of choice.

0097–6156/85/0273–0479$06.00/0

Table I.   Selected Symptoms Of Organophosphorus Ester-Induced
Delayed Neuropathy

Early (First few days) Inhibition of NTE, a special carboxy-esterase activity	Later (First few weeks) Aggregation of neurotubules Axonal swelling proximal to distal nodes of Ranvier

Still Later
(Two-three weeks)
Interruption of axoplasmic flow; axonal demyelination
Cell body damage in brain and spinal cord
Progressive ataxia and paralysis of lower limbs.

Much Later
(Months)
Slow recovery of movement may occur.

Agriculture has been fortunate to be relatively free of mass outbreaks of OPIDN. The major chemical offender has been the plasticizer and lubricant tri-ortho-cresyl phosphate (TOCP). Contamination of various products with TOCP has paralyzed thousands of people since the turn of the century (2). OPs in use in agriculture that have been shown to be neuropathic include the cotton defoliant DEF and the pesticides EPN, haloxon and leptophos (not registered in the US). Neuropathic OPs used experimentally include DFP and mipafox; one nerve gas (sarin) has been shown to cause OPIDN and there is evidence another (soman) is also a delayed neuropathic agent (3). Recently, Wilson et al. (4) found that isofenphos (IFP) caused OPIDN in hens.

EPA guidelines specify a two-stage test for identifying neuropathic OPs using laying hens (5,6). In the first step OPs are screened with a single acute dose (usually near the LD50) and observed for three weeks. If OPIDN appears, a 90 day subchronic repeated exposure study is performed to determine a no-effect level (NOEL).

The cause of OPIDN is unknown; there is no cure. A special carboxyesterase enzyme test developed by Johnson (7) quantifies the inhibition of the hydrolysis of phenyl valerate due to a neuropathic OP that occurs in addition to the inhibition in the presence of a non-neuropathic OP. Although the existence of a single enzyme corresponding to NTE activity is not universally accepted (1), inhibitions of NTE activity greater than 70-80% are fairly reliable predictors of the appearance of OPIDN weeks later. NTE activity is especially high in nervous tissue and lymphocytes (8) and its inhibition is thought by some to be the initiating step in the disorder (9).

OPs are also known to damage muscles. Dettbarn and colleagues (10) propose that injury to skeletal muscle of rats brought about by parathion is due to an excess of ACh at the neuromuscular junction. Not all muscles are severely damaged by the agent (perhaps no more than 10 per cent of the muscles are affected) and the phenomenon has been mainly studied in rodents. It is

important that it be examined in animals prone to OPIDN such as
chickens, cats and man.

There is increasing concern but little knowledge concerning
subtle effects of OP's on behavior. One study of field workers
poisoned badly enough by OPs to be hospitalized indicated that a
memory deficit could be found as long as ten years after an
episode (11).

Research Levels

Research on agricultural chemicals falls naturally into several
categories reflecting the order of events that occur when a
pesticide is used. The rows in Table II are a list of a loose
hierarchy of levels of pesticide action from environment to gene;
the columns in the table separate topics appropriate to research
(factors) and regulation (actions).

Different research factors and regulatory actions are
associated with each level of organization. Each of these,
environment, body surface, metabolism, cells and molecules, and
nucleic acids, present special features. Although outside the
hierarchy of organization of living systems, the major problem of
identification of OPs that cause OPIDN is also included in the
diagram.

Table II.   Research and Regulation of Use of Organophosphorus
Esters

Categories	Factors	OP Examples	Actions
Workplace and Environment	Residues Reactions Who's at Risk?	DEF & IFP EPN & DFP Mixer/Loaders Homeowners	Restrict Use Reentry Times Revise Instructions
Body Surfaces	Permeability Solubility	Parathion DEF Others	Protective Clothing
Metabolism	Conversions to Active/Inactive Forms. Depots.	Oxons, Cyclics Detoxification	Monitor Damage in Blood
Target Cells Molecules	Serum, Tissue Levels. Kinetics Acute Effects	Muscle Nerve AChE NTE	Give Antidotes Prevent Aging
Gene Regulation	Long-Term Damage Protein, Nucleic Acid Syntheses	Neuropathy Myopathy MEP Damage	Stimulate Reinnervation Therapy
Identify Toxicities	Animal, Tissue Molecule Screens	Cholinergic or Neuropathic	Revise Registration Procedures

Workplace and Environment: Isofenphos Residues on Tomatoes

$$ET-O-\overset{\overset{S}{\|}}{\underset{\underset{O}{|}}{P}}-NH-CH(CH_3)_2$$

$$CO_2CH(CH_3)_2$$

IFP

Isofenphos (IFP) is the active ingredient of the registered pesticide Oftanol; last fall it was applied as a granular formulation to soil in a part of Sacramento County, California, as part of an eradication program against the Japanese Beetle. Since the infested area included yards and private dwellings, there was some concern over exposures of persons to residues in soil, water and air, and, potentially, from fruits and vegetables grown in the yards nearby. To evaluate the latter possibility, tomatoes were analyzed from soil from an experimental plot treated with Oftanol at the rate, and 5 times the rate used in the eradication program. IFP was both relatively persistent in soil and converted into its oxon (Table III). However, no detectable residues were found in whole tomatoes, and only traces of residue were present in surface rinses of tomatoes even when treatments were 5 times the normal rate.

Table III.   IFP Residue in Soils and Tomatoes Treated on 8/28/83

Sample	Treatment lb/acre	Sampling Date	IFP		IFP Oxon	
Soil *	2	9/4/83	1.90	0.35	1.08	0.45
ppm	10	9/4/83	14.0	1.0	0.92	0.07
	10	10/28/83	10.8	3.8	2.53	0.50
Tomato **	2	9/4/83	0.047	0.012	0.057	0.015
Surface	10	9/4/83	0.23	0.19	0.170	.0096
pg/cm2	2	10/28/83	<0.04		<0.04	
	10	10/28/83	<0.04		0.67	1.06

*: Three composites sampled to 2.5 cm soil depth were analyzed. **: Three samples consisting of the surface rinse from 15 red tomatoes were analyzed. Whole tomatoes yielded <0.01 ppm of IFP and IFP oxon at both sampling dates. IFP applied as 5% granular formulation.

The data in Table III represent an example of the type of exposure information used by regulatory agencies to assess risk. In this case, the data show that likelihood of exposure to IFP is minimal from consumption of tomatoes grown in IFP treated soils. A more likely route of exposure in this case might be from contacting the soil itself (e.g. by children at play). Extensive exposure data of this type are summarized in an FAO monograph (12). As with all registered pesticides, the manufacturer is required to submit exposure information (residues remaining on foliage, in soil and foodstuffs) as a part of the registration process.

Technically, residue analyses may be the best worked out and most satisfactory data obtained for assessment of worker risk. However, there has been little direct study of the relationships between residue levels of neuropathic OPs and the risk from OPIDN to humans and other animals such as wildlife.

Body Surfaces

Dermal absorption is a major problem in assessing risk with OPs. Research seeking general rules for their penetrability make up an important part of this conference including a paper presented elsewhere in the Symposium by Dr. Knaak. Neuropathic OPs seem to pose no special problem in penetration compared to other OPs. However, this does not mean they are not deserving of special attention.

Research on OPs is often performed by subcutaneous injection because of factors of cost, safety and perhaps habit even though inhalation, oral and dermal routes are all important avenues of exposure in the real world. EPA regulations emphasize testing by the oral route. Short term studies are often performed with gavage; repeated exposures may involve capsules. However, there is evidence that dermal exposure may lead to altered toxicities compared to oral routes (13). In the future, more consideration may have to be given to which route is best for studying agricultural chemicals.

A few years ago, we performed an experiment in which featherless chicken mutants were put in various locations in and around a cotton field in which the neuropathic OP DEF was being sprayed (14). There was an excellent correlation between the amounts of DEF residues deposited near the chickens and levels of their blood cholinesterase (Figure 1). None became neuropathic in the acute test. Tests in the laboratory later showed that featherless chickens developed OPIDN at levels similar (but somewhat higher) than normal chickens. The idea (using experimental animals as sentries in fields) may be one whose time has not yet come. Even so, work like this may point the way to a more sophisticated use of experimental animals in real-life situations.

Metabolism

Many commercial OPs are merely precursors of their active forms, being converted in the body, particularly by the liver, into their active toxic agents. (A common conversion is P=S to P=O for

production of anticholinesterase OPs.) Delayed neuropathic OPs
also are often converted into active agents in the body (e.g.
conversion of TOCP to o-cresyl saligenin phosphate), and these
conversions are not necessarily monitored by anticholinesterase
activity. Indeed, lack of definitive evidence for the primary
molecular site of action of neuropathic OPs precludes our being
certain of their active neuropathic metabolic products.

Target Cells and Molecules

The finding that NTE activity is high in lymphocytes, and that
NTE levels are decreased after acute exposure to neuropathic OPs
in hens offers a way to sample experimental animals and humans
for exposure to such agents (Table IV).
        Measurements of the NTE activities of farmworkers in
California exposed to DEF conducted by Lotti et al. (15)
suggested that decreases in worker lymphocyte NTE levels may have
occurred (Figure 2). However, the small number of workers, and
the variability of the values in this preliminary study preclude
drawing definitive conclusions until more studies are performed.
        Inhibition of blood ChE enzymes are used to estimate the
actions of the OPs on the nerve/muscle junctions that are
inaccessible to sampling. Interestingly, birds do not have AChE
activity in their RBC's, making it possible to use serum CHE
activity as a crude estimate of OP intoxication.
        Blood cholinesterase levels of farmworkers have been the
subject of several studies including one of mixer-loaders and
applicators in California (17); fewer studies have been done of
the appearance of tissue enzymes in blood which would suggest
tissue damage had occurred somewhere in the body. The two studies
summarized are drawn from studies of farmworkers in Florida
(Table V) and alcoholics (a group known to suffer damage to
muscle, liver and other tissues) in a VA hospital in Pennsylvania
(Table VI). In farmworkers, there was a significant decrease in
blood ChE levels indicating exposure to OPs. In both farmworkers
and alcoholic patients, there were increases in serum glutamic-
oxalacetic transferase (SGOT) levels suggesting damage to tissues
(such as liver or kidney).
        We have been examining blood enzyme levels in experimental
animals, demonstrating that exposure to neuropathic chemicals
like TOCP result in increases in enzymes such as CK and LDH,
indicative of tissue damage, that do not occur with exposure to a
non-neuropathic compound like paraoxon (19) (Table VII).
        Research with IFP offers a recent example of the use of NTE
as a predictor of OPIDN. While examining the effectiveness of
antidotes to protecting experimental animals from the
anticholinergic effects of isofenphos, Wilson and his colleagues
obtained evidence that the agricultural chemical is neuropathic
to the hen at single doses of 100 mg/kg and beyond (4). The data
in Table VIII of brain NTE levels versus dose show that levels of
the compound that cause the neuropathy inhibit NTE greater than
80%, and that the results could have been predicted from studies
at lower doses of the agent. For example, of 14 hybrid hens
injected with 100 mg/kg IFP s.c. (a dose 20 x the unprotected
LD50), half (7) developed Stage 4 (paralyzed), 4 developed Stage

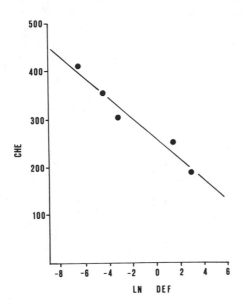

Figure 1. Plasma ChE activity in scaleless chickens after field applications of DEF. ChE in nmoles/min/ml; DEF in ln ug/cm². (Reproduced with permission from Ref. 14. Copyright 1980 Springer-Verlag, New York, Inc.)

Table IV. NTE Activities in Hen Tissues

Tissue	Total			NTE		
	Activity Mean	SEM	Percent of Brain	Activity Mean	SEM	Percent of Brain
Brain	14.9	1.2	100	2.43	0.10	100
Spinal Cord	5.93	0.14	40	0.51	0.05	21
Heart	6.95	0.45	47	0.33	0.05	14
Spleen	7.51	0.66	50	1.69	0.02	70
Spleen Lymphocytes	1.61	0.16	11	0.63	0.06	26
Blood Lymphocytes	1.78	0.07	12	0.59	0.04	24

Means & SEM; activities in umoles/min/g weight. Total, phenyl valerate hydrolysis without inhibitors; NTE, hydrolysis difference after paraoxon and mipafox.
Source: Adapted from Ref. 5.

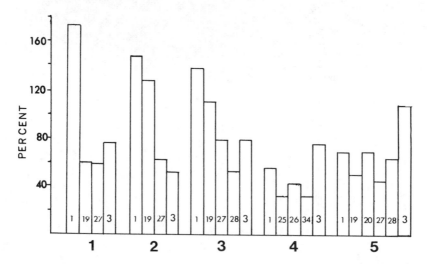

Figure 2. NTE activity in lymphocytes of workers during and after exposure to DEF. Values are expressed as percent of baseline (100%) NTE activity determined for each worker (1-5) before exposure. Sampling times are 1, 19, 20, 25, 26, 27, 28 days during and 3 weeks after exposure. (Adapted from Ref. 15.)

Table V. Blood Enzyme Levels of Florida Farmworkers

Enzyme	Control Mean	SD	Exposed Mean	SD	E/C	P
RBC AChE	0.80	0.14	0.70	0.11	0.88	>0.001
Δ pH		(51)		(253)		
Plasma ChE	0.94	0.19	0.76	0.17	0.81	>0.001
Δ pH		(49)		(215)		
Creatinine	1.08	0.14	1.18	0.18	1.09	>0.001
mg %		(58)		(178)		
Urea N	16.12	2.86	15.50	4.10	0.96	NS
mg %		(66)		(103)		
Alk.Ptase	9.76	2.38	10.55	3.41	1.08	NS
Units		(53)		(78)		
SGOT	18.68	5.64	24.32	9.50	1.30	>0.001
Units/ml		(61)		(154)		

Means and standard deviations ( ) are sample numbers. P are t-test results.
Source: Adapted from Ref. 16.

Table VI. Blood Enzymes, Muscle Damage and Alcoholism

Situation	CPK		SGOT		LDH	
	Mean	SD	Mean	SD	Mean	SD
No Recent	0.21	0.20	47	41	450	181
Drinking		(11)		(7)		(5)
Acute Muscle	7.9	2.7	193	321	923	1000
Complaints		(6)		(6)		(4)
Delerium	13	11	169	158	758	448
Tremens		(24)		(19)		(7)

Means & Standard Deviations. Activities in units/ml.
Normal upper limits: CPK, 1.5-2.0; SGOT, 35; LDH, 350.
Source: Adapted from Ref. 18.

Table VII. Plasma Enzymes of Hens And OPIDN

Treatment	Score	AChE	BChE	CK	LDH
Parathion	0	0.35	1.15	0.91	1.17
TOCP	3.4	1.57	0.28	7.04	2.63

Blood samples from hens 22 days after treatment with 10
mg/kg parathion and 500 mg/kg TOCP s.c., protected with
40 mg/kg atropine sulphate. Mean values (n=5) expressed
as fractions of untreated controls. Score is estimate of
locomotion from 0 (normal) to 4 (paralyzed).
Source: Adapted from Ref. 19.

Table VIII. Dose-response of Brain NTE After Isofenphos

Treatment	Total Hydrolysis		NTE	
	Activity	Percent	Activity	Percent
Control	12.6	100	2.45	100
30 mg/kg	11.7	92.9	1.49	60.8
70 mg/kg	7.47	59.2	0.603	24.6
100 mg/kg	7.44	59.0	0.291	11.9

10 percent homogenates of chicken brain assayed for
total phenyl valerate hydrolysis and NTE activity 3 days
after injection s.c. with IFP; umoles/ min/mg protein x
10-2. Means from duplicate samples from two chickens.

3 symptoms (severe ataxia), 1 showed Stage 2 (stumbling) and 2
showed no gross symptoms of OPIDN. Histological examination of
Stage 4 birds showed the lesions characteristic of the disorder
(Figure 3).

Gene Regulation

Many scientists are accustomed to thinking of toxic agents as

antimetabolites, interrupting the orderly processes of the body
at the levels of proteins or their metabolic products. Gene
level toxicities are often thought of in terms of cancers and
malignancies, interruptions to the process of DNA replication.
Another possibility is that a compound is acting to interrupt the
orderly synthesis of proteins, blocking in subtle ways the

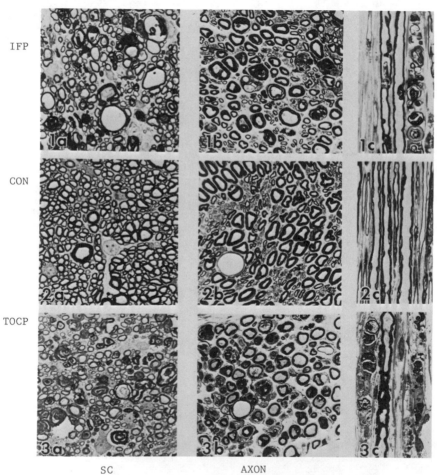

Figure 3. Microphotographs of cervical spinal cord (a), cross
(b) and longitudinal (c) sections of lateral metatarsal nerve
from IFP (1), antidote-treated (2) and TOCP-treated (3) hens.
Note axonal swellings, necrosis and myelin degeneration in TOCP
and IFP samples. Tissues embedded in epoxy, stained with
toluidine blue. 160X. (Reproduced with permission from Ref. 4.
Copyright 1984 Springer-Verlag, New York, Inc.)

production of housekeeping molecules like LDH or specialized proteins like neurofilaments. For example, there is evidence that DDT acts as a hormone during the development of birds to impair, but not prevent, the development of the reproductive system (20).

OPs act by irreversibly altering cellular proteins; one hypothesis we are seriously considering is that the "delay" in OPIDN is a clue that the cause of the abnormality is the interruption of protein synthesis in the nerve cell body by a phosphorylated protein that was transported there from the periphery by reverse axonal transport (19).

Identification of Neuropathic OPs

Regardless of the cellular and molecular mechanisms bringing about OPIDN, OPs must be screened for their ability to cause OPIDN and decisions must be reached on whether or not they are too dangerous to be registered. Some toxicologists think that no neuropathic OP should be put into widespread use; others think that safe levels can be established; for example, that OPs that are neuropathic at levels in excess of their LD50s are suitable candidates for registration.

The roles of the research scientist and the regulation officer differ. Laboratory scientists are obligated to "get the facts" and not prejudge the situation; worst-case experiments may be their stock-in-trade. Regulatory decisions are difficult to make, and demand the best and most comprehensive data base available.

Two important issues at the interface of research and regulation with regard to neuropathic OPs are "How high is too high?" and "How long is too long?" The EPA two-step test for OPIDN is set up in such a way that compounds do not need to be tested at levels beyond their LD50s in the hen; thus, OPs that may be neuropathic at higher acute doses do not need to be subjected to repeated exposures to establish a NOEL. ("The selected dose level of the test substance should not be less than the unprotected LD50 dose"; 5). Such a process means that OPs like IFP will be registered as "non-neuropathic," leading to their detection at a later date in other ways.

There are data to indicate that the NOEL with repeated exposure of neuropathic OPs is much lower than the neuropathic acute exposure levels (Table IX). The problem of the researcher is to unravel the relationships between toxic levels of different experimental animals, and the time-frames involved. The predictive value of tests like the NTE assay may be a great help in this research. The problem of the regulatory agencies is to sort out what data is important for setting regulatory decisions. Whatever processes are ultimately established, it is safe to say that OPs that cause delayed neuropathy will not disappear from the scene; those that have been registered in the United States have not been removed from the marketplace and toxicologists, regardless of their jobs, face the problem of dealing with their toxicities.

Table IX.   Comparison of OPIDN-Causing Chemicals

Compound	LD50 mg/kg	Acute Dose	Subchronic Low	NOEL
EPN	10	25	0.1	0.01
Leptophos	4700	100	1.0	0.5
DEF	NA	100	0.5	0.1
Isofenphos	5-20	100-150	ND	ND

EPN, leptophos and DEF given orally; isofenphos s.c. All doses in mg/kg. Acute is lowest single dose causing OPIDN. Subchronic based on daily doses; Low is lowest dose causing ataxia; NOEL is no-effect level.
Source: Adapted from Ref. 4, 21, 22, 23.

Nontechnical Summary

Some organophosphates used in industry, agriculture and the military cause insidious delayed nerve damage, appearing days after an animal is poisoned by them.   Research aimed at identification of these delayed neurotoxicants, and blood tests to monitor exposure to them are reviewed.   Evidence that isofenphos (the active ingredient of Oftanol, a registered pesticide) causes delayed nerve damage in laying hens is presented and the EPA regulations for screening for neuropathic agents are discussed.

Acknowledgments

The authors are grateful to Dr. M.G. McNamee, Dr. R. Higgins, and Mr. M. McChesney. The data and encouragement of Dr. M. Lotti is particularly acknowledged.   Supported in part by NIH ES 00202 (BWW), contracts to BWW and JNS from CDFA, the Western Regional Pesticide Impact Reassessment Program, the Northern California Occupational Health Center and (with regard to basic nerve/muscle relations, the Muscular Dystrophy Association). IFP was a gift of the Mobay Corp, Kansas City, Mo.

Literature Cited

1.   Abou-Donia, M.B. Ann. Rev. Pharmacol. Toxicol. 1981, 21, 511-548.
2.   Metcalf, R.L. NeuroTox. 1982, 3, 269-284.
3.   Willems, J.L.; Nicaise, M.; DeBisschop, H.C. Arch. Toxicol. 1984, 55, 76-77.
4.   Wilson, B.W.; Hooper, M; Chow, E.; Higgins, R.; Knaak, J.B. Bull. Environ. Contam. Toxicol. 1984, In Press.
5.   "Acute Delayed Neurotoxicity of Organophosphorus Substances," Office of Toxic Substances, EPA, 1982.
6.   "Subchronic Delayed Neurotoxicity of Organophosphorus Substances," Office of Toxic Substances, EPA, 1982.
7.   Johnson, M.K. Arch. Toxicol. 1977, 37, 113-115.

8. Dudek, B.R.; Richardson, R.J. Biochem. Pharmacol. 1982, 31, 1117-1121.
9. Johnson, M.K.; Richardson, R.J. NeuroTox. 1983, 4, 311-320.
10. Wecker, L.; Dettbarn, W.D. Exp. Neurol. 1976, 57, 281-291.
11. Savage, E.P.; Lewis, J.A.; Parks, L.H. "Chronic Neurological Sequelae of Acute Organophosphate Pesticide Poisoning: A Case Control Study. EPA 540/9-80-003. 1980.
12. "Pesticide Residues in Food: 1981 Evaluations" FAO Plant Production and Protection Paper 42. 1982.
13. Francis, B.M. NeuroTox. 1983, 4, 139-146.
14. Wilson, B.W.; Cisson, C.M.; Randall, W.R.; Woodrow, J.E.; Seiber, J.N.; Knaak, J.B. Bull. Environ. Contam. Toxicol. 1980, 24, 921-928.
15. Lotti, M.; Becker, C.E.; Aminoff, M.J.; Woodrow, J.E.; Seiber, J.N.; Talcott, R.E.; Richardson, R.J. J. Occup. Med. 1983, 25, 517-522.
16. Tocci, P.M.; Mann, J.B.; Davies, J.E.; Edmundson, W.F. Ind. Med. 1969, 38, 188-195.
17. Knaak,. J.B.; Maddy, K.T.; Jackson, T.; Frederickson, A.S.; Peoples, A.; Love, R. Tox. Appl. Pharmacol. 1978, 45, 755-770.
18. Lafair, J.S.; Myerson, R.M. Arch. Int. Med. 1968, 122, 417-422.
19. Wilson, B.W.; Ishikawa, Y.; Chow, E.; Cisson, C.M. NeuroTox. 1983, 4, 143-156.
20. Fry, D.M.; Toone, C.K. Science, 1981, 922-924.
21. Abou-Donia, M.B. Science, 1979, 205, 713-715.
22. Abou-Donia, M.B.; Graham, D.G.; Abdo, K.M.; Komeil, A.A. Toxicol. 1979, 14, 229-243.
23. Abou-Donia, M.B.; Preissig, S.H. Tox. Appl. Pharm. 1976, 38, 595-606.

RECEIVED December 3, 1984

Pesticide Drift: Toxicological and Social Consequences

JAMES M. WITT

Department of Agricultural Chemistry, Oregon State University, Corvallis, OR 97331

The drift of pesticides in the forestry
environment has the potential for greater
environmental impact than in an agricultural
environment and results in a greater social
concern for their impact on human health. The
factors affecting drift transfer of pesticide,
especially herbicides, will be examined, the
probable deposit and exposure level identified,
and the risk of probability of injury to human
health calculated.

The role of an Extension Specialist in chemistry is somewhat
different than that of a research chemist. A research chemist
produces data; an Extension chemist utilizes this data,
interpreting it, applying it to specific problems, and
presenting the conclusion to the public. The research data you
have presented here and elsewhere, to ultimately be of value,
must contribute to making social decisions, such as, to use a
pesticide or disdain its use. When such decisions are made in
the social, political, or even jurisprudical arena, the research
data must be simplified--often to the point that it will not be
easily recognizable even by its originators. It must, however,
continue to be correct and never be simplified to the point
where it will support misleading conclusions.
    As research chemists, you may be interested in how your
data are sometimes used and how they are presented to the
concerned public. Conclusions or simplified research data may
be presented by public agencies--such as state or federal
departments of agriculture, forestry, public health, or
occasionally the EPA or a Department of Environmental Quality,
and by citizens or public interest groups (especially by those
groups which are opposed to the use of pesticides in general),
and also by university research, teaching, or extension faculty.
    I represent the extension faculty in Oregon. I frequently
must discuss the risk to human health from pesticide spray

Reprinted from "Chemical and Biological Controls in Forestry";
Willa Y. Garner and John Harvey, Jr., Editors; ACS SYMPOSIUM
SERIES 238.

drift. This information is most often presented in situations
where confrontation, and even antagonism, exists; where one
group is pitted against another regarding the issue of whether a
particular pesticide should be used in a pest control program,
or whether such a program should even proceed at all. In this
atmosphere it is often difficult for the persons involved to
direct their attention to a thorough examination of the research
available and make a careful assessment of the risk.

I shall present a perception of the public concerns and a
little of how I evaluate and how I present the risks. I will
present information on pesticide use, public concerns as they
are expressed in the news, allegations of harm, toxicity of a
forest pesticide--2,4-D, human exposure to drift of this
pesticide, and the margins of safety which exist when this
exposure occurs.

It is interesting to compare the concerns expressed about
pesticide use with the actual types, locations, and pesticide
use levels. Table I shows pesticide use in Oregon. These data
are the result of a pesticide use survey, or census, carried out
in Oregon for 1981 and shows the ten pesticides used in largest
amounts in Oregon. Some surprises are revealed by this survey.

Table I. Oregon Pesticide Use Estimates, 1981

Rank	Pesticide	Pounds
	A. THE TOP TEN	
1	Creosote	15,000,000
2	Dichloropropane/dichloropene (D-D, Telone)	2,938,000
3	Pentachlorophenol (Penta)	1,590,000
4	2,4-D	1,169,050
5	Spray oil	1,065,700
6	Chromated copper arsenate	1,000,000
7	Diuron (Karmex)	520,000
8	Metam-sodium (Vapam)	440,000
9	Dinoseb (Dow General)	423,000
10	EPTC (Eptam)	395,000
	B. AGRICULTURAL AND FORESTRY USE	
1	Dichloropropane/dichloropropene (D-D, Telone)	2,938,000
2	2,4-D	1,169,050
3	Diuron (Karmex)	520,300
4	Metam-sodium (Vapam)	440,000
5	Dinoseb (Dow General)	423,400
6	EPTC (Eptam)	395,500
7	Sulfur	360,500
8	Captan	320,000
9	Bromoxynil (Brominal, Buctril)	308,400
10	Carbaryl (Sevin)	305,000

The most commonly used pesticide is not one we normally
call to mind when we consider pesticide use to control insects,
weeds and plant diseases in agriculture and forestry. It is
creosote, a wood preservative. Its use exceeds that of all
other pesticides combined, being used in an amount of
approximately 15 million pounds per year. Other wood
preservatives in the top ten are pentachlorophenol and chromated
copper arsenate, the third and sixth most used pesticides,
respectively. The second most commonly used pesticide is a soil
fumigant, DD or telone, used at about 3 million pounds per year.

Finally, in fourth place we find 2,4-D, which is used at a
little over 1 million pounds per year. This is the first
pesticide which we might normally think of when considering the
most common pesticides. This is followed in 7th-10th positions
by four other herbicides, Diuron, Vapam, Dinoseb, and Eptam.

Table II shows pesticides used by the US Forest Service and
the amounts used in 1980. On this list 2,4-D is in first place,
being used at in an amount of 215,000 pounds per year. In 1980
the second most commonly used pesticide by the USFS was the
insecticide malathion at in an amount of 102,000 pounds. There
are only three insecticides on this list of the nine most
commonly used pesticides in the USFS. The insecticide use rate
will vary considerably from year to year as its use is dependent
on insect outbreaks, whereas herbicides are used at a more
constant rate because the appearance of weeds and brush, as they
affect forest management, do not occur as periodic outbreaks.

Table II. Oregon Pesticide Use Estimate

Pesticide	Pounds
A. PESTICIDE USE BY THE USFS, 1980	
2,4-D	215,000
Malathion	102,000
Picloram	40,000
Atrazine	30,000
Carbaryl	30,000
Azinophos Methyl	18,000
Glyphosate	10,000
Dalapon	9,000
Fosamine	8,000
B. USE ON OREGON FORESTLAND, 1981 **(25,000,000 acres)**	
2,4-D	130,000
Glyphosate (Roundup)	37,000
Atrazine (Aatrex)	22,000
Fosamine ammonium (Krenite)	21,000
Hexazinone (Velpar)	20,000
Picloram (Tordon)	16,000
2,4-DP	16,000
Dicamba (Banvel)	6,400

Pesticide use in private forestry will more-or-less
parallel that in the USFS, with one exception. They will not
use malathion, carbaryl, or azinophos-methyl, the insecticides
shown in Table II, because nearly all insect outbreaks are
managed by either a federal or other public agency rather than
by private forestry. Although 2,4-D is the principal pesticide
used in forest management, Table III shows that its use in
Oregon for 1979 in forestry is only about 10 percent of the
total use in the State. The principal use is in wheat and other
grains, which utilized nearly 3/4 of a million pounds, while
forestry used 147,000 pounds.

Table III. 2,4-D Use in Oregon, 1979

Crop	1979
Cereal grains	731,000
Range and pasture	185,000
Forestry	147,000
Grass Seed	97,000
Home and garden	70,000
Rights-of-way	43,000
Miscellaneous	13,000
TOTAL	1,287,000

If we combine the use on grass grown for seed with home and
garden use, both of which are principally in the Willamette
Valley, we find that the total used in the Valley, 167 thousand
pounds, exceeds the amount used in forestry by a small margin.
Nevertheless, we find the principal public concern about 2,4-D
use does not focus on its Willamette Valley use, the region of
highest population density in Oregon, nor its use in wheat and
cereal grains, which is the principal use of 2,4-D, but is used
in eastern Oregon where there are far fewer people, but with few
exceptions focuses almost solely on its use in forestry.

Public concern over 2,4-D use is reflected by a constant
parade of newspaper articles and headlines, such as "200 Fleeing
Herbicide Spraying", and expressions of concern in these
articles, such as "I am nursing a five-month-old baby this time
and I am even more scared. There is no way they can tell me it
is not dangerous to babies," or, "The last time the Forest
Service sprayed here, they didn't tell us, and our children
immediately contracted extreme nausea." The newspaper stories
are not confined to quotations from concerned citizens, but
sometimes involve agency officials, such as the following
quotation from the recent head of the EPA Office of Toxic
Substances, Steve Jellenik, who stated, "Now we have a lot of
dead bodies, a lot of dead fetuses in Alsea." It is small
wonder that a very large segment of the public are very
concerned and very fearful of 2,4-D use when all they know is
what they have read in the newspapers. This is a good example
of the kind of information they most frequently receive.

We frequently find that newswriters add to the confusion
concerning the possible effects of pesticides. For example, in

newspaper discussions of the EPA "Alsea II" study, articles
frequently leaped from a discussion of 2,4,5-T, which was the
pesticide at issue, to all "phenoxy herbicides" and from there
to simply "herbicides".

The news headlines show varying stories of 2,4-D
controversy outcomes, such as "BLM Ordered to Halt Herbicide
Spraying Effort", "Environmentalists Fail in Attempt to Stop
Spraying of 2,4-D", and "Ozark Forest Spraying Stopped".
Sometimes the stories carry humorous headlines, such as "Spray
Protestors Didn't Run Naked in Woods, Leader Says".   Sometimes
stories are of a more grave nature, "No Cause for Civil
Disobedience".   The result of many persons concerns have ranged
from civil disobedience to violence, much of it with grave
overtones.   These vary from sitting or standing in spray areas
to prevent the spraying from proceeding, attempting to
physically block the spraying, threatening personnel involved,
armed confrontations, burning and destruction of spray
helicopters, and firing shots at low-flying spray aircraft.

The technical basis for this high, even agitated, level of
concern over herbicide use, can be well expressed by a news
story quotation of an attorney representing plaintiffs in a suit
against BLM herbicide use in the forests, "There are good
studies on the other side of that question that suggest there is
no safe exposure level to any of the herbicides.   And, if you
take those studies and combine them with the 20-mile spray
drifts and the mutagenic and carcinogenic properties of the
chemicals, ..."   It is this perception and these fears which
provide the basis for public concerns reflected in the news
stories quoted above.

There are many episodes or allegations of harm from
pesticide use.   The roster is a litany of place names: Alsea,
Ashford, Broken Bow, Lincoln City, Orleans, Rose Lodge,
Roseburg, Swan Valley.   The list could go on and on.   Although
much of this concern has been expressed in Northern California,
Oregon and Washington, it ranges from the Pacific states through
Montana, Arkansas, and all the way to Newfoundland.   All over
the United States and Canada there are many citizen groups who
fear herbicide use and actively oppose their use through the
courts, and hearings of governmental bodies from school boards
to county commissioners, on county and statewide ballots, and,
as indicated, through confrontation and violence.

The allegations of harm are not so very different than
those effects we know can be caused by the herbicide 2,4-D.   The
allegations of acute effects include headaches, shortness of
breath, substernal pain, gastrointestinal distress, nausea,
bloody diarrhea, skin rash, parathesis of the extremities, and
hysterical anxiety or tachycardia.   Parathesis of the
extremities is generally exhibited as a numbness or tingling in
the fingers and has been observed in cases of extreme or
high-level exposures to 2,4-D.   Hysterical anxiety is not a
comment, but a medical condition which is associated with
tachycardia.

The allegations of chronic effects include spontaneous
abortion, birth defects, cancer, mutation, and peripheral

neuropathy. Peripheral neuropathy is a chronic condition which is a sequela of the acute effect of parathesis of the extremities. Some allegations are categorized as "bizarre" and these are burning and blisters in the mouth, first and second degree skin burns, and coughing of blood. These effects are categorized as bizarre on the basis that when the patient presents himself or herself to a physician's office complaining of these effects, they cannot be detected by the examining physician even though these should be objective, easily identifiable clinical effects. For example, the person will insist they have blisters in their mouth, yet none are present. They may insist they had them yesterday, and they must be gone now. If this were so, there would be evidence of recent mouth blisters. And so on for the other effects.

Many of the concerns are not expressed as allegations of harm to health, but as philosophical positions. Some of these are that there is not a "no-effect level" or such a thing as a safe exposure level. There is a strong philosophical position which states that a person wishes to experience "zero risk". This will take the form of "I don't care if you just proved that this herbicide will not harm us, we don't want to be exposed to any. We want zero risk."

This also takes the form of objection to "chemical trespass". It is, of course, not an unreasonable position to hold that people and things should be prevented from trespassing upon your private property. But when one deals with the concept of chemicals being carried by the air over your property, whether they be herbicides, automobile exhaust, or chemicals emitted by trees in the forest, the concept of zero chemical trespass is difficult to encompass. It might be more useful to determine how much chemical is trespassing, whether there is enough chemical present to cause any biological or biochemical effect, and whether these effects are adverse, rather than holding the concept of zero trespass and zero risk. These philosophies often culminate in a distrust of institutions, whether these be chemical companies, universities, or regulatory agencies, such as the EPA.

The outcome of these concerns and philosophies is that pesticides are no longer being regulated on a national basis by a single agency--the EPA. They are being regulated at all political levels by a great many institutions--from court appeals to county government, from park boards to school boards, from state agencies to congressional committees. These bodies or institutions often usurp the role of EPA in regulation and evaluation of the toxicology of a pesticide and determination of the risk associated with a particular use pattern. At each of these political jurisdiction levels, it is expected by the public that the political body, be it a judge in the courtroom or a park board, have the expertise, the chemical knowledge, and the toxicological knowledge to make or assess a pesticide hazard evaluation which will result in imposing restrictions intended to result in public safety.

I believe that much of this concern has its genesis in the fact that many persons in the public have difficulty in distinguishing between and properly utilizing the concepts of toxicity, hazard, and safety.

Toxicity is the inherent ability of a chemical to cause injury. It is a property of the molecule and does not change. Hazard, on the other hand, involves toxicity but also involves exposure. And exposure involves many factors, some of them difficult to quantify. However, it can be said that hazard is the probability that a chemical will cause injury. The distinction between toxicity and hazard is often omitted in public discussions of risk from the use of herbicides in the forest.

Many people will correctly identify the toxicity or toxic effects which can be elicited from a particular chemical, and leap to the conclusion that there is a hazard without any intervening attempt to identify the exposure levels, and thus the likelihood that enumerated effects will in fact occur. Toxic effects are often hung out like a laundry list, eliciting concern on the part of the public with no attempt to relate toxic effect to dose or exposure levels.

Safety is a difficult concept to deal with and absolute safety is probably impossible to prove. We define safety as the practical certainty that a chemical will not cause injury. We cannot absolutely demonstrate that safety exists, because in a sense it is a negative entity. You can demonstrate through many laboratory experiments that toxicity exists. But, you cannot demonstrate that one further experiment will not reveal an unexpected toxic effect, and therefore you cannot demonstrate that safety is absolute.

Undergirding this confusion is that the first and simplest law of toxicology, that there is such a thing as a dose-response relationship, seems to be a most difficult concept to present to the public. That an increasing exposure or increasing dose will result in increasing severity and frequency of effects, and that conversely decreasing the dose level will result in a decreasing frequency and severity of effects and that there is a dose level below which no effects will occur has been demonstrated so often that it is routinely taken by granted by all of us working in the field.

However, many of the public are not comfortable with this as a concept and do not use it in their evaluation of pesticide risk. Part of the difficulty in their acceptance of the dose-response relationship and threshold concepts in toxicology has to do with the fact that there is, of course, a debate in toxicology as to whether there is a threshold for chemical injury in the self-replicating diseases such as cancer and mutagenesis. This has been rapidly extended in the minds of many people to include all chemical injury and not just restricted to self-replicating disease. That we can assume there is no threshold with regard to chemical carcinogenesis, and still calculate a safe dose level, is not a concept easily accepted by many of the public. The knowledge that carcinogenesis follows a dose-response relationship, with or without a threshold, and that the result of this is that lower and lower doses result in fewer tumors per individual, a lower frequency amongst individuals, and, perhaps most importantly, a longer time to tumor, is not well understood. This results in the possibility of determining a dose level of a carcinogen

which will not result in the onset of a tumor within the
lifetime of an exposed individual.

A brief summary of the toxicity of the forest herbicide
2,4-D can be presented as follows. Table IV shows the acute
LD-50 values of most of the phenoxy herbicices. These range
from 300 mg/kg for 2,4,5-T and 375 mg/kg for 2,4-D up to 6400
mg/kg for Bifenox. It is useful to set the acute oral toxicity
for 2,4-D in the context of other phenoxy herbicides and in
relation to other pesticides so the public can gain a perception
of where 2,4-D fits on a scale of relative values with regard to
the onset of acute toxicity symptoms and to show that all
phenoxies are not identical in their acute toxicity but cover a
wide range of toxicities.

Table IV. Acute Oral LD_{50} Values (mg/kg)

PHENOXY HERBICIDES

Herbicide	Value	Herbicide	Value
2,4,5-T	300	MCPA	700
2,4-D	375	MCPB	680
2,4,5-TP	375	MCPP	930
2,4-DB	500	Bifenox	6,400

The acute toxicity values for 2,4-D are expanded to cover a
number of species in Table V and show that the 375 mg/kg we
commonly use is the acute oral toxicity for the mouse. The
chemical is not that toxic to nearly all other species, from the
rat, to the rabbit, to the guinea pig. The one exception to
this is 2,4-D toxicity to the dog, which is greater than to the
mouse, having a toxicity of 100 mg/kg. It is considered that
this is because dogs, as a species, do not excrete aryl acids as
do the rodents--the mouse, rat, and rabbit-- nor do they excrete
these acids as readily as does man. Sometimes we find that
pesticide users are resistant to accepting the knowledge that a
herbicide such as 2,4-D is a toxic chemical and that it can kill
animal organisms as well as plants. It should be obvious that
any chemical which has an LD-50 (for any laboratory test
animal), is capable of causing death to animals.

Table V. Median Lethal Doses of 2,4-D

Mouse	375 mg/kg
Rat	666 mg/kg
Rabbit	800 mg/kg
Guinea Pig	1,000 mg/kg
Dog	100 mg/kg
Monkey	ca. 400 mg/kg
Chicken	ca. 900 mg/kg

Table VI shows that the toxicity of 2,4-D is not restricted to mammals which are commonly used as test organisms in the laboratory, but is also capable of being lethal to birds, fish, aquatic insects, and aquatic crustaceans. This point must sometimes be made quite strongly to this chemical's users so that they will want to use safeguards in its application to prevent injury to these organisms.

Table VI. 2,4-D Toxicity to Environmental Organisms

Species	Toxicity
Mammals	375 – 1,000 mg/kg
Birds	540 – 2,000 mg/kg
Fish	1 – 435 ppm--48 hr
Aquatic Insects	2 – ppm--96 hr
Crustacean	60 – ppm--48 hr

It is interesting to consider the symptoms which are known to occur in humans and have been demonstrated in cases of overexposure, particularly in cases of deliberate ingestion of 2,4-D, and have been demonstrated with laboratory animals. These symptoms are irritation at the point of contact: the skin, respiratory tract and the gastrointestinal tract. 2,4-D can also cause nausea, vomiting, muscle twitching and pain, muscle stiffness (myotonia), fatigue, and nerve damage. It is important to realize these symptoms occur usually at only high doses; that is, high in relation to the LD-50 values. The onset of symptoms is usually at or over 100 mg/kg for 2,4-D, or approximately 1/3 of the LD-50 value. This is a rather high exposure value.

However, most public concern does not center around death or other acute intoxication symptoms, but rather those chronic injuries which we term as irreversible. These are carcinogenesis (cancer), teratogenesis (birth defects), or mutagenesis (genetic defects). There have been three good studies involving the ability of 2,4-D to cause cancer. The conclusion by the authors of these three studies is that there is no evidence that 2,4-D causes cancer. However, the study design was such that they were not adequate to prove that 2,4-D could not cause cancer, and as a result, further cancer studies were required by the EPA which should provide a definitive answer.

Since the discovery by Dr. Bruce Ames of the Ames test for mutagenesis of chemicals, there has been a proliferation of a great many types of laboratory tests to discover whether a chemical is mutagenic. Examination of 2,4-D mutagenicity tests, reveal that of 18 tests, 15 were negative and 3 were positive. This places 2,4-D in the category of being a weak mutagen and it has an insufficient number of positive responses to trigger action against it on the basis of its being a mutagenic chemical.

There is in the public mind a misperception as to the implication of a chemical being determined to be a mutagenic chemical. This term raises fear of a production of monsters arising from mutation or the production of a new genetic or biochemical disease such as Tay-Sachs disease or Sickle-cell anemia. To reach such a conclusion is a long leap from a positive mutagenic assay. The principle piece of information gained from a mutagenic assay is the probability that the chemical will be a carcinogen and should be thoroughly tested for carcinogenicity. But, our knowledge of this field is insufficient to reach firm conclusions about the possibility or probability of an increasing rate of mutations.

An important and recurrent concern on the part of the public is that of birth defects and miscarriages and whether they can be caused by herbicides such as 2,4-D. 2,4-D most certainly can cause birth defects, and has in tests with laboratory animals. It is a teratogenic chemical and the onset of teratogenic effects will occur at a dose level of about 75 mg/kg, repeated daily, in rats from the 6th to the 15th day of pregnancy. The corresponding human dose time would be the 15th through the 60th day of pregnancy. At a dose level of 20 mg/kg, there is no teratogenic effect, and this is considered to be the no-observable- effect level, NOEL, for 2,4-D. This is the most sensitive NOEL. We use this NOEL in all of our risk calculations and believe that it pertains to birth defects, spontaneous abortions, and miscarriages, even though it only applies to only a small portion of the population: those persons who are pregnant and in their 15th to 60th day of pregnancy. There is no argument in the field of toxicology as to whether there is a threshold for the onset of teratogenesis.

The principle public concern with regard to risk from herbicide application in the forest is not the overt, or occupational, exposure to pesticide applicators or to persons who might be in the spray zone. It is the possible injury from pesticide drift at a distance of a few hundred yards or a quarter of a mile, up to 5 to 20 miles. All aerially-applied pesticides will drift for some distance, whether they be applied by fixed-wing craft or helicopter.

It is sometimes difficult for pesticide applicators to realize that chemical spray will drift farther than it appears to be drifting from observation of the spray. One might observe a spray drifting for a few tens or hundreds of feet at most, but chemical analysis can reveal that some small amount of the spray, unobserved by the eye, can continue to drift for long distances. This distance has often been measured to be up to a mile, and in many cases, several miles. The question is not how far the chemical drifts, but how much drifts and what is the effect of the amount that drifts a given distance.

There are many variables affecting deposit from drift of pesticide spray and these variables will seldom be quantified or known in advance at a given spray site. This makes it difficult to predict exactly the amount of exposure to expect from a proposed treatment. One can, at the minimum, show a range of deposit or exposure levels arrived at in different circumstances. Table VII presents three types of results:

drift levels from a single experiment in Oregon under high wind
conditions, an average of a number of experiments with coarse
sprays under typical agricultural spray conditions, and the
average of a few (four) trials under forest conditions on steep
slopes with a five (insecticide) spray application.

Table VII. Drift Deposit

Distance Downwind	Single Trial Flat Land Medium Spray High Wind Small Target		Multiple Trials Flat Land Coarse Spray Small Target		Multiple Trials Steep Land Fine Spray Large Target	
	% of Dep.	ng/ft^2	%	ng/ft^2	%	ng/ft^2
1/4 mi.	0.01	1	0.001	100	2	200
1/2 mi.	0	0	0.0005	20	0.5	50
1 mi.	0.0	0	0.0001	10	0.15	15

The first column of drift data is from the medium spray
(300-400μ) experiment conducted mainly under wind conditions of
10 to 15 mph, or high wind conditions in Dallas, Oregon by
Phipps, Montgomery and Witt. (1). The drift in the first 50
feet downwind is 250 millipounds per acre, or 25% of amount
deposited on target. The level of deposit drops off rapidly and
is about 10% of that value at 165 feet (20 millipounds). As
shown in Table VII, the deposit at 1/4 mi. is 0.1
millipounds/acre or 1 μg/square foot and decreases to zero, or
less than 1 μg/square foot at 1/2 mile and beyond. This
experiment shows less drift for the longer distances than
expected, and is probably because of the high wind. Although a
high wind velocity will cause more drift, it may result in less
deposit from drift (beyond the first 200 feet or so) because the
short transit time over a given point results in less time of
exposure to the drift cloud.
     For the purpose of attempting to predict the amount of
drift one might expect in general from a spray operation, it is
more useful to composite the data from a number of drift
experiments into a generalized curve and extrapolate from that
to the operation being considered. Table VII shows such data
developed by Dr. Norman Akesson from the University of
California, Davis. (2,3,4). This data is for a coarse spray
with a diameter of 900 microns used on agricultural, or level,
crop lands.
     The expected levels of drift deposit are from 10 ng/square
foot at 1/4 mile to 1 ng/square foot at 1 mile. In utilizing
averaged data it must be understood that variations in drop
size, application methods, meteorological conditions, or terrain
can increase or decrease the drift deposition by 10 fold or one
can imagine, in oder to be ultra conservative, even as much as
1,000 fold.
     Another factor that will increase the drift is the target
size or number of spray swaths. If the spray block is more than

about 200 yards wide, then the expected deposit amount could
increase by a factor of 2- to 10-fold. There is a need for a
great deal more drift data and for it to be summarized into
generalized drift curves with some limitations placed on them as
to the upper and lower limits of expected spray drift amounts
under a variety of conditions so that they can be applied to
various spray situations. There is not a great deal of drift
data specific to forest spraying.

One set of good spray experiments was also conducted by Dr.
Norm Akesson and reported in 1979 and 1982. (5,6). Table VII
shows the deposit levels for the mean drift values in a set of
experiments in forest land conducted by him with a fine spray of
75-150 microns median diameter on steep terrain which had a
slope of 700 to 1000 feet per mile. These data result from
spraying very large tracts, up to three miles in diameter, and
apply to insecticide sprays, rather than herbicide sprays.

It is important for the public to recognize that there is
no fixed distance or buffer zone for a safe distance to provide
protection from spray drift. This will be a function of the
pesticide being used, its toxicity and environmental behavior
such as bioaccumulation, the nature and sensitivity of the
downwind sites, and the nature of the application method,
meteorological conditions, and so on.

The interpretation of the effects of such drift,
particularly its potential for adverse effects on human health,
is dependent on some of the parameters of environmental behavior
shown on Table VIII. The dose is given at 2 lbs/acre and
translated into a deposit level of 20 mg/square foot, which is
more useful in the interpretation of exposure data. The figures
given for the deposit amount from spray drift at 100 yards and
1/2 mile are the figures for drift from a coarse spray on flat
land for small target areas and are average drift amounts. The
figure of 20 mg/kg is the NOEL for 2,4-D.

Table VIII. Environmental Behavior

Dose	–		20 mg/square foot
Deposit	–		10-100 ppm
T-1/2	–	plants, litter, soil	2 weeks-2 months
		water	1 week
		mammals	1 day
Drift	–	total	0.25 - 4.0%
		100 yards (avg.)	1 μg/square foot
		1/2 mile (avg.)	20 ng/square foot
NOEL	–		20 mg/kg/day

The exposure for a person standing directly under a spray
plane with 50% of their skin area exposed is shown in Table IX.
This results in a risk calculation giving a margin of safety of
100. Or, more exactly, 100 per day if repeated daily, because
the margin of safety assumes a daily exposure for a given period
of time during the pregnancy. This calculation does not include
exposure from inhalation of drift particles because, as shown by
Akesson, this is a negligible amount in drift exposures.

Exposure from inhalation in occupational exposure by a sprayman
handling a spray nozzle may be as high as 1-3% of his dermal
exposure, but generally is well below that from inhalation from
drift exposures.

Table IX. 2,4-D Risk of Birth Defects or SAB

Direct Deposit - under a spray plane

Assumptions	- 2 lb/acre (20 mg/ft^2) female, enceinte, 15-60th day 50% of skin exposed (10 ft^2) weight, 110 lb (50 kg)
Calculations	- 20 mg/ft^2 x 10 ft^2 ÷ 50 kg = 4 mg/kg Dermal penetration = 5%; 0.05 x 4 mg/kg = 0.2 mg/kg

NOEL for 2,4-D = 20 mg/kg

$$\text{Margin of Safety} = \frac{\text{NOEL}}{\text{Dose}} = \frac{20 \text{ mg/kg}}{0.2 \text{ mg/kg}} = 100/\text{day}$$

Exposure from deposit directly under a spray plane would
have to be considered an unusual exposure situation. A more
common situation would be that resulting from drift. Table X
shows a summary of a similar risk calculation resulting from the
subject being 1/2 mile downwind. That results in a margin of
safety of 100,000,000. Again, one should caution the reader
that you can make different assumptions about the deposit of
drift than those made herein and arrive at deposits from drift
being 20 to 1000 times greater, which would result in a margin
of safety of only 100,000.

Table X. 2,4-D Risk -- Drift

Deposit	- 2 lb/acre = 20 mg/ft^2 VDM =900 μ
Distance	- 1/2 mile Downwind = 20 ng/ft^2
Subject	- female, pregnant, 15-60th day, 50 kg, 10 ft^2 dermal surface
Dose	- 10 x 200 x 0.05 x 1/50 = 0.2 ng/ft^2
Margin of Safety =	$\dfrac{\text{NOEL}}{\text{Dose}}$ $\dfrac{20 \text{ mg/kg/day}}{0.2 \text{ mg/kg}}$

An area of concern with regard to 2,4-D which is commonly
encountered, is the drift of 2,4-D into surface water to be used
for drinking water. Table XI shows a calculation of risk
involving drinking water which has been subject to direct spray
from aircraft at the rate of 20 mg/ft^2 and, given the
assumptions shown, results in a margin of safety of about 700.

The same water exposed to drift with a 200 foot buffer zone
would have a margin of safety of 7,000,000. It should be
pointed out that these are maximum concentrations that would
exist in a plug of water that would pass by a given water-intake
point within 10 minutes. The possibility of using that water,
contaminated at those levels over a period of time sufficient to
replicate the chronic exposure experiments on which the NOEL is
based would be very slight to non-existent.

Table XI. 2,4-D Risk -- Water

Direct Spray - Overflight, 1/2 mile of stream

Stream   - 1 foot deep, velocity 3 mph
Deposit   - 20 mg/ft^2 = 700 ppb = 0.7 ppm
Consume   - 2 qt/day, 50 kg = 0.028 mg/kg

Margin of Safety = $\dfrac{\text{NOEL}}{\text{Dose}}$ = $\dfrac{230 \text{ mg/kg/day}}{0.028 \text{ mg/kg}}$ = 714

DWS = 0.1 ppm = 100 ppb, MOS = 5,000
Drift 200' downwind
DG, JB and Visc. Ag.
Deposit 2 μg/ft^2 = 0.07 ppb
Margin of Safety = 7,140,000

We have shown in three scenarios that the margin of safety
for 2,4-D exposure could range from 100 to 10,000,000, and yet
we have not related the magnitude of these values to other
common margins of safety which people might encounter in their
daily life.

Table XII shows some margins of safety calculated by Dr.
Sheldon Wagner of Oregon State University, for a set of common
prescription medicines. These include caffeine when prescribed
at the dose level for which it is prescribed as a medicine,
antibiotics, tranquilizers, vitamins, and other drugs. Notice
that the margins of safety range from 1/2 through 100, 200, and
up to 1000.

Table XII. Comparative Margin of Safety

Chemical	Teratogenic Dose	Clinical Dose	MOS by Dose
Caffeine	75 mg/kg	2.5 mg/kg	30
Chlorotetracycline	10 mg/kg	20 mg/kg	0.5
Diazepam	200 mg/kg	0.8 mg/kg	250
Phenytoin	75 mg/kg	6 mg/kg	12.5
Vitamin A	35,000 I.U.	8,000 I.U.	1,000*
Prednisolone	2.5 mg/kg	0.2 mg/kg	125
Reserpine	1.5 mg/kg	0.02 mg/kg	75
Tetracycline	40 mg/kg	20 mg/kg	2
Salicylate	300 mg/kg	50 mg/kg	6

*Adjusted to I.U./kg

When one compares the risk of caffeine as taken in one cup of
coffee to that from the forest herbicide, 2,4-D, one finds that
the margin of safety for teratogenesis or birth defects ranges
from 5 to 16 (Table XIII).

Table XIII. Comparative Risk -- Coffee

Caffeine is a teratogen
  MDL = 75 mg/kg   (2,4-D = 75 mg/kg)
  NOEL = 25 mg/kg   (2,4-D = 20 mg/kg)
  Dose = one cup of coffee
        Bertrand 25 mg/kg/liter = 5 mg/kg/cup

Margin of Safety = $\dfrac{25}{1.5 - 5}$ = 5 - 16

Many persons consider such comparisons invidious because they
feel that they have a choice as to whether or not to drink a cup
of coffee, but not as to whether they will be exposed to a
herbicide spray drift. The point is not to enter a discussion
of that philosophy, but to compare a commonly encountered
phenomena by carrying out the same type of analysis as we do for
pesticides, and thereby obtain comparable Margin of Safety
values, independent of philosophical differences. Philosophy
does not change toxic action, or the lack of it.
     The value of 100 is generally considered a good margin of
safety. This value may be increased depending on the quality of
data undergirding the risk evaluation, or the type of injury
sustained from exposure to the chemical. A socially acceptable
margin of safety may be increased for unwilling exposure over
the margin of safety acceptable for occupational exposure.
However, a comparison of the margin of safety from drinking one
cup of coffee or any other common activity allows the public to
compare what may be an unusual exposure to them, herbicide
drift, to a common phenomenon in our society.
     One can also compare the margin of safety of a herbicide
such as exposure to 2,4-D from direct spray at 2 lbs/acre to
another common experience, taking aspirin according to the label
directions, 2 tablets every 4 hours. Table XIV shows that the
margins of safety for aspirin taken at this rate are
considerably smaller than the margins of safety for direct spray
exposure to 2,4-D. These comparisons of MOS should assist the
public in developing a frame of reference for what constitutes a
large or small Margin of Safety.

Table XIV. Comparative Margins of Safety

| Chemical | Exposure | Margin of Safety | |
		Death	Birth Defects
Aspirin	2 tab./4 hours	3.5	1.3-6.8
2,4-D	direct spray	625	100
2,4-D/Aspirin	RATIO	178:1	15:1

Identification of risk levels and margins of safety in comparisons with other commonly encountered chemicals do not finally solve the problem whether a particular chemical risk constitutes a socially acceptable risk. This must finally be determined in the social institutions mentioned earlier at the various political jurisdictions. Whether a risk will be socially acceptable depends not only on the level of risk, which we have dealt with here, but on the nature of the risk, on who assumes the risk, who receives the benefit, and one's personal philosophy of accepting any risk versus zero risk.

Perhaps the dilemna is best summed up and its timeliness underscored by an editorial which appeared in this city on the first day of this symposium in which the mayor of Seattle, in relation to a local controversy regarding the spraying of carbaryl (Sevin) for gypsy moth eradication, was quoted as saying, "Carbaryl poses no significant public health hazard--even to children, the elderly, or the pregnant." Nonetheless, he opposed aerial spraying of carbaryl, stating in effect, "It is harmless, but lets not use it." The editorial continued, "In politics, perception, not reality, is everything."

The lesson for scientists involved in these issues is that we must present what we learn here in a clear enough way so that public perceptions of pesticide application, toxicity, and risk are congruent with reality. The public's social decisions regarding pesticide use will then be based on a careful appraisal of the risk or margin of safety, and not on fear and fear alone.

Literature Cited

1. Phipps, Frank, in "A Study of Drift of Aqueous and Propylene Glycol 2,4-D Amine Formulation from Aerial Application"; Montgomery, M.M.; Witt, J.M.; Oregon State University, Dept. of Agricultural Chemistry, 1981; Unpublished data.

2. Akesson, N.B., in "What's Happening in Aerial Application Research"; Yates, W.E.; Cowden, personal communication.

3. Wilce, S.E., in "Drop Size Control and Aircraft Spray Equipment"; Akesson, N.B.; Yates, W.E.; Christensen, P.; Cowden, R.E.; Hudson, D.C.; Weigt, G.I.; Agricultural Aviation, 1974; Vol. 16 (1), p. 7-16.

4. "A Study of the Efficiency of the Use of Pesticides in Agriculture", Von Rumker, R.; Kelso, G.L.; 1975, EPA-540/9-75-025.

5. Yates, W.E., in "Atmospheric Transport of Sprays from Helicopter Applications in Mountainous Terrain"; Akesson, N.B.; Cowden, R.E.; Am. Soc. Agric. Engineers, 1978; p. 78-1504.

6. Gharserni, M., in "Estimating Drift and Exposure Due to Aerial Application of Insecticides in Forests"; Painter, P.; Powers, M.; Akesson, N.B.; DeLarco, M.; Env. Sci. & Tech., 1982; Vol. 16 (8), p. 510.

RECEIVED October 12, 1984

Author Index

Subject Index

509

Production by Meg Marshall
Indexing by Susan F. Robinson
Jacket design by Pamela Lewis

Elements typeset by Hot Type Ltd., Washington, D.C.
Printed and bound by Maple Press Co., York, Pa.

DATE DUE